Health-Related Emergency Disaster Risk Management (Health-EDRM)

Health-Related Emergency Disaster Risk Management (Health-EDRM)

Special Issue Editors

Emily Ying Yang Chan
Holly Ching Yu Lam

MDPI • Basel • Beijing • Wuhan • Barcelona • Belgrade • Manchester • Tokyo • Cluj • Tianjin

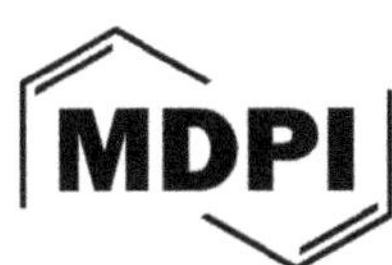

Special Issue Editors
Emily Ying Yang Chan
The Chinese University of Hong Kong
China

Holly Ching Yu Lam
Imperial College London
UK

Editorial Office
MDPI
St. Alban-Anlage 66
4052 Basel, Switzerland

This is a reprint of articles from the Special Issue published online in the open access journal *International Journal of Environmental Research and Public Health* (ISSN 1660-4601) (available at: https://www.mdpi.com/journal/ijerph/special_issues/Health-EDRM).

For citation purposes, cite each article independently as indicated on the article page online and as indicated below:

LastName, A.A.; LastName, B.B.; LastName, C.C. Article Title. *Journal Name* **Year**, *Article Number*, Page Range.

ISBN 978-3-03936-314-8 (Hbk)
ISBN 978-3-03936-315-5 (PDF)

Contents

About the Special Issue Editors

Emily Ying Yang Chan serves as Professor and Assistant Dean (External Affairs) at Faculty of Medicine, and Head of Division of Global Health and Humanitarian Medicine at JC School of Public Health and Primary Care, at The Chinese University of Hong Kong (CUHK). She is Director of the Collaborating Centre for Oxford University and CUHK for Disaster and Medical Humanitarian Response (CCOUC), the Centre for Global Health (CGH), and the Centre of Excellence (ICoE-CCOUC) of Integrated Research on Disaster Risk (IRDR). Professor Chan is also Co-chairperson of the WHO Thematic Platform for Health Emergency & Disaster Risk Management (H-EDRM) Research Network, Co-Chair of World Health Organization COVID-19 Research Roadmap Social Science working group, and a member of the Asia Pacific Science Technology and Academia Advisory Group (APSTAAG) of the United Nations Office for Disaster Risk Reduction (UNDRR). She concurrently serves as Visiting Professor (Public Health Medicine) at Oxford University Nuffield Department of Medicine and Fellow at FXB Center, Harvard University. She was also appointed CEO of the GX Foundation for two years in 2019. Her research interests include disaster and humanitarian medicine, climate change and health, global and planetary health, human health security, health emergency and disaster risk management (Health-EDRM), remote rural health, implementation and translational science, ethnic minority health, injury and violence epidemiology, and primary care. Awarded the 2007 Nobuo Maeda International Research Award of the American Public Health Association, Professor Chan has published more than 300 international peer-reviewed academic/technical/conference articles. She also had extensive experience as a frontline emergency relief practitioner in the mid-1990s, which spanned across 20 countries.

Holly Ching Yu Lam is an environmental epidemiologist. She completed her PhD study in the Jockey Club School of Public Health and Primary Care, Chinese University of Hong Kong (CUHK), in which she investigated the association between meteorological factors and respiratory hospital admissions in Hong Kong using time series analysis. Afterwards, she continued on environmental health studies at the school and participated in disasters and humanitarian studies in Collaborating Centre for Oxford University and CUHK for Disaster and Medical Humanitarian Response (CCOUC), CUHK. At CCOUC, Holly worked with Prof. Emily Chan and focused on studies in exposure–health–outcomes associations, risk perception assessments, and knowledge–attitude–practice of health issues caused in Hong Kong and among ethnic minorities in China by emergencies/disasters. She is currently a Medical Research Council (MRC) Early Career Research Fellow at the National Heart and Lung Institute, Imperial College London, where she studies the association between environmental exposures and allergic conditions. Dr. Lam's research interests include effects of ambient exposures and climate change on human health and factors for formulating disease-prevention/health-improvement strategies against environmental exposures.

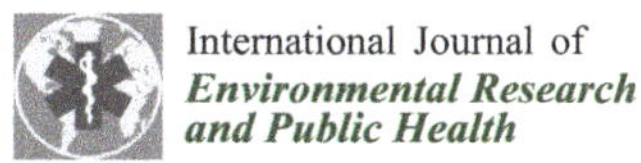
International Journal of
Environmental Research and Public Health

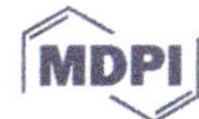

Editorial

Research Frontiers of Health Emergency and Disaster Risk Management: What Do We Know So Far?

Emily Ying Yang Chan [1,2,*] and Holly Ching Yu Lam [3]

1 JC School of Public Health and Primary Care, Faculty of Medicine, The Chinese University of Hong Kong, Hong Kong, China
2 Nuffield Department of Medicine, University of Oxford, Oxford OX3 7BN, UK
3 Genomic and Environmental Medicine, National Heart and Lung Institute, Imperial College London, London SW7 2AZ, UK; ching.lam@imperial.ac.uk
* Correspondence: emily.chan@cuhk.edu.hk

Received: 28 February 2020; Accepted: 3 March 2020; Published: 10 March 2020

Health-Emergency Disaster Risk Management (Health-EDRM) emerged as the latest knowledge, research and policy paradigm shift from response to preparedness and health risk management in non-emergency times [1]. This approach attempts to enlist and empower communities to invest and emphasize their disaster health risk reduction efforts, thereby strengthening health systems and supporting community health resilience building. This Special Issue has collected 20 scientific papers that attempt to examine the research frontier in Health-EDRM.

Major Health-EDRM research evidence gaps were found during a global research agenda setting meeting of the 2018 WHO Health-EDRM global research group in Kobe. Kayano, Chan, Murry et al. [2] highlighted the development need for relevant research methodologies, risk communication approaches, health data management strategies, practical health emergency study ethical guidelines, bridging global research capacity disparities, and infrastructure constraints, to ensure knowledge advancement in Health-EDRM. The authors also pointed out the lack of understanding of psychosocial health risk profiling in population subgroups. Reifel's analysis showed a better understanding of current doctrines and practices in both clinical mental health practices and policy, which will help to bridge the conceptual interlinkages between the preventive-based disaster risk reduction policy agenda and the curative-focused disaster mental health discipline [3]. Genereux, Schluter, Tamahashi et al. [4] argued that standardizing psychometrically robust instruments would also be urgently needed to identify at-risk patients throughout—before, during, and after emergencies and disasters—to ensure that mental and social health needs are addressed throughout the pathway of care (prevention, screening, diagnosis, treatment, and rehabilitation). Aung, Murry and Kayano [5] discussed the need for new research and ethical guidelines to harmonize research efforts in Health-EDRM and Kubo, Yanasan, Herbosa et al. [6] described the challenges in the standardization of health data collection throughout the research processes.

Existing surveillance databases, new study tools, and innovation methodologies may help to identify population health risks and support Health-EDRM policy development. Using a syndromic surveillance database in the Philippines, Salazar, Law, Winkler [7] showed how an existing clinical based database might be useful in assisting emergency health service planning decision making during outbreaks in armed conflict. Even with the database limitations to report injuries and death, this existing data system was nevertheless useful to support non-communicable diseases' service caseload planning. Using the computerized random digit dialling methods for rapid data collection after a major urban subway fire incident, Chan, Huang, Hung et al. [8] captured health risk perception, misconceptions, and community first-aid response knowledge in urban man-made emergency incidents. Using social media data from Twitter, Gruebner, Lowe, Sykora et al. [9] showed how the spatio-temporal distribution of negative emotions varied in New York City after a natural disaster. Their study showed that pre-disaster status could be used as a significant predictor of post-disaster emotional outcomes in communities. Using a disturbance management model to estimate logistics constraints in medical supplies during natural disasters, Shi and He [10] examined how medical supplies, which required cold-chain support (e.g., blood and vaccines), might be optimized after natural disasters when transport might be disturbed. Using a three-phase methodology and the online, global, and publicly available databases, Chan, Huang, Lam et al. [11] developed a health vulnerability index (HVI) that captures seven main health dimensions with nine indicators. This index allows the inclusion of non-communicable disease burden of countries/communities into the disaster risk assessment and may reflect underlying health needs and the capacity requirement to address Health-EDRM at the country level.

This Special Issue also presents studies that attempted to capture health consequences of less reported extreme events and identify at-risk communities. With the increased frequency of climate-induced disasters and weather events [12], household preparedness is regarded as an important means of bottom-up resilience. Yet, limited research evidence is currently available to understand how climate events might affect megacities in Asia. Chan, Man, Lam et al.'s [13] paper of health risks and impact after the 2018 Super Typhoon Mangkhut in Hong Kong SAR China showed that education status, risk perception, routine household emergency preparedness, and previous experience of direct disaster impact are factors associated with the uptake of typical typhoon-specific preparedness measures (TSPM). Belleville, Ouellet, Morin [14] documented the post-traumatic stress symptoms reported and experienced by evacuees after the 2016 Fort McMurray wildfires in Canada. Their study findings showed that a significant proportion of the study participants reported post-traumatic stress symptoms that might warrant clinical attention and argued that the mental health at-risk population should be identified to protect psychosocial well-being after large-scale disaster events.

Translation of research evidence to programme and policy agenda has been a major constraint to ensure evidence-based practices. Genereux, Lafontaine and Eukelbosh [15] identified some key determinants that facilitate knowledge-to-action strategies for better community health risk preparedness. The team argued that blending traditional and modern approaches, fostering community engagement, cultivating relationships, investing in preparedness and recovery, putting knowledge into practice, and availability of human and financial resources are key successful factors for integrating expertise and research in disaster management practice. Yet, a lack of emergency preparedness often exacerbates the underlying community health risks in resource-deficit minority-based areas in times of crisis and emergencies. Ho, Chan, Lam et al. [16] showed indicators capturing perceived water security in the non-emergency/normal period might not be associated with Health-EDRM preparedness attitude and coping ability in a water-stressed rural context of PRC China. Chan, Lam, Lo et al. [17] showed food-labelling and perceptions of food-related health risk might be influenced by face-to-face health education interventions and should be considered as a core emergency preparedness and health risk reduction management strategy to strengthen bottom-up resilience in minority communities. Kamara, Akombi, Agho et al. [18] conducted a systematic review of resilience and well-being evidence in southern Africa and showed disaster risk reduction interventions that were based only on Western modelled or scientific warning systems might undervalue traditional warning insights and undermine intrinsic and community capacities. To strengthen resilience and well-being outcomes, efforts should be invested to ensure household, community/indigenous knowledge, and government-level capabilities are harnessed. Public health planning models might be instrumental in facilitating the planning for Health-EDRM-related risk reduction efforts in both emergency and non-emergency situations [19,20].

Perhaps one of the most important global health emergency incidents for 2020 would be the global response to COVID-2019 [21]. With their proposed influenza A simulation model that considered the three main routes of transmission—long–range airborne, fomites, and close contact—Zhang and Li [22] found in a non-clinical office setting that mask wearing and regular cleaning of high-touch surfaces were more useful than hand-washing for viral-related disease transmission control. Through their retrospective public health response policy analysis of SARS and MERS in South Korea, Lee and Jung [23] showed that legislation and leadership influenced the overall emergency response process and the establishment of intergovernmental response systems and the success of risk communications during infectious-related events. Meanwhile, although new technology platforms (e.g., smartphones and internet) had generated interests and showed promises in efficiency and speed in mass communication in emergencies and crises, community receptivity of communication channels might differ with the nature of the emergency events [24]. For major infectious disease-based event such as the H7N9 outbreak in 2014 in Hong Kong, Tam, Huang and Chan [19] showed traditional risk communication channels (television and telephone) might still be the preferred channels of the general public.

New scientific evidence will be generated from the research studies for the 2019 novel coronavirus global epidemic. Not only will such knowledge facilitate a better understanding of new emerging diseases, but also identify treatments, enable a better uptake of community health protection behaviours, examine the usefulness of modern public health measures, and evaluate the effectiveness of technology innovation in health protection; it will also serve to remind researchers, academic, and policy makers that the landscape of Health-EDRM-related research is constantly evolving with global crises and emergencies.

Funding: This research received no external funding.

Acknowledgments: Our special thank goes to Sherry Cao and Chi Shing Wong for their facilitation and coordination in this special issue in Health-EDRM.

Conflicts of Interest: The authors declare no conflict of interest.

References

1. World Health Organization. *Health Emergency and Disaster Risk Management Framework*; World Health Organization: Generva, Switzerland, 2019.
2. Kayano, R.; Chan, E.Y.Y.; Murray, V.; Abrahams, J.; Barber, S.L. WHO thematic platform for health emergency and disaster risk management research network (TPRN): Report of the Kobe expert meeting. *Int. J. Environ. Res. Public Health* **2019**, *16*, 1232. [CrossRef] [PubMed]
3. Reifels, L. Reducing the future risk of trauma: On the integration of global disaster policy within specific health domains and established fields of practice. *Int. J. Environ. Res. Public Health* **2018**, *15*, 1932. [CrossRef] [PubMed]
4. Généreux, M.; Schluter, P.J.; Takahashi, S.; Usami, S.; Mashino, S.; Kayano, R.; Kim, Y. Psychosocial management before, during, and after emergencies and disasters—results from the Kobe expert meeting. *Int. J. Environ. Res. Public Health* **2019**, *16*, 1309. [CrossRef] [PubMed]
5. Aung, M.N.; Murray, V.; Kayano, R. Research methods and ethics in health emergency and disaster risk management: The result of the Kobe expert meeting. *Int. J. Environ. Res. Public Health* **2019**, *16*, 770. [CrossRef] [PubMed]
6. Kubo, T.; Yanasan, A.; Herbosa, T.; Buddh, N.; Fernando, F.; Kayano, R. Health data collection before, during and after emergencies and disasters—The result of the Kobe expert meeting. *Int. J. Environ. Res. Public Health* **2019**, *16*, 893. [CrossRef] [PubMed]
7. Salazar, M.A.; Law, R.; Winkler, V. Health consequences of an armed conflict in Zamboanga, Philippines using a syndromic surveillance database. *Int. J. Environ. Res. Public Health* **2018**, *15*, 2690. [CrossRef] [PubMed]
8. Chan, E.Y.Y.; Huang, Z.; Hung, K.K.C.; Chan, G.K.W.; Lam, H.C.Y.; Lo, E.S.K.; Yeung, M.P.S. Health emergency disaster risk management of public transport systems: A population-based study after the 2017 subway fire in Hong Kong, China. *Int. J. Environ. Res. Public Health* **2019**, *16*, 228. [CrossRef] [PubMed]
9. Gruebner, O.; Lowe, S.R.; Sykora, M.; Shankardass, K.; Subramanian, S.V.; Galea, S. Spatio-temporal distribution of negative emotions in New York city after a natural disaster as seen in social media. *Int. J. Environ. Res. Public Health* **2018**, *15*, 2275. [CrossRef] [PubMed]
10. Shi, Y.; He, Z. Decision analysis of disturbance management in the process of medical supplies transportation after natural disasters. *Int. J. Environ. Res. Public Health* **2018**, *15*, 1651. [CrossRef] [PubMed]

11. Chan, E.; Huang, Z.; Lam, H.; Wong, C.; Zou, Q.; Chan, E.Y.Y.; Huang, Z.; Lam, H.C.Y.; Wong, C.K.P.; Zou, Q. Health Vulnerability Index for Disaster Risk Reduction: Application in Belt and Road Initiative (BRI) Region. *Int. J. Environ. Res. Public Health* **2019**, *16*, 380. [CrossRef] [PubMed]
12. Chan, E.Y.Y. *Essentials for Health Protection: Four Key Components*; Oxford University Press: Oxford, UK, 2020.
13. Chan, E.Y.Y.; Man, A.Y.T.; Lam, H.C.Y.; Chan, G.K.W.; Hall, B.J.; Hung, K.K.C. Is urban household emergency preparedness associated with short-term impact reduction after a super typhoon in subtropical city? *Int. J. Environ. Res. Public Health* **2019**, *16*, 596. [CrossRef] [PubMed]
14. Belleville, G.; Ouellet, M.C.; Morin, C.M. Post-traumatic stress among evacuees from the 2016 Fort Mcmurray Wildfires: Exploration of psychological and sleep symptoms three months after the evacuation. *Int. J. Environ. Res. Public Health* **2019**, *16*, 1604. [CrossRef] [PubMed]
15. Généreux, M.; Lafontaine, M.; Eykelbosh, A. From science to policy and practice: A critical assessment of knowledge management before, during, and after environmental public health disasters. *Int. J. Environ. Res. Public Health* **2019**, *16*, 587. [CrossRef] [PubMed]
16. Ho, J.Y.E.; Chan, E.Y.Y.; Lam, H.C.Y.; Yeung, M.P.S.; Wong, C.K.P.; Yung, T.K.C. Is "perceived water insecurity" associated with disaster risk perception, preparedness attitudes, and coping ability in rural China? (A health-EDRM pilot study). *Int. J. Environ. Res. Public Health* **2019**, *16*, 1254. [CrossRef] [PubMed]
17. Chan, E.Y.Y.; Lam, H.C.Y.; Lo, E.S.K.; Tsang, S.N.S.; Yung, T.K.C.; Wong, C.K.P. Food-related health emergency-disaster risk reduction in rural ethnic minority communities: A pilot study of knowledge, awareness and practice of food labelling and salt-intake reduction in a Kunge community in China. *Int. J. Environ. Res. Public Health* **2019**, *16*, 1478. [CrossRef] [PubMed]
18. Kamara, J.K.; Akombi, B.J.; Agho, K.; Renzaho, A.M.N. Resilience to climate-induced disasters and its overall relationship to well-being in southern Africa: A mixed-methods systematic review. *Int. J. Environ. Res. Public Health* **2018**, *15*, 2375. [CrossRef] [PubMed]
19. Tam, G.; Huang, Z.; Chan, E. Household Preparedness and Preferred Communication Channels in Public Health Emergencies: A Cross-Sectional Survey of Residents in an Asian Developed Urban City. *Int. J. Environ. Res. Public Health* **2018**, *15*, 1598. [CrossRef] [PubMed]
20. Chan, E.Y.Y. *Building Bottom-Up Heath and Disaster Risk Reduction Programmes*; Oxford University Press: Oxford, UK, 2018.
21. Yazdanpanah, Y. 2019 Novel Coronavirus Global Research and Innovation Forum: Towards a Research Roadmap. 2019. Available online: https://www.who.int/blueprint/priority-diseases/key-action/Overview_of_SoA_and_outline_key_knowledge_gaps.pdf?ua=1 (accessed on 6 March 2020).
22. Zhang, N.; Li, Y. Transmission of influenza a in a student office based on realistic person-to-person contact and surface touch behaviour. *Int. J. Environ. Res. Public Health* **2018**, *15*, 1699. [CrossRef] [PubMed]
23. Lee, K.M.; Jung, K. Factors influencing the response to infectious diseases: Focusing on the case of SARS and MERS in South Korea. *Int. J. Environ. Res. Public Health* **2019**, *16*, 1432. [CrossRef] [PubMed]
24. Chan, E.Y.Y.; Huang, Z.; Mark, C.K.M.; Guo, C. Weather information acquisition and health significance during extreme cold weather in a subtropical city: A cross-sectional survey in Hong Kong. *Int. J. Disaster Risk Sci.* **2017**, *8*, 134–144. [CrossRef]

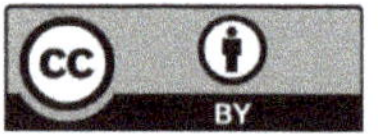

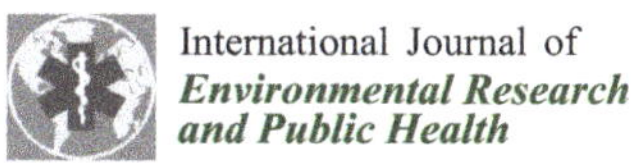
International Journal of
Environmental Research and Public Health

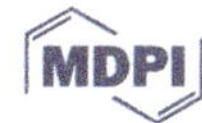

Article

Household Preparedness and Preferred Communication Channels in Public Health Emergencies: A Cross-Sectional Survey of Residents in an Asian Developed Urban City

Greta Tam [1], Zhe Huang [2] and Emily Ying Yang Chan [1,2,*]

1 Jockey Club School of Public Health and Primary Care, The Chinese University of Hong Kong, Hong Kong, China; gretatam@cuhk.edu.hk
2 Collaborating Centre for Oxford University and CUHK for Disaster and Medical Humanitarian Response, The Chinese University of Hong Kong, Hong Kong, China; huangzhe@cuhk.edu.hk
* Correspondence: emily.chan@cuhk.edu.hk; Tel.: +852-22528411

Received: 14 June 2018; Accepted: 14 July 2018; Published: 27 July 2018

Abstract: Disaster awareness and household preparedness are crucial for reducing the negative effects of a disaster. This study aims to examine the citizens' preparedness level in the event of a general disaster or outbreak of infectious disease and to identify suitable channels for community disease surveillance and risk communication. We used a stratified random design to conduct a digit-dialed telephone survey in Hong Kong during February 2014. Level of disaster preparedness was examined according to the possession of disaster kit items. Associations between socio-demographic factors and good household preparedness were assessed using multiple logistic regression models. Preferences for infectious disease surveillance were collected and analyzed. There were 1020 respondents. Over half of the respondents (59.2%) had good household preparedness. After adjustment, female respondents, having higher education and higher household income were significantly associated with good household preparedness. Television and telephone were the preferred channels to obtain and report infectious disease information, respectively. In conclusion, general and specific infectious-disease household preparedness levels in Hong Kong were generally good. Tailored preparedness programs targeted to specific communities are necessary for those lacking preparedness. Risk communication and public health surveillance should be conducted through television and telephone, respectively.

Keywords: disaster; household preparedness; infectious diseases

1. Introduction

Disaster awareness and household preparedness are crucial for reducing the negative effects of a disaster [1]. According to the Center for Disease Control and Prevention (CDC), in the United States of America, disaster awareness is associated with household preparedness, which includes possessing an emergency kit [2]. Globally, campaigns have emphasized the importance of disaster kits. For example, the Australian government has guidelines on emergency kits, updates of alerts and warnings, as well as carrying out disaster education through schools and ongoing research [3]. The American government holds a 'Get10' campaign that publicizes a disaster kit [4]. The Canadian government provides guidelines of household emergency kits and organized a national Emergency Preparedness Week annually to promote emergency preparedness through local events and media coverage [5,6]. In Nepal, organized training programs and guidelines are provided on the preparation of emergency kits and family emergency planning [7,8].

Hong Kong is the city most at risk of natural hazards in Asia, ranking third in the world. As one of the wettest cities within the Pacific Rim region [9], Hong Kong is prone to typhoons, floods, and fires. Also, Hong Kong has a history of infectious disease epidemics due to a dense population and close connection to mainland China [10,11]: Avian influenza A (H5N1) in 1997 and 2003, SARS epidemic in 2003, and swine influenza H1N1 in 2009 [12–15]. Frequent travelers from and to the Mainland increase the risk of transmission of such viruses such as human influenza A H7N9 and H5N6, causing significant morbidity and mortality [16].

The Hong Kong government has attempted to reduce the injuries and damages caused by natural hazards by implementing early hazard warnings and emergency planning, such as the weather warning system and storm protection plans [17,18]. Nevertheless, individual household preparedness is also necessary to build a bottom up disaster resilient community. Although disaster household preparedness guidelines have been issued through leaflets by the government [19], no general campaigns have been conducted to increase awareness, as evidenced by a study that showed Hong Kong citizens had low perceived susceptibility and awareness of disasters [10]. This might be because few have endured any physical harm or loss of personal property caused by disasters. Regarding infectious disease emergencies, the Hong Kong government has mass media materials on influenza, which includes TV and radio announcements, pamphlets, and booklets [20]. Despite this, a study showed that Hong Kong citizens had low anxiety level towards A/H7N9, misconceptions such as mixing up A/H7N9 and seasonal flu as well mistaking the transmission routes. They were also lacking in preventive practices [21].

Suitable channels for risk communication are critical in targeting health promotion, raising disaster awareness and preparedness. Major channels available for Hong Kong citizens to obtain information on household preparedness for diseases include television, internet, and telephone. For the preparation for an outbreak of infectious diseases, the Center for Health Protection of the Department of Health has given advice to the public (e.g., clean hands with alcohol-based hand rub and put on surgical masks when infectious disease is prevalent [22]) through television advertisements and their official website to promote personal hygiene and reduce the chances of an infectious disease outbreak through public health education.

Our study aims to assess the level of household preparedness for general disaster and infectious disease outbreak and preferred communication channels during 2014 when the A/H7N9 outbreak occurred in Hong Kong, an Asian developed urban city facing the double risks of natural hazards and infectious disease epidemics. Household preparedness levels are assessed based on whether households have an adequate supply of necessary items in their disaster kit in preparation for natural hazards and infectious disease epidemics. We also assess the likelihood of each item being stocked. We investigate what sociodemographic factors are associated with good household preparedness and whether vulnerable populations have better household preparedness. We examine the channels preferred by citizens for risk communication, according to different socio-demographic groups and for community disease surveillance. In addition, we explore citizens' expectations of the government in risk communication and their willingness to co-operate with the government in community disease surveillance.

2. Materials and Methods

2.1. Study Design and Study Population

A cross-sectional, randomized, population-based landline telephone survey was conducted on February 2014 in Hong Kong. A total of 2500 calls were made to the Cantonese-speaking population aged over 15 years who resided in Hong Kong including valid work or study visa holders. The flow of participant selection is shown in Figure 1.

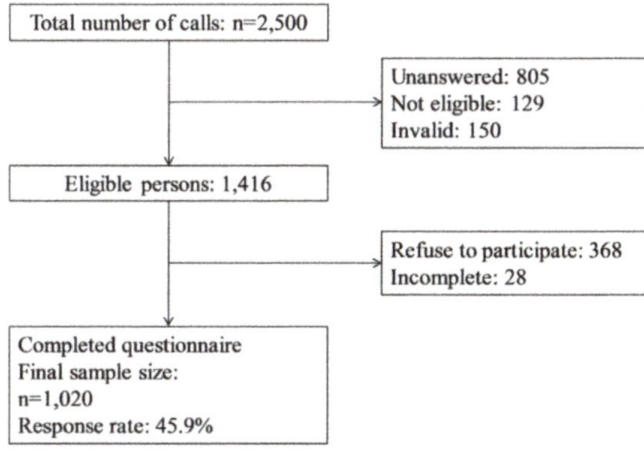

Figure 1. Study flow of the telephone survey.

Each interview lasted 15 to 25 min. A pilot study was conducted in January 2014 (n = 50) to test the practicability and validity of answers to the survey questionnaire. Wording and format were slightly modified based on the results of the pilot study.

The survey was completed when the second wave of the A/H7N9 epidemic occurred in Hong Kong. During this time, the total number of cases had risen to 320, compared to 135 in the first wave [23]. Confirmed case fatality rate was around 20% while the estimated symptomatic case fatality risk was lower [24]. Meanwhile, the infection rate of seasonal influenza was high in Hong Kong according to the Government Center for Health protection sentinel surveillance system [23]. The anxiety level of Hong Kong citizens was reported low in the first wave of the A/H7N9 outbreak [25].

2.2. Instrument

A structured questionnaire was constructed and comprised of 78 closed-ended questions related to the information below:

- Socio-demographic and background information, including age, gender, district of residence, occupation and employment status, educational attainment, type and size of housing, and household income (21 questions). Vulnerable population referred to the elderly (>60 years old), those with respiratory or chronic diseases including asthma and hypertension and those who had flu in the past 2 weeks from the day of the interview.
- Knowledge, attitudes, and practices of preventive measures against A/H7N9 influenza infections (26 questions), reported elsewhere [21].
- Figure 2 summarizes the categories of household preparedness, the items for each category and the definition of household preparedness levels.

A cut-off of five items was used because two of the items may not necessarily be applicable to all citizens. As antivirals for influenza (e.g., Tamiflu) are prescription medicines, it would be unrealistic to expect all citizens to obtain this [26]. In addition, only households with members suffering from chronic disease would be expected to possess long-term medication. Thus, a household could still be termed as having good preparedness if they did not possess antivirals and long-term medication but possessed the remaining five essential items. Three of these essential items were derived from CDC recommendations and were chosen to represent a category: First aid kit represented "safety supplies", food and water was itself a separate category, while basic medication represented "health supplies" [27]. These items were also included in similar surveys of disaster preparedness in Hong Kong [10,28] so that the findings were comparable. The remaining two essential items were specific to infectious diseases: masks and alcohol hand rubs were included as "cleaning hands with alcohol-based hand rubs and putting on surgical masks" were advice given to the Hong Kong public by the government [22].

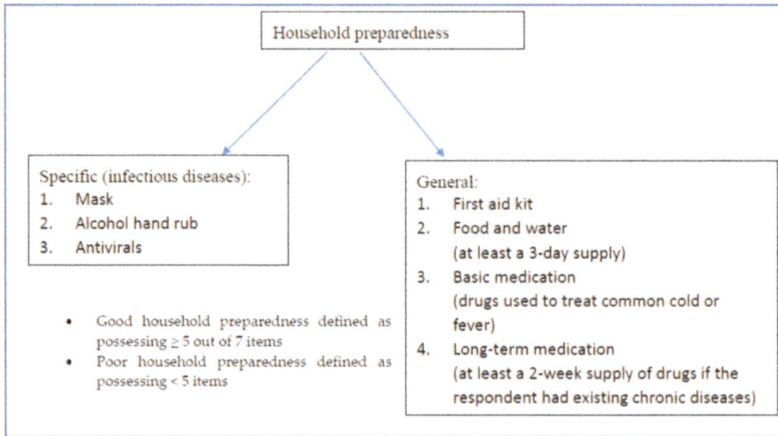

Figure 2. Definition of household preparedness levels and items.

Channel preference for obtaining and providing information to officials for surveillance and preference of internet use (total 30 questions) and a five-point Likert-type scale were used to ascertain the level of agreement or disagreement for the questions (from 1 to 5, 1 = strongly disagree, 2 = disagree, 3 = uncertain, 4 = agree, 5 = strongly agree).

2.3. Data Collection

Telephone numbers were generated randomly from the Hong Kong 2014 population telephone directory. Telephone interviews were conducted by trained interviewers from 6 p.m. to 10 p.m. on weekdays and 10 a.m. to 10 p.m. on weekends to prevent the under-representation of the employed population. Participants were chosen using the "last birthday method", referring to the household member with the birthdate and month, ignoring year of birth, closest to the interview date [29,30]. Subjects were invited in proportion to the age, gender, and living district of the 2011 Hong Kong Population Census data. The sampling stopped when each stratum reached the limits. Selected participants were followed up by a maximum of four calls before classifying as unanswered.

2.4. Statistical Analysis

Descriptive statistics of the household preparedness level and suitable channels for community disease surveillance and risk communication were presented. Likert-type scale results were collapsed to binary outcomes for analysis. Cut off point for questions with 5-point scales were defined as >3 and for questions with 4-point scale as >2. Univariate analysis was conducted by a logistic regression model to identify the association between the socio-demographic characteristics of respondents and good household preparedness. Subsequently, backward selection multivariable analysis determined factors that remained significantly associated with actual household preparedness. The association between a vulnerable population and good household preparedness was also examined. The results were presented in an adjusted odds ratio with 95% confidence intervals and p-values. All statistical analyses were conducted in R (R Core Development Team, version 3.0.3).

3. Results

The final number of respondents included in the study was 1020, and the response rate was 45.9% (1020/2223). Table 1 shows the socio-demographic characteristics of the study population in comparison to the general population in Hong Kong in 2011.

Table 1. Socio-demographic characteristics of respondents and the general population in Hong Kong 2011.

Demographics	Sample Population		Hong Kong Population 2011	Sample vs. Census p-Value [a]
	n	%	%	
Age (n = 1020)				
15–24	143	14.0	14.0	0.99
25–44	348	34.1	35.5	
45–64	363	35.6	35.4	
≥65	166	16.3	15.1	
Gender (n = 1020)				
Male	461	45.2	46.0	1.00
Female	559	54.8	54.0	
Education (n = 1019)				
Primary education or below	138	13.5	22.7	0.18
Secondary education	517	50.7	50.0	
Post-secondary education (including diploma and certificate)	364	35.7	27.3	
Occupation (n = 1006)				
White collar	411	40.9	NA	
Blue collar	96	9.5	NA	
Housewife, retired or unemployed	393	39.1	NA	
Students	106	10.5	NA	
Area of residence (n = 1020)				
Hong Kong Island	185	18.1	18.0	1.00
Kowloon	308	30.2	29.8	
New Territories	527	51.7	52.2	
Marital status (n = 1018)				
Single	355	34.9	42.2	0.36
Married	663	65.1	57.8	
Household income (n = 969)				
<$10,000	135	13.9	23.8	0.30
$10,000–19,999	220	22.7	23.8	
$20,000–39,999	346	35.7	29.0	
≥$40,000	268	27.7	23.5	
Type of housing (n = 1017)				
Public housing	387	38.1	30.3	0.61 [b]
Subsidized homeownership housing	160	15.7	15.9	
Private permanent housing	455	44.7	52.3	
Others	15	1.5	1.4	

[a] Chi-square test was used to measure the overall difference in proportions between this survey and the 2011 Hong Kong Population Census data. p-Value < 0.05 indicates a significant difference. [b] Fisher-exact test p-value was used.

3.1. Preparedness Level in General Disasters and Infectious Diseases Outbreaks

Most participants (59.2%) had good household preparedness (Figure S1), although only 3.4% of participants had a complete household preparedness kit. Although only 46.6% of general population possessed long-term medication, 157/206 (76.2%) respondents with chronic diseases possessed long-term medication (Figure 3).

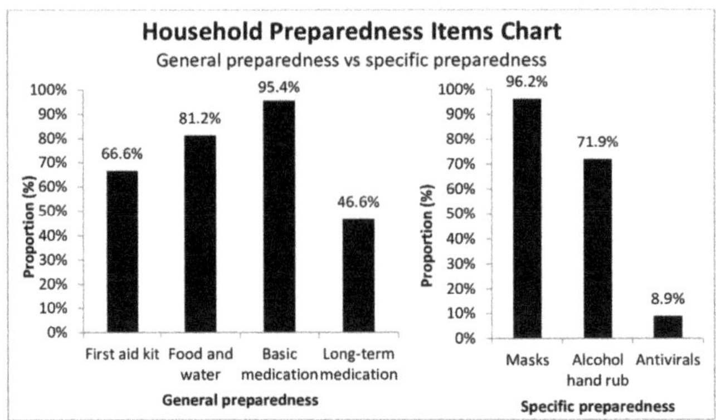

Figure 3. Proportion of respondents with household preparedness items (general and specific).

3.2. Characteristics of Respondents Lacking Household Preparedness

Univariate analysis of socio-demographics associated with good household preparedness was included in multivariable analysis. The remaining socio-demographic factors analyzed involved household-level characteristics: (Table 2).

Table 2. Socio-demographic characteristics of respondents associated with good household preparedness.

Characteristics	Household Preparedness		[a] COR (95% CI)	[b] p-Value	[c] AOR (95% CI)	[b] p-Value
	Poor	Good				
	N (%)	N (%)				
Respondents						
Gender						
Male	214 (46.4)	247 (53.6)	1		1	
Female	202 (36.1)	357 (63.9)	1.53 (1.19, 1.97)	**<0.01**	1.63 (1.25, 2.21)	**<0.01**
Occupation						
White collar	156 (38.0)	255 (62.0)	1			
Blue collar	56 (58.3)	40 (41.7)	0.44 (0.28, 0.69)	**<0.01**		
Unemployed	162 (41.2)	231 (58.8)	0.87 (0.66, 1.16)	0.34		
Student	38 (35.8)	68 (64.2)	1.09 (0.70, 1.71)	0.69		
Education						
Primary education or below	75 (54.3)	63 (45.6)	1		1	
Secondary education	213 (41.2)	304 (58.8)	1.70 (1.16, 2.48)	**0.01**	1.68 (1.12, 2.53)	**0.01**
Post-secondary education (including diploma and certificate)	127 (34.9)	237 (65.1)	2.22 (1.49, 3.31)	**<0.01**	1.92 (1.21, 3.02)	**0.01**
Household characteristics: Type of housing						
Public housing	176 (45.5)	211 (54.5)	1			
Subsidized home ownership housing	71 (44.4)	89 (55.6)	1.05 (0.72, 1.51)	0.81		
Private permanent housing	164 (36.0)	291 (64.0)	1.48 (1.12, 1.95)	**0.01**		
Household income						
<$10,000	70 (51.9)	65 (48.1)	1		1	
$10,000–19,999	104 (47.3)	116 (52.7)	1.20 (0.78, 1.84)	0.40	1.12 (0.78, 1.73)	0.60
$20,000–39,999	140 (40.5)	206 (59.5)	1.58 (1.06, 2.36)	**0.02**	1.40 (0.93, 2.11)	0.11
≥$40,000	83 (31.0)	185 (69.0)	2.40 (1.57, 3.67)	**<0.01**	2.01 (1.27, 3.17)	**<0.01**
Family size						
1	38 (61.3)	24 (38.7)	1			
2	80 (40.8)	116 (59.2)	2.30 (1.28, 4.12)	**0.01**		
3–4	233 (39.9)	351 (60.1)	2.39 (1.39, 4.08)	**<0.01**		
≥5	65 (36.5)	113 (63.5)	2.75 (1.52, 4.99)	**<0.01**		

[a] COR: Crude odds ratio; [b] Boldface indicates statistical significance; [c] AOR: Adjusted odds ratio; model was adjusted with gender, occupation, education, living quarters, household income, family size, and area of residence.

We analyzed whether households with vulnerable members had better household preparedness, but found no significant association (Table S1).

3.3. Suitable Channels for Community Disease Surveillance and Risk Communication

The preferred channels to obtain infectious disease information were from television (56%) and internet (16%). Meanwhile, smartphone/apps were one of the least popular sources. (Figure S2).

Preferred channels according to demographics were analyzed (Figure 4: television was the most popular regardless of age, gender, occupation, education level, living quarters, household income, family size, and area of residence (not shown), while most respondents (75%) thought there was a need to have official indices that could easily communicate to the public the level of health risk of an infectious disease outbreak. Around 66% showed a willingness to cooperate with local officials for infectious disease data collection if needed.

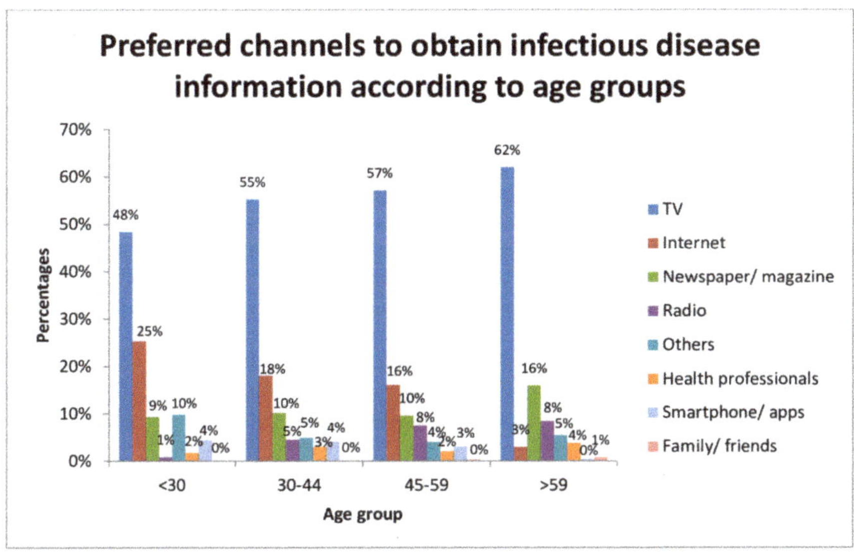

Figure 4. Preferred channels to obtain infectious disease information according to age groups.

Preferred channels for providing health information to officials for surveillance purposes were telephone (61%) and online forms (48%) (Figure S3).

4. Discussion

We examined general and infectious disease-specific household preparedness levels and communication channel preferences. Most respondents had good household preparedness. Television and telephone were the preferred media for the Hong Kong public to obtain and report infectious disease information, respectively.

4.1. Household Preparedness Level

In this study, 59.2% of participants had good household preparedness (possessing at least five items. The kit items in our survey differed from the Security Bureau of Hong Kong guidelines [19], since infectious disease outbreaks were also considered. A similar study in Hong Kong examined the risk perception at the individual level and household level and assessed the household disaster preparedness level according to five measures among 1002 respondents: basic supplies, first aid kit, basic medication, non-perishable food, drinking water and fire extinguisher [10]. Half of the respondents reported being equipping with a first aid kit, 57.3% were equipped with non-perishable food and drinking water while 95.3% and 89.2% reported possessing basic and long-term medications, respectively. Our study was unique from the 2016 study of Chan et al. as infectious disease preparedness items (masks, antivirals, and alcohol hand rub) were incorporated in this study and *Chan* et al. only considered general disaster preparedness. A lower number of respondents possessed a first aid kit, food, and drinking water compared to our study. *Chan* et al.'s study was conducted two years before our study, and may indicate an improved general disaster preparedness over the years. Furthermore, similar findings were found in a previous study assessing families with young children in Hong Kong [28]. In Australia, a similar proportion of respondents possessed a first aid kit for preparedness against regular natural hazards such as bushfires, storms, and tropical cyclones [31]. In the USA and Canada, however, few had a good household preparedness level. In a USA study, only 8% had adequate food, water, and medication for 3-day survival in spite of significant frequency in hurricanes [32]. In Canada, few respondents possessed a 5-item disaster kit including a 3-day supply of canned food and water for each member of the household, a family evacuation plan, a portable battery-operated radio, a flashlight with functioning batteries, and home or apartment insurance for winter power-outages, fires, and medical emergencies [33]. The natural hazards anticipated in the USA and Canada include earthquakes, hurricanes, and tornadoes. The type of Hong Kong natural hazard differed, and correspondingly so did the necessary disaster kit items. Differing preparedness levels might be due to other countries' perception that household preparedness was the government's responsibility [33].

For infectious disease preparedness, few (8.9%) had antiviral medications in the present study. We were interested to see what proportion of the population possessed antivirals because although it is not currently a recommended practice, a study showed that antivirals for prophylaxis in the household might eliminate pandemic outbreaks [34]. Antivirals were important drug agents recommended by the WHO in promptly treating viral infections for high-risk individuals including seasonal influenza and preventing serious complications such as pneumonia [35]. They can be used as an alternative to vaccination. If vaccination cannot cover the circulating flu strain, such as A/H7N9, the chance of widespread transmission increases. Early detection and delivery of antivirals within 24 hours are crucial for reducing transmission and reducing complications [36]. Citizens might also be showing interest in obtaining antivirals because of anxiety over influenza outbreak: A study in Australia showed that 35% of respondents would store antivirals in preparation for pandemic influenza [37]. Although globally Tamiflu is only available as a prescription medicine [26], there have been reports of over the counter and online purchase of Tamiflu in Hong Kong [38] and other countries [39–41]. 8.9% of respondents may, therefore, reflect the eagerness of citizens to store antivirals at home. Further research is needed to explore how respondents obtain antivirals and the attitude of citizens towards the availability of antivirals.

Several determinants of health were associated with good household preparedness, consistent with previous studies [33,42–45]. In the current study, female respondents, having higher income and higher education level were associated with good household preparedness. Apart from differences in gender associated with good household preparedness [43,44], higher education and socioeconomic status (including higher income level) have been consistently associated with completion of disaster preparedness tasks such as storing food, water or first-aid supplies [33,42,45,46]. This demographic subgroup of individuals might possess greater self-efficacy, which has been shown to encourage disaster preparedness [47].

4.2. Preferred Channels in Different Countries

In Hong Kong, the penetration rate of licensed domestic free television service is 99%, which may explain the popularity of this channel for obtaining infectious disease information. USA citizens preferred obtaining health information on television news and newspapers [48]. Most in the UK also preferred television [49], as did Australians (31%). Only 13.9% of Australians preferred the internet, with 68.1% of respondents reporting home access [50]. Similar to Hong Kong, in the USA, internet popularity differs markedly between generations: 62% aged 18–29 preferred the internet compared to only 28% aged 60 or over [49]. This might be due to a divide of internet usage among age groups regarding skills including formal and operational skills [51]. Particularly low utilization of the internet in those aged over 65 in Hong Kong could explain why the internet was not preferred [52]. For information reporting, the telephone was preferred in the present study in spite of technology advancement. In the USA, internet was also not the most popular choice for reporting health information to healthcare providers [53]. The elderly seemed to prefer face-to-face interactions rather than using technology. In Australia, preferred channels of providing information for public health surveys varied across demographic characteristics. Younger individuals preferred online interviews while older ones preferred written questionnaires [54]. Only a few participants across age groups and sex preferred telephone questionnaire. In the instance of a pandemic, television and telephone should be feasible channels of communication. However, there are limitations in relation to natural hazards disabling such channels due to a lack of power or signal.

Our results show that Hong Kong citizens have relatively good household preparedness compared to other countries. Despite the relative self-sufficiency of citizens, many nevertheless hoped the government could do more in terms of risk communication for infectious disease. This could be because the risk of natural hazards is easily communicated through the Hong Kong Observatory's weather warnings, using warning signals in their warning system, which are accompanied by suggested precautionary measures. In contrast, there are no official indices to indicate the risk of infection in a disease outbreak in Hong Kong. Citizens are exposed to media reports on the bi-yearly seasonal influenza and frequent reports on avian and swine flu waves. The information overload could cause pandemic fatigue and an inability to differentiate between influenza types. Official indices for infectious disease outbreaks, along with recommended precautionary measures specific to the disease, could be broadcast over television to simplify risk communication messages.

5. Limitations

This study is limited by methodological limitations of a cross-sectional telephone survey. Firstly, there may have been selection bias due to non-contact and non-response bias. Households that did not possess a land-based telephone service may be missed. The finding that most respondents preferred telephone for providing information to officials for surveillance may be influenced by selection bias. Nonetheless, the penetration rate of residential fixed line service in Hong Kong was 102.6% in November 2013, which implied that almost all households had at least one home-based telephone service in Hong Kong. To reach households that do not use landlines to communicate, alternative survey methods could be used; e.g., postal survey, online survey, or mobile phone survey. The sample population were more highly educated and had a higher household income than the general population. Thus, overestimation of the overall results may occur. Results may not be generalized, as other countries or cities have not experienced the same epidemiology of disasters. Reporting bias may be present due to self-reported data and missing data from non-respondents. Some factors that may be positively associated with participants' household preparedness level including whether the participants ever receive any education or training for disaster preparedness before and or whether participants or their families or friends had negative experience related to disaster are missing for this survey. Finally, the consistency of the responses may be influenced by external factors during the survey period. Nevertheless, the field data collection was completed within a short period of two weeks to produce a consistent response.

6. Conclusions

In conclusion, the general and specific infectious-disease household preparedness level in Hong Kong was generally good, with a small proportion of households possessing antivirals, despite over-the-counter unavailability. A tailored preparedness program to targeted communities is necessary for those lacking preparedness [31]. Educational program has been shown to increase both infectious disease and general disaster preparedness through talks and group discussions led by health promoters [55]. Since low-income households showed poorer preparedness, health campaigns should target them. Health campaigns could be held at public housing estates, as these households had poorer preparedness. Risk communication campaigns need to use the appropriate channels to increase effectiveness. As most citizens are willing to provide information to officials for surveillance, more frequent telephone surveys could be carried out during an infectious disease outbreak to strengthen surveillance. The results would also provide information for conducting tailored health campaigns. Health campaign efforts could focus on television, as this is by far the most popular channel across all demographic groups for obtaining information. There is also a demand for official indices, which would provide a direct and timely summary of the relevant health risk of infectious disease to the public.

Supplementary Materials: The following are available online at http://www.mdpi.com/1660-4601/15/8/1598/s1, Figure S1: The proportion of individuals against the number of household preparedness items (mask, alcohol hand rub, antivirals, first aid kit, food and water, basic medication, and long-term medication) at home. Figure S2: Preferred channels (TV, internet, newspaper/magazine, radio, others, health professionals, smartphone/apps, family/friends) to obtain infectious disease information. Figure S3: Preferred channels for providing health information to officials for surveillance Appendix: survey questionnaire. Table S1: Household preparedness of vulnerable population.

Author Contributions: Conceptualization, G.T. and E.Y.Y.C.; Data curation, G.T. and Z.H.; Formal analysis, G.T. and Z.H.; Funding acquisition, E.Y.Y.C.; Investigation, Z.H.; Methodology, Z.H.; Project administration, E.C.; Resources, E.Y.Y.C.; Software, Z.H.; Supervision, E.Y.Y.C.; Writing—original draft, G.T.; Writing—review & editing, G.T.

Funding: This research was funded by the Research Fund for the Control of Infectious Disease, Food and Health Bureau, Government of the Hong Kong SAR grant number CU-13-01-01.

Conflicts of Interest: Emily Y. Y. Chan is an editor of this journal. The founding sponsors had no role in the design of the study; in the collection, analyses, or interpretation of data; in the writing of the manuscript, and in the decision to publish the results

References

1. Landesman, L.Y. *Public Health Management of Disasters: The Practice Guide*; American Public Health Association: Washington, DC, USA, 2005.
2. Thomas, T.N.; Leander-Griffith, M.; Harp, V.; Cioffi, J.P. Influences of preparedness knowledge and beliefs on household disaster preparedness. *MMWR Morb Mortal Wkly. Rep.* **2015**, *64*, 965–971. [CrossRef] [PubMed]
3. Australian Government. Department of Health. Health Emergency Preparedness and Response. Available online: www.health.gov.au/internet/main/publishing.nsf/content/health-pubhlth-strateg-bio-index.htm (accessed on 13 July 2016).
4. The Alabama Department of Public Health. Get 10—The Campaign. Available online: http://adph.org/get10/Default.asp?id=2290 (accessed on 9 July 2016).
5. Emergency Preparedness Week Toolkit. Available online: http://www.getprepared.gc.ca/cnt/rsrcs/ep-wk/tlkt-en.aspx (accessed on 13 July 2016).
6. Get Prepared. Emergency Kits. Available online: http://www.getprepared.gc.ca/cnt/kts/index-en.aspx (accessed on 9 July 2016).
7. National Society for Earthquake Technology. Prepare Earthquake Emergency Kit. Available online: http://www.nset.org.np/nset2012/index.php/menus/menuid-62/submenuid-115 (accessed on 10 July 2016).
8. National Society for Earthquake Technology. Nepal Earthquake Risk Management Program II (NERMP 2). Available online: http://www.nset.org.np/nset2012/index.php/programs/programdetail/programid-80 (accessed on 13 July 2016).
9. Prevention Web. Hong Kong has the Highest Natural Disasters Risk in Asia—Study. Available online: https://www.preventionweb.net/news/view/44503 (accessed on 13 July 2016).
10. Chan, E.Y.; Yue, J.; Lee, P.; Wang, S.S. Socio-demographic Predictors for Urban Community Disaster Health Risk Perception and Household Based Preparedness in a Chinese Urban City. *PLoS Curr. Disasters* **2016**, *8*. [CrossRef] [PubMed]
11. Hong Kong SAR Census and Statistics Department. Population—Overview | Census and Statistics Department. Available online: http://www.censtatd.gov.hk/hkstat/sub/so20.jsp (accessed on 13 July 2016).

12. Hong Kong SAR Information Services Department. Avian Flu: Frequently Asked Questions. Available online: http://www.info.gov.hk/info/flu/chi/faq.htm (accessed on 14 July 2016).
13. World Health Organization. Avian Influenza. Available online: http://www.who.int/mediacentre/factsheets/avian_influenza/en/ (accessed on 14 July 2016).
14. Hung, L.S. The SARS epidemic in Hong Kong: What lessons have we learned? *J. R. Soc. Med.* **2003**, *96*, 374–378. [CrossRef] [PubMed]
15. Hong Kong SAR Centre for Health Protection—Number of Notifiable Infectious Diseases by Month in 2009. Available online: http://www.chp.gov.hk/en/data/1/10/26/43/375.html (accessed on 13 July 2016).
16. Bao, C.-J.; Cui, L.-B.; Zhou, M.-H.; Hong, L.; Gao, G.F.; Wang, H. Live-animal markets and influenza A (H7N9) virus infection. *N. Engl. J. Med.* **2013**, *368*, 2337–2339. [CrossRef] [PubMed]
17. Hong Kong Observatory. Tropical Cyclone Warning System for Hong Kong. Available online: http://www.weather.gov.hk/informtc/tcService.htm (accessed on 5 December 2016).
18. Hong Kong Jockey Club Disaster Preparedness and Response Institute. Hong Kong's Emergency and Disaster Response System. Available online: http://www.hkjcdpri.org.hk/policy-brief-hong-kong\T1\textquoterights-emergency-and-disaster-response-system (accessed on 14 July 2016).
19. Hong Kong SAR Security Bureau. Simple Guidelines in the Event of Major Mishaps. Available online: http://www.sb.gov.hk/eng/emergency/mishaps/guidelines_mishaps.pdf (accessed on 4 November 2016).
20. Hong Kong SAR Centre for Health Protection. E-resources-Avian Influenza. Available online: http://www.chp.gov.hk/en/her_list/463/24/13.html (accessed on 14 July 2016).
21. Chan, E.Y.; Cheng, C.K.; Tam, G.; Huang, Z.; Lee, P. Knowledge, attitudes, and practices of Hong Kong population towards human A/H7N9 influenza pandemic preparedness, China, 2014. *BMC Public Health* **2015**, *15*, 1. [CrossRef] [PubMed]
22. Hong Kong SAR Centre for Health Protection—Frequently Asked Questions on Influenza (Flu). Available online: http://www.chp.gov.hk/en/view_content/38225.html (accessed on 21 July 2016).
23. Hong Kong SAR Centre for Health Protection. Seasonal Influenza. Available online: https://www.chp.gov.hk/en/features/14843.html (accessed on 26 July 2018).
24. Yu, H.; Cowling, B.J.; Feng, L.; Lau, E.H.; Liao, Q.; Tsang, T.K.; Peng, Z.; Wu, P.; Liu, F.; Fang, V.J.; et al. Human infection with avian influenza A H7N9 virus: An assessment of clinical severity. *Lancet* **2013**, *382*, 138–145. [CrossRef]
25. Wu, P.; Fang, V.J.; Liao, Q.; Ng, D.M.; Wu, J.T.; Leung, G.M.; Fielding, R.; Cowling, B.J. Responses to threat of influenza A (H7N9) and support for live poultry markets, Hong Kong, 2013. *Emerg. Infect. Dis.* **2014**, *20*, 882. [CrossRef] [PubMed]
26. Tamiflu. Fever, Aches, Chills. *Check Your Symptoms and Learn More about a Prescription Flu Treatment.* Available online: http://www.tamiflu.com/ (accessed on 8 August 2016).
27. Centers for Disease Control and Prevention. Emergency Preparedness and Response. Available online: https://emergency.cdc.gov/preparedness/kit/disasters/index.asp (accessed on 14 January 2016).
28. Fung, O.W.M.; Loke, A.Y. Disaster preparedness of families with young children in Hong Kong. *Scand. J. Public Health* **2010**, *38*, 880–888. [CrossRef] [PubMed]
29. Chan, E.Y.; Kim, J.H.; Griffiths, S.M.; Lau, J.T.; Yu, I. Does living density matter for nonfatal unintentional home injury in Asian urban settings? Evidence from Hong Kong. *J. Urban Health* **2009**, *86*, 872–886. [CrossRef] [PubMed]
30. Chan, E.Y.; Kim, J.H.; Ng, Q.; Griffiths, S.; Lau, J. A descriptive study of nonfatal, unintentional home-based injury in urban settings: Evidence from Hong Kong. *Asia-Pac. J. Public Health* **2008**, *20*, 39–48. [PubMed]
31. Nicolopoulos, N.; Hansen, E. How well prepared are Australian communities for natural disasters and fire emergencies? *Aust. J. Emerg. Manag.* **2009**, *24*, 60.
32. Kapucu, N. Culture of preparedness: Household disaster preparedness. *Disaster Prev. Manag.* **2008**, *17*, 526–535. [CrossRef]
33. Phillips, B.D.; Metz, W.C.; Nieves, L.A. Disaster threat: Preparedness and potential response of the lowest income quartile. *Glob. Environ. Chang. Part B Environ. Hazards* **2005**, *6*, 123–133. [CrossRef]
34. Ferguson, N.M.; Cummings, D.A.; Cauchemez, S.; Fraser, C.; Riley, S.; Meeyai, A.; Iamsirithaworn, S.; Burke, D.S. Strategies for containing an emerging influenza pandemic in Southeast Asia. *Nature* **2005**, *437*, 209–214. [CrossRef] [PubMed]

35. World Health Organization. WHO Guidelines on the Use of Vaccines and Antivirals during Influenza Pandemics. 2004. Available online: http://www.who.int/csr/resources/publications/influenza/11_29_01_A.pdf (accessed on 14 July 2016).
36. Black, A.J.; House, T.; Keeling, M.J.; Ross, J.V. Epidemiological consequences of household-based antiviral prophylaxis for pandemic influenza. *J. R. Soc. Interface* **2013**, *10*, 20121019. [CrossRef] [PubMed]
37. Marshall, H.; Ryan, P.; Roberton, D.; Street, J.; Watson, M. Pandemic influenza and community preparedness. *Am. J. Public Health* **2009**, *99*, S365–S371. [CrossRef] [PubMed]
38. Hong Kong SAR Information Services Department. Concern over Sale of Antiviral Drug Tamiflu. Available online: http://archive.news.gov.hk/isd/ebulletin/en/category/healthandcommunity/041228/html/041228en05003.htm (accessed on 14 July 2016).
39. Rosenthal, E. Healthy Public Is Hoarding a Drug to Fight a Distant Threat. The New York Times. Available online: http://www.nytimes.com/2005/10/28/world/europe/healthy-public-is-hoarding-a-drug-to-fight-a-distant-threat.html (accessed on 28 October 2005).
40. Davis, A.; Moore-Bridger, B. Flu Drug Distribution in Chaos as Patients Ignore Rules. Evening Standard. Available online: http://www.standard.co.uk/news/flu-drug-distribution-in-chaos-as-patients-ignore-rules-6745719.html (accessed on 12 April 2015).
41. Hong Kong SAR Information Services Department. LCQ 17: Stockpiling of Antiviral Drugs. Available online: http://www.info.gov.hk/gia/general/200901/14/P200901140138.htm (accessed on 4 November 2016).
42. Tomio, J.; Sato, H.; Matsuda, Y.; Koga, T.; Mizumura, H. Household and Community Disaster Preparedness in Japanese Provincial City: A Population-Based Household Survey. *Adv. Anthropol.* **2014**, *4*, 68. [CrossRef]
43. DeBastiani, S.D.; Strine, T.W.; Vagi, S.J.; Barnett, D.J.; Kahn, E.B. Preparedness Perceptions, Sociodemographic Characteristics, and Level of Household Preparedness for Public Health Emergencies: Behavioral Risk Factor Surveillance System, 2006–2010. *Health Secur.* **2015**, *13*, 317–326. [CrossRef] [PubMed]
44. Mohammad-pajooh, E.; Ab Aziz, K. Investigating factors for disaster preparedness among residents of Kuala Lumpur. *Nat. Hazards Earth Syst. Sci. Discuss.* **2014**, *2*, 3683–3709. [CrossRef]
45. Botzen, W.; Aerts, J.; Van Den Bergh, J. Dependence of flood risk perceptions on socioeconomic and objective risk factors. *Water Resour. Res.* **2009**, *45*. [CrossRef]
46. Smith, D.L.; Notaro, S.J. Personal emergency preparedness for people with disabilities from the 2006–2007 Behavioral Risk Factor Surveillance System. *Disabil. Health J.* **2009**, *2*, 86–94. [CrossRef] [PubMed]
47. Becker, J.S.; Paton, D.; Johnston, D.M.; Ronan, K.R. Salient beliefs about earthquake hazards and household preparedness. *Risk Anal.* **2013**, *33*, 1710–1727. [CrossRef] [PubMed]
48. Ofcom. News Consumption in the UK—2014 Reportjuly 13, 2016. Available online: http://stakeholders.ofcom.org.uk/binaries/research/media-literacy/media-lit-10years/2015_Adults_media_use_and_attitudes_report.pdf (accessed on 14 July 2016).
49. Manganello, J.A.; Gerstner, G.; Pergolino, K.; Graham, Y.; Strogatz, D. Understanding Digital Technology Access and Use Among New York State Residents to Enhance Dissemination of Health Information. *JMIR Public Health Surveill.* **2016**, *2*. [CrossRef] [PubMed]
50. Eastwood, K.; Durrheim, D.; Francis, J.L.; d'Espaignet, E.T.; Duncan, S.; Islam, F.; Speare, R. Knowledge about pandemic influenza and compliance with containment measures among Australians. *Bull. World Health Organ.* **2009**, *87*, 588–594. [CrossRef] [PubMed]
51. Van Deursen, A.J.; van Dijk, J.A. Internet skill levels increase, but gaps widen: A longitudinal cross-sectional analysis (2010–2013) among the Dutch population. *Inf. Commun. Soc.* **2015**, *18*, 782–797. [CrossRef]
52. Chan, E.Y.; Huang, Z.; Mark, C.K.; Guo, C. Weather information acquisition and health significance during extreme cold weather in a subtropical city: A cross-sectional survey in Hong Kong. *Int. J. Disaster Risk Sci.* **2017**, *8*, 134–144. [CrossRef]
53. Hill, J.H.; Burge, S.; Haring, A.; Young, R.A. Communication technology access, use, and preferences among primary care patients: From the Residency Research Network of Texas (RRNeT). *J. Am. Board Fam. Med.* **2012**, *25*, 625–634. [CrossRef] [PubMed]

54. Glass, D.C.; Kelsall, H.L.; Slegers, C.; Forbes, A.B.; Loff, B.; Zion, D.; Fritschi, L. A telephone survey of factors affecting willingness to participate in health research surveys. *BMC Public Health* **2015**, *15*, 1017. [CrossRef] [PubMed]
55. Bradley, D.T.; McFarland, M.; Clarke, M. The Effectiveness of Disaster Risk Communication: A Systematic Review of Intervention Studies. *PLoS Curr. Disasters* **2014**, *6*. [CrossRef] [PubMed]

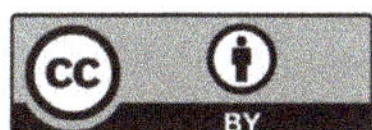

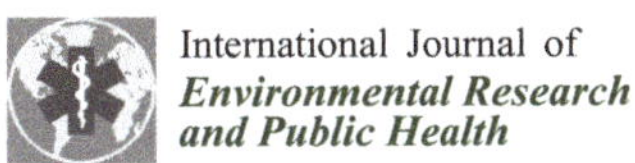

International Journal of
Environmental Research and Public Health

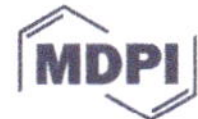

Article

Decision Analysis of Disturbance Management in the Process of Medical Supplies Transportation after Natural Disasters

Yuhe Shi and Zhenggang He *

School of Transportation and Logistics, Southwest Jiaotong University, Chengdu 610031, China; SHI681242@163.com

* Correspondence: hezhenggang@swjtu.edu.cn; Tel.: +86-028-8763-4338

Received: 19 June 2018; Accepted: 31 July 2018; Published: 3 August 2018

Abstract: Public health emergencies, such as casualties and epidemic spread caused by natural disasters, have become important factors that seriously affect social development. Special medical supplies, such as blood and vaccines, are important public health medical resources, and the cold-chain distribution of medical supplies is in a highly unstable environment after a natural disaster that is easily affected by disturbance events. This paper innovatively studies the distribution optimization of medical supplies after natural disasters from the perspective of disturbance management. A disturbance management model for medical supplies distribution is established from two dimensions: time and cost. In addition, a hybrid genetic algorithm is introduced to solve the model. Disturbance recovery schemes with different weight coefficients are obtained through the actual numerical experiments, and experimental results show the effectiveness of the proposed model and algorithm. Finally, we discuss the formulation of weight coefficients in the case of emergency distribution and general distribution, which provide a reference for emergency decisions in disturbance events.

Keywords: natural disasters; medical supplies transportation; cold-chain distribution; disturbance management; hybrid genetic algorithm

---

1. Introduction

In recent years, various natural disasters have occurred frequently, such as Hurricane Katrina in 2005, the Wenchuan Earthquake in 2008, and the Typhoon in the Philippines in 2013 [1–4]. After natural disasters, special medical supplies such as blood and vaccines are the key to reducing casualties and fighting infectious diseases. The efficient distribution of these special medical supplies is of great importance to public health and individual health. In general, special medical supplies, such as blood and vaccines, are extremely sensitive to temperature, and the quality of their cold-chain distribution is positively correlated with medical efficacy [5]. Only under specific temperatures or external environment conditions can it be ensured that medical supplies will not lose efficacy or deteriorate. In the circulation process of medical supplies, the cold-chain logistics are clearly important for ensuring the immune efficacy and safety of medical supplies [6]. However, the process of cold-chain distribution, which has the characteristics of high uncertainty, dynamics, and interactions, is easily affected by a multitude of disturbance events, including demand changes, road interruptions caused by natural disaster, vehicle refrigeration equipment failure, and so on, thus leading to the original distribution plan being affected, and even interruptions to the cold-chain.

Therefore, it is important to address disturbance events scientifically after the occurrence of natural disasters. After a disturbance event occurs, the distribution order of the remaining service objects should be adjusted, which is bound to result in a chain reaction and cause system confusion.

At this point, we need to consider the impact of the disturbance on the entire cold-chain logistics and distribution system to generate an adjustment program that minimizes the system disturbance. Based on this, if the distribution quality and efficiency of medical supplies need to be ensured simultaneously, the medical supplies' cold-chain distribution problem will become more complicated. How to effectively address disturbance events that lead to the interruption of the cold-chain and maintain the safety and efficiency of medical supplies are urgent problems that need to be solved in medical supply cold-chain distribution after natural disasters.

The remaining parts of this paper are organized as follows. In the next section, a literature review on the disturbance management problem as well as the logistics and distribution of medical supplies is presented. Section 3 discusses the construction of the disturbance management model for medical supplies distribution (DMMSD). The hybrid genetic algorithm is introduced to solve the model in Section 4. Section 5 gives a numerical experiment and results analysis. Finally, Section 6 concludes this paper and presents expectations for future work.

2. Literature Review

Since the main idea of the current research is to study the distribution optimization of medical supplies after natural disasters from the perspective of disturbance management, we review the studies in two fields: disturbance management in transportation and distribution optimization of medical supplies.

2.1. Disturbance Management in Transportation

There have been a large number of disturbance events across all walks of life. At present, disturbance management has become a hot issue for scholars to study, including aspects such as aviation disturbance management [7,8], supply chain disturbance management [9,10], machine scheduling disturbance management [11,12], railway scheduling disturbance management [13], and so on. As early as the 1970s and 1980s, research on disturbance had begun. The disturbance management was first applied in the aviation field by Yu [14], and since then, many research results have been produced on this classical optimization problem. There have also been many achievements in research on the disturbance management of logistics distribution. Zeimpekis et al. [15] classified the disturbance problem in logistics distribution and set up a mathematical model with the objectives of minimizing the delay cost and serving the largest number of customers. A disturbance recovery model of logistics distribution was established by Potvin et al. [16] to solve the problems of new customer demand and travel time disturbance, and they introduced an insertion algorithm for this model. Tiguiguchi and Shimamoto [17] studied the influence of uncertain vehicle traveling time on formulating a distribution plan and conducted an experiment that introduced changeable traveling time as the disturbance variable. Ruan and Wang [18] constructed a disturbance recovery model for the joint delivery of emergency medical supplies to analyze the disturbance of an emergency logistics system due to transfer point changes, and they designed a genetic algorithm to solve the model. Ding et al. [19] measured disturbance based on the prospect theory, and a multi-objective disturbance management model was proposed. Combined with related theories in behavioral science, Liu et al. [20] discussed the influence of disturbance events on an emergency logistics system from three aspects: demand point, decision maker, and logistics worker. In conclusion, many scholars have studied disturbance management in different transportation environments, but there is no literature related to disturbance events in the transportation of medical supplies.

2.2. Distribution Optimization of Medical Supplies

Another study related to this article is the logistics and distribution of medical supplies which requires high safety and punctuality. Based on the needs of theoretical research and practical application, scholars have conducted a great deal of research on this pertinent problem. According to the characteristics of emergency medical blood, Ramezanian et al. [21] proposed an optimization model for blood supply chain design in both deterministic and robust environments, and the application of the proposed model was evaluated by a case study in Tehran. The target functions in the integrated optimization model for the selection of emergency blood transfer points and transport routes proposed by Wang et al. [22] included having a minimum arrival time for emergency blood, maximum freshness at the time of reception, and minimization of the total transportation cost. A genetic algorithm for local neighborhood optimization was designed in their study. Chen et al. [23] considered the time constraints from the perspective of joint distribution and established an optimization model for multi-species cold-chain vaccine distribution. To minimize the maximum arrival time and the average arrival time, Campbell et al. [24] set up a path optimization model for vehicles with emergency supplies and used a local search algorithm to solve the model. Taking the Haiti earthquake in 2010 as an example, Battini et al. [25] developed a last mile distribution optimization model for emergency supplies and analyzed the optimization results under different scenarios. Ruan et al. [26] presented a two-stage approach for the intermodal transportation of medical supplies by "helicopters and vehicles" in large-scale disaster responses. Although there has been a large number of studies on the distribution optimization of medical supplies, few scholars have studied the distribution optimization of special medical supplies after natural disasters based on the perspective of disturbance management.

In short, as important medical supplies that are relevant to public health, the cold-chain distribution environments of blood and vaccine are highly unstable and vulnerable to disturbance. However, there have been few studies on the disturbance management of medical supply distribution. Taking vehicle breakdown (failure of refrigerating equipment) in the distribution process as an example, the idea of disturbance management is used to study the disturbance events in the cold-chain distribution of medical supplies in this paper. In contrast to the single-objective optimization model, we measure the disturbance from two dimensions, time and cost, and establish a disturbance management model for medical supply distribution (DMMSD) with minimum cost and time disturbance as the objective functions, and we design a hybrid genetic algorithm to solve this problem. Then, based on an actual case, the distribution schemes of disturbance recovery under different weights are obtained by our model and algorithm, thus providing a reference for the decision-making process of medical supply cold-chain distribution disturbance management.

3. Model Formulation

3.1. Problem Description

After a disaster, the rescue work in the first phase mainly involves the repair of basic facilities, such as road traffic and communication, as well as the simultaneous rescue of survivors. Then, on the basis of unimpeded communication and roads, a large number of medical materials are transported into the disaster area to reduce casualties and reduce the risk of secondary disasters caused by the outbreak of an epidemic situation [27,28]. This is called the second phase of post-disaster rescue [26,29], which is the background of this paper and the application environment for the DMMSD.

The problem studied in this paper can be described as follows. In the second phase of rescue after a natural disaster, the Medical Supplies Distribution Center (MSDC) distributes medical supplies to a number of temporary medical points (TMPs) through refrigerated trucks, and the locations of TMPs are known. There are same types of refrigerated vehicles, and medical supplies that require the same distribution temperature are transported by the same vehicle. Each refrigerated vehicle starts from the MSDC and will return to the MSDC after delivering the medical supplies to the designated TMPs along a known distribution route. The TMPs have time windows in which they receive services, which means the medical supplies are required to reach the TMP within a certain time interval. In the absence of any disturbances, the initial known delivery schemes can meet the requirements of the TMPs and the load limits of the vehicles. When a disturbance event occurs (taking vehicle breakdown and refrigeration equipment failure during the delivery process as an example), the problems that need to be resolved are as follows: the recovery of normal operation of the system as soon as possible, the completion of the distribution tasks with consideration of the interests of multiple stakeholders, and the minimization of the time disturbance and cost at the same time.

After a natural disaster, during the process of cold-chain distribution, any one of many factors, such as vehicles, cargoes, paths, demands and others, may be disturbed, which will influence the distribution task. Disturbance events can interrupt the cold-chain. If we continue to deliver medical supplies according to the initial schemes formulated before the occurrence of the disturbance event, inevitably some of the demand points will not receive the expected service, and the immune efficacy of the medical supplies will be affected. Therefore, it is necessary to construct a disturbance management model and to adjust the distribution schemes according to the disturbance event to utilize adjustment schemes that minimize the disturbance of the system. In this paper, disturbance management in the cold-chain logistics distribution of medical supplies is studied with the example of vehicle breakdown in the distribution process.

In short, the real environment after natural disasters is more complicated. In order to model the situation after a natural disaster and make scientific quantitative decision analysis, we refer to the literature [30–42], and make the following assumptions:

- As mentioned above, after a natural disaster, any one of a number of factors, such as vehicles, cargoes, paths, demands, and others, may be disturbed in the process of cold-chain distribution, which will influence the distribution task. In this paper, we assume that the transport capacity is disturbed (vehicle breakdown) to study the distribution optimization after a single type of disturbance event occurs.
- After a natural disaster, the rescuers dispatched by the government restore basic communication and traffic as soon as possible and rescue the survivors simultaneously. On the basis of unimpeded communication and roads, medical supply distribution can be carried out to ensure timely medical assistance to the injured and to reduce the risk of secondary disasters caused by the outbreak of epidemic situation. So, in this paper, we assume that the communication and roads are basically unimpeded during the distribution process of medical supplies.
- The location and service time windows of TMPs are known.
- The initial distribution scheme is known, and the same type of refrigerated vehicle is used.
- In a distribution task, each TMP is only served once.

3.2. Disturbance Processing Strategy

In the distribution process of medical supplies, a vehicle is not able to continue driving and the refrigerator cannot continue to work normally—the vehicle breaks down and the issue cannot be resolved in a short period of time. After the vehicle fails, the pending delivery cargoes and unfinished delivery tasks will be affected. The subsequent rescue mission includes picking up the cargoes and completing the unfinished delivery tasks of the disturbed vehicle. If a disturbance occurs to a distribution vehicle while the vehicle is on its way to the next TMP or the vehicle is servicing a TMP, it is assumed that the location of the disturbed vehicle is the pseudo demand point and the rescue vehicle needs to reach this location for rescue. If the vehicle fails when it is still at the MSDC, only new vehicles can be dispatched to service the affected demand points.

The problem studied in this paper involves the disturbance management of the vehicle routing problem with time window (VRPTW); the cargoes need to be delivered in the time window required by TMPs. Furthermore, because of the characteristics of the medical supplies, it is necessary to store and transport them under certain temperature conditions. Thus, there are two kinds of rescue strategy: (1) the additional vehicle rescue strategy, which means new vehicles in the MSDC are dispatched for rescue in accordance with the original path, and (2) the near vehicle rescue strategy, which assumes that the locations of the vehicles on the way to deliver cargoes are pseudo distribution centers when the disturbance event occurs, and that the vehicles in the pseudo distribution centers are deployed to assist the disturbed vehicle to complete the remaining tasks. A schematic diagram of vehicle breakdown rescue is shown in Figure 1.

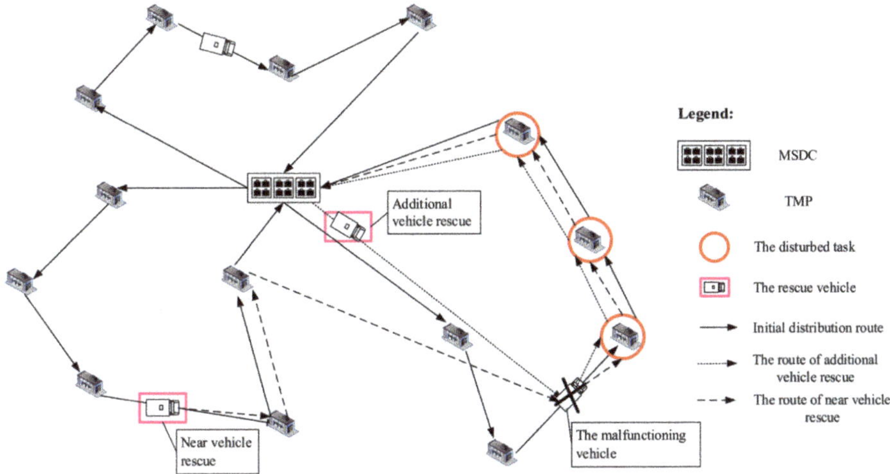

Figure 1. A schematic diagram of vehicle breakdown rescue.

3.3. Parameters and Variables

According to the needs for building the model, this paper uses the following parameters and variables, as shown in Table 1.

Table 1. The meanings of parameters and variables.

Parameters and Variables	Meaning
E	Collection of temporary medical points (TMPs)
CE	Collection of TMPs that have been served when a disturbance event occurs
UE	Collection of TMPs that have not been served when a disturbance event occurs
VE	Collection of pseudo demand points
V	Collection of distribution vehicles
R	Collection of vehicles on their way to deliver cargoes
D	Collection of vehicles at the Medical Supplies Distribution Center (MSDC)
0	Starting point of the vehicle
F	End point of the vehicle after the delivery service is completed
$V = R \cup D$	Collection of all available vehicles
$RF = UE \cup VE$	Collection of task points after the disturbance event occurs
$OP = \left\{ (i,j,k) \middle\vert \begin{array}{c} i,j \in E \cup 0 \cup F, \\ k \in V \end{array} \right\}$	Original distribution scheme
EP	New distribution scheme, the collection of network nodes changes as $E_0 = RF \cup \{0, F\}$
a	Total number of TMPs that have not been served
b	Total number of the vehicles on the way to deliver cargoes in the original distribution scheme

Table 1. *Cont.*

Parameters and Variables	Meaning
P	Collection of points, $P = \{p_1, p_2, \ldots, p_{a+b+1}\}$, where $\{p_1, p_2, \ldots, p_a\}$ represents the TMPs that have not been served; p_{a+1} is the location of the disturbed vehicle; $\{p_{a+2}, \ldots, p_{a+b}\}$ represents the location of the vehicles on the way to deliver cargoes when a disturbance event occurs, that is, the pseudo distribution centers; p_0 is the location of the MSDC, which is the initial distribution center
d_{ij}	Distance between p_i and p_j
s	Speed of the refrigerated vehicles
t_0	Time that the temperature inside the refrigerated box goes up by 1 °C when the refrigeration equipment fails to work
T_0	Critical temperature at which the medical supplies approach deterioration
T_n	Temperature inside the refrigerated box when the refrigerated vehicle is normal working
w_i	Service time of the vehicle for p_i
t_s	Moment of the disturbance event occurs
DT_{ki}	Time for vehicle k to reach TMP i in the original plan
DT_{ki}'	Time for vehicle k to reach TMP i after adjusting the distribution scheme
$[ET_i, LT_i]$	Time window of TMP i, including the beginning and end point of the arrival time required by the TMP
g_i	Medical supply demands of TMP i in the original distribution scheme
g_i^{EP}	Medical supply demands of TMP i after the disturbance event occurs
Q_k	Maximum load allowed for refrigerated vehicle k
Q_k^{EP}	Available load of vehicle k that is on its way to deliver cargo
C_{ij}	Transportation cost for a unit of distance for a refrigerated vehicle from TMP i to TMP j
$L(EP)$	Collection of distribution path edge in the new scheme
$L(OP)$	Collection of distribution path edge in the original scheme
L_{ijk}	The deviation parameter of the path, when $(i,j,k) \in L(OP)/L(EP)$, $L_{ijk} = -1$ indicates the path edge between TMP i and TMP j is shown in the original scheme but not in the new scheme; when $(i,j,k) \in L(EP)/L(OP)$,$L_{ijk} = 1$ indicates the path edge between TMP i and TMP j is shown in the new scheme but not in the original scheme; when $(i,j,k) \in L(EP) \cap L(OP)$, $L_{ijk} = 0$ indicates the path edge between TMP i and TMP j is shown in both the original and new schemes
x_{ijk}	A 0–1 variable, $x_{ijk} = 1$ represents that vehicle k is driven from TMP i to TMP j, otherwise $x_{ijk} = 0$
z_{ijk}	A 0–1 variable, $z_{ijk} = 1$ represents that vehicle k is driven from the pseudo distribution center p_i to demand point p_j, otherwise $z_{ijk} = 0$
z_{0jk}	A 0–1 variable, $z_{0jk} = 1$ represents that vehicle k is driven from the MSDC p_0 to demand point p_j, otherwise $z_{0jk} = 0$

3.4. Measurement of Disturbance

In this paper, the disturbance of vehicle breakdown is measured from two aspects: the arrival time disturbance of the medical supplies and the cost disturbance of the distribution. Then, a multi-objective function model with minimum cost and time disturbances is established.

3.4.1. The Cost Disturbance

After a disturbance event occurs, the original distribution plan is terminated, and a new distribution plan is started. The cost disturbance is composed of the cost of the path change, the cost of the additional new vehicle rescue, and the penalty cost that includes the penalty cost of failing to serve the TMPs and the cost of breaking the required time window. We set C_1 as the unit cost for a new vehicle; C_2 as the unit penalty cost for distribution failure; μ_1 as the waiting cost per unit of time when the vehicle arrives at the TMP in advance; and μ_2 as the penalty cost per unit of time when the vehicle is late to the TMP. The expression for cost disturbance is

$$\begin{aligned}\min C &= \sum_{k\in R}\sum_{i\in RF}\sum_{j\in E_0} z_{ijk}C_{ij}d_{ij}L_{ijk} + \sum_{k\in D}\sum_{j\in RF} z_{0jk}C_1L_{0jk} + \sum_{k\in V}\sum_{i\in RF}\sum_{j\in E_0} C_2\left(1-x_{ijk}\right) \\ &+ \sum_{k\in V}\sum_{i\in RF}\left(\mu_1\max\{ET_i - DT_{ki}{}',0\} + \mu_2\max\{DT_{ki}{}' - LT_i,0\}\right)\end{aligned} \tag{1}$$

In Formula (1), $\max\{ET_i - DT_{ki}{}',0\}$ indicates the advanced arrival time for vehicle k with service TMP i, and $\max\{DT_{ki}{}' - LT_i,0\}$ indicates the amount of time by which vehicle k is late to service TMP i.

3.4.2. The Time Disturbance

After a natural disaster, there are three situations for the time disturbance of medical supplies arriving at the TMP: (1) the arrival time after adjusting the distribution scheme ($DT_{ki}{}'$) is exactly the same as the original planned arrival time (DT_{ki}); (2) the arrival time after adjusting the distribution scheme ($DT_{ki}{}'$) is later than the original planned arrival time (DT_{ki}); or (3) the arrival time after adjusting the distribution scheme ($DT_{ki}{}'$) is earlier than the original planned arrival time (DT_{ki}). The third situation has a positive impact on the TMP, but it is likely generated by delaying the delivery time of other TMPs or increasing delivery vehicles, so we also regard it as a disturbance.

According to the analysis presented above, the disturbance of the medical supplies' arrival time for TMP i can be expressed as

$$\lambda(DT_{ki} - DT_{ki}{}'),\ \lambda \in \{-1,0,1\} \tag{2}$$

where λ is a symbolic variable. When $DT_{ki}{}' = DT_{ki}$, there is no arrival time disturbance in TMP i ($\lambda = 0$); when $DT_{ki}{}' > DT_{ki}$, that is, the arrival time after adjusting the distribution scheme is later than the originally planned arrival time ($\lambda = 1$); when $DT_{ki}{}' < DT_{ki}$, that is, the arrival time after adjusting the distribution scheme is earlier than the originally planned arrival time ($\lambda = -1$). Then, the arrival time disturbance of all of the TMPs can be obtained.

$$\min T = \sum_{k\in RF}\sum_{i=E^{ki}} \lambda(DT_{ki} - DT_{ki}{}'),\ \lambda \in \{-1,0,1\} \tag{3}$$

where E^{ki} is a collection of TMPs serviced by vehicle k in the original scheme.

3.5. The DMMSD Model Setting

In the second phase of post-disaster rescue, time and cost are the main targets followed by the three subjects of medical supplies distribution (MSDC, TMP, and distribution operator) in the face of a disturbance. Based on the analysis of disturbance in Section 3.4, the DMMSD model was constructed as follows:

$$\begin{aligned}\min C &= \sum_{k\in R}\sum_{i\in RF}\sum_{j\in E_0} z_{ijk}C_{ij}d_{ij}L_{ijk} + \sum_{k\in D}\sum_{j\in RF} z_{0jk}C_1L_{0jk} + \sum_{k\in V}\sum_{i\in RF}\sum_{j\in E_0} C_2\left(1-x_{ijk}\right) \\ &+ \sum_{k\in V}\sum_{i\in RF}\left(\mu_1\max\{ET_i - DT_{ki}{}',0\} + \mu_2\max\{DT_{ki}{}' - LT_i,0\}\right)\end{aligned} \tag{4}$$

$$\min T = \sum_{k\in RF}\sum_{i=E^{ki}} \lambda(DT_{ki} - DT_{ki}{}'),\lambda \in \{-1,0,1\} \tag{5}$$

subject to

$$\sum_{i\in RF}\sum_{j\in E_0} x_{ijk} * g_i^{EP} \le Q_k^{EP}\forall k \in V \tag{6}$$

$$\sum_{j\in E_0}\sum_{k\in V} x_{ijk} \le 1\forall i \in RF \tag{7}$$

$$\sum_{k\in V}\sum_{j\in RF} z_{0jk} \leq |D| \tag{8}$$

$$L_{ijk} = \begin{cases} 1(i,j,k) \in L(EP)/L(OP) \\ 0(i,j,k) \in L(EP) \cap L(OP) \\ -1(i,j,k) \in L(OP)/L(EP) \end{cases} \tag{9}$$

$$\sum_{i=1}^{a+b+1} x_{i(a+b+1)k} = 1k = 1,2,\ldots,b \tag{10}$$

$$(T_0 - T_n)/t_0 \geq DT_{ki}{'} - t_s, T_n \leq T_0 \tag{11}$$

$$\sum_{i=1}^{a+b+1}\sum_{k=1}^{b} x_{ijk}\left[t_i + w_i + \left(d_{ij}/s\right)\right] = t_j j = 1,2,\ldots,a+1 \tag{12}$$

$$ET_i \leq t_i + w_i \leq LT_i i = 1,2,\ldots,n \tag{13}$$

The model indicates that the objective of our problem is to minimize the deviation between the adjusted and initial schemes, which means that the degree of disturbance to the system is minimal, as shown in Expressions (4) and (5). Constraint (6) represents that the demands of TMPs cannot exceed the current load capacity of the rescue vehicle after the disturbance event occurs. Each task point can only be served once, and its operation is shown in constraint (7). The maximum number of available vehicles for rescue is emphasized in constraint (8). Constraint (9) imposes the notion of the definition of a path deviation parameter in the original and new schemes, including the path added in the new scheme, the path deleted in the original solution, and the changeless path. Constraint (10) shows the vehicle returning to the initial distribution center after finishing its service to the TMPs. Constraint (11) ensures that the disturbed vehicle is rescued before the medical supplies lose efficacy or deteriorate. The time window set for the TMPs must be met, which is imposed by constraints (12) and (13).

4. Algorithm Design

Based on the idea of the genetic algorithm [43–48], a hybrid genetic algorithm (HGA) for solving the DMMSD model is designed in this section. The specific process is shown in Figure 2.

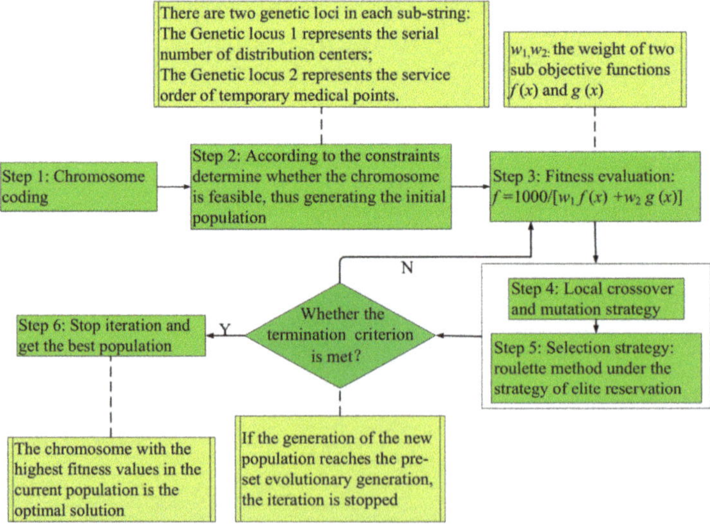

Figure 2. The specific process of the hybrid genetic algorithm.

Step 1: Chromosome coding. One chromosome represents a solution to the problem; each chromosome consists of n gene strings, and each gene string represents the service status of a TMP. There are two genetic loci in each substring: genetic locus 1 represents the serial number of the distribution center and genetic locus 2 represents the service order of TMP. Taking the chromosome in Figure 3 as an example, substring 1 indicates that TMP 1 is served by pseudo distribution center 3 in the second order, and substring n indicates that TMP n is served by pseudo distribution center 2 in the first order.

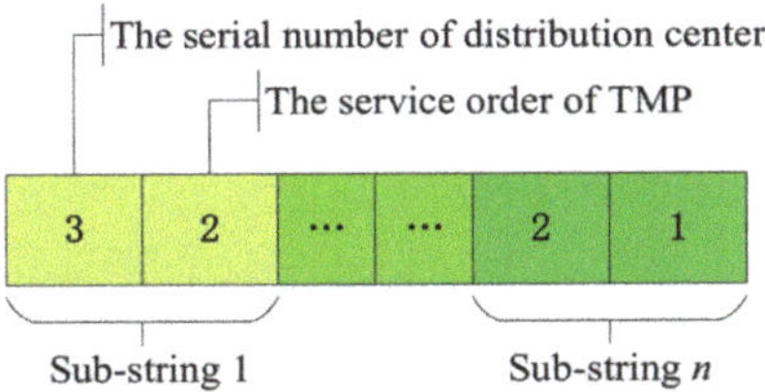

Figure 3. Example of chromosome coding.

Step 2: Initializing the population. To ensure that the algorithm performs the optimization in a feasible solution space, each chromosome is decoded after it is generated in the process of population initialization. The chromosome is judged by constraints (6)–(13). If all of the constraints are satisfied, the chromosome is viable. Otherwise, new chromosomes will be regenerated through population initialization or genetic evolution until M chromosomes are obtained.

Step 3: Evaluation of population fitness. In order to intuitively see the subtle changes in the fitness value in the algorithm convergence graphs, we set the numeric value of the numerator to 1000. The fitness function set in the HGA is as follows:

$$f = \frac{1000}{w_1 f(\mathrm{x}) + w_2 g(\mathrm{x})} \tag{14}$$

where w_1 and w_2 represents the weights of two sub-objectives, respectively.

Step 4: Crossover and mutation operation. According to the characteristics of the DMMSD model, we designed a local crossover and mutation method to improve the evolutionary efficiency of the algorithm. First, gene strings affected by disturbance are identified in two parent chromosomes. Then, the identified gene strings and unidentified gene strings are implemented in the local crossover (cross-probability, PC) and mutation operations (mutation probability, PM) separately to form progeny chromosomes. Finally, it is determined whether the newly generated progeny chromosomes meet the constraints until sufficient progeny chromosomes are constructed.

Step 5: Selection strategy. The roulette method under the strategy of elite reservation was chosen as the selection strategy in this paper. When generating the next-generation population, the parental population and the best individuals in the temporary population generated by crossover and mutation operations are directly reserved to the offspring. The other individuals in the new population are chosen from the parental and temporary populations by the roulette method.

Step 6: Termination conditions of the algorithm. The maximum iteration number of the genetic algorithm LS is set. The algorithm stops iterating when $gen > \mathrm{LS}$, where gen is the algorithm iteration.

5. Numerical Experimental Design

The numerical experiments include the following three parts: First, the example data from the medical supplies distribution are used to verify the effectiveness of the DMMSD model in Section 5.1. Second, we obtain the experimental results and import them into the actual map to analyze the results in Section 5.2. Finally, the experimental results are discussed in Section 5.3.

This paper used MATLAB R2014a to implement the HGA, and all experiments in this paper were evaluated on PCs with Intel® Core™ (Santa Clara, CA, USA) i7-3610QM CPU@ 2.10 GHz and 4 GB memory.

5.1. Model Experiment

5.1.1. Experimental Parameters

We used a batch of medical supplies distribution data from a county MSDC that provides service for 20 township TMPs (due to the particularity of natural disasters, the acquisition of real data is difficult). Information about the MSDC and TMPs, such as the location, demand, and time window is shown in Table 2 (the MSDC is numbered 1 and the overall mass of the medical supplies is 47 kg per case). The parameters of the refrigerated vehicles are shown in Table 3 (the maximum load capacity, maximum travel speed, maximum load volume and other parameters of the vehicle will affect the final distribution plan), and the model parameters are set in Table 4. The average speed of the refrigerated vehicles was 30 km/h in the distribution process; 3 CNY/km was the transport cost for per unit mileage, and the maximum load of the refrigerated vehicle was 670 kg.

Table 2. Required information for MSDC and TMPs.

Number	Longitude (° E)	Latitude (° N)	Demand (Box)	Acceptable Time Window	Service Time (min)
1	105.385	30.871	0	5:30–17:00	0
2	105.439	31.012	1.5	6:00–8:00	10
3	105.396	30.983	0.5	7:30–9:00	5
4	105.535	30.885	1.5	6:00–8:00	10
5	105.396	30.791	1.5	6:30–8:20	10
6	105.346	30.816	1	7:40–9:30	8
7	105.287	30.989	1	7:00–9:00	8
8	105.243	30.896	0.5	7:20–9:00	5
9	105.396	30.923	1	7:30–9:00	8
10	105.236	30.855	0.5	7:00–8:30	5
11	105.250	30.803	1	7:30–9:30	8
12	105.312	30.755	2	7:30–9:30	15
13	105.237	30.752	0.5	7:30–9:30	5
14	105.233	30.697	1.5	7:30–9:30	10
15	105.352	30.680	1.5	7:30–9:00	10
16	105.418	30.720	1.5	6:50–8:30	10
17	105.618	30.911	1.5	7:00–8:40	10
18	105.572	30.958	1.5	7:00–8:40	10
19	105.395	31.063	0.5	7:50–9:00	5
20	105.172	31.009	1	6:30–8:30	8
21	105.133	30.956	1	7:50–9:00	8

Table 3. Vehicle Parameters.

Parameter	Parameter Value	Parameter	Parameter Value
Outline dimension	4845 × 2000 × 2500 (mm)	Container volume	3 m^3
Fastest speed	135 km/h	Rated load capacity	670 kg
Engine type	SOFIM8140.43S4	Fuel type	diesel oil
Engine power	95 kw	Engine emission volume	2798 mL

Table 4. Model parameter settings.

Parameter	Parameter Value
t_0	15 min
T_0	8 °C
T_n	2 °C
t_s	133 min
C_1	300 CNY
C_2	1000 CNY
μ_1	60 CNY/h
μ_2	80 CNY/h
PC	0.8
PM	0.2
LS	200

5.1.2. Initial Distribution Scheme

The initial distribution scheme is shown in Table 5 and Figure 4.

Table 5. The initial distribution service order.

Route Number	Service Order
1	1-5-16-15-14-12-6-1
2	1-3-19-2-18-17-4-9-1
3	1-7-20-21-8-10-11-13-1

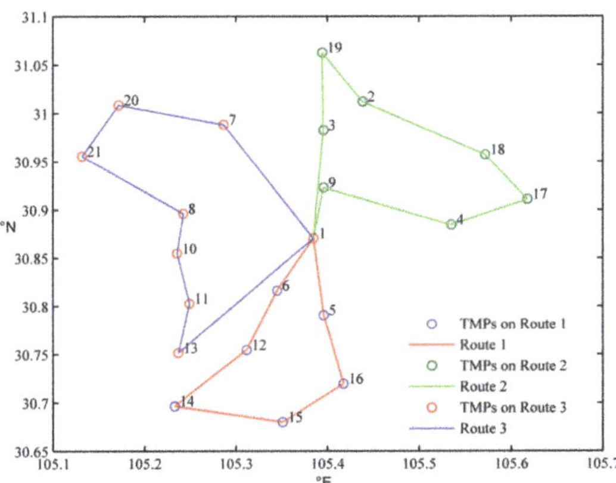

Figure 4. The initial distribution scheme.

5.1.3. A Disturbance Occurs

The simulated situation was as follows: at 133 min after starting the delivery tasks, refrigerated vehicle 3 breaks down at position AP (105.242° E, 30.833° N), which is en route from TMP 10 to 11. CE represents the collection of TMPs that have been served when the disturbance event occurs; UE represents the collection of TMPs that have not been served when the disturbance event occurs; and VE represents the collection of pseudo demand points ($AP \in VE$). The state when the disturbance occurs is shown in Figure 5.

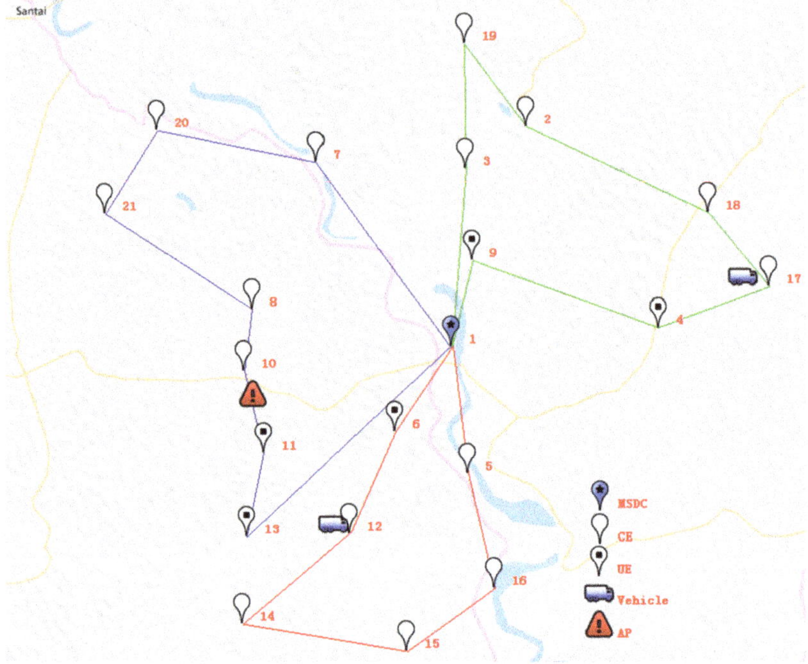

Figure 5. The state when the disturbance occurs.

5.2. Experimental Results

5.2.1. Results under Different Objective Weights

After the disturbance event occurs, the DMMSD model proposed in this paper was used to obtain a rescue scheme for the TMPs that had not been served. The transfer time of the medical supplies was 10 min. The results under different weights of the objective functions were obtained, which are presented in Table 6 and Figure 6. Each group of data is iterated ten times, and the best solution is obtained as shown in Table 6.

Table 6. Results under different objective weights.

Weights	$w_1 = 0.5, w_2 = 0.5$	$w_1 = 0.4, w_2 = 0.6$	$w_1 = 0.3, w_2 = 0.7$	$w_1 = 0.2, w_2 = 0.8$
The number of vehicles that complete the remaining distribution Tasks	2	2	3	3
Path of Vehicle 1	12-AP-11-13-6-1	12-13-AP-11-6-1	12-AP-11-1	12-11-AP-1
Path of Vehicle 2	17-4-9-1	17-4-9-1	17-4-9-1	17-4-9-1
Path of Vehicle 3	AP	AP	AP	AP
Path of Vehicle 4	/	/	1-13-6-1	1-13-6-1
$f(x)$/CNY	1526.1	1819.7	2400.4	3627.5
$g(x)$/min	153.7	103.4	99.7	80.5
Average time for solving (s.)	8.4	8.1	8.9	10.2

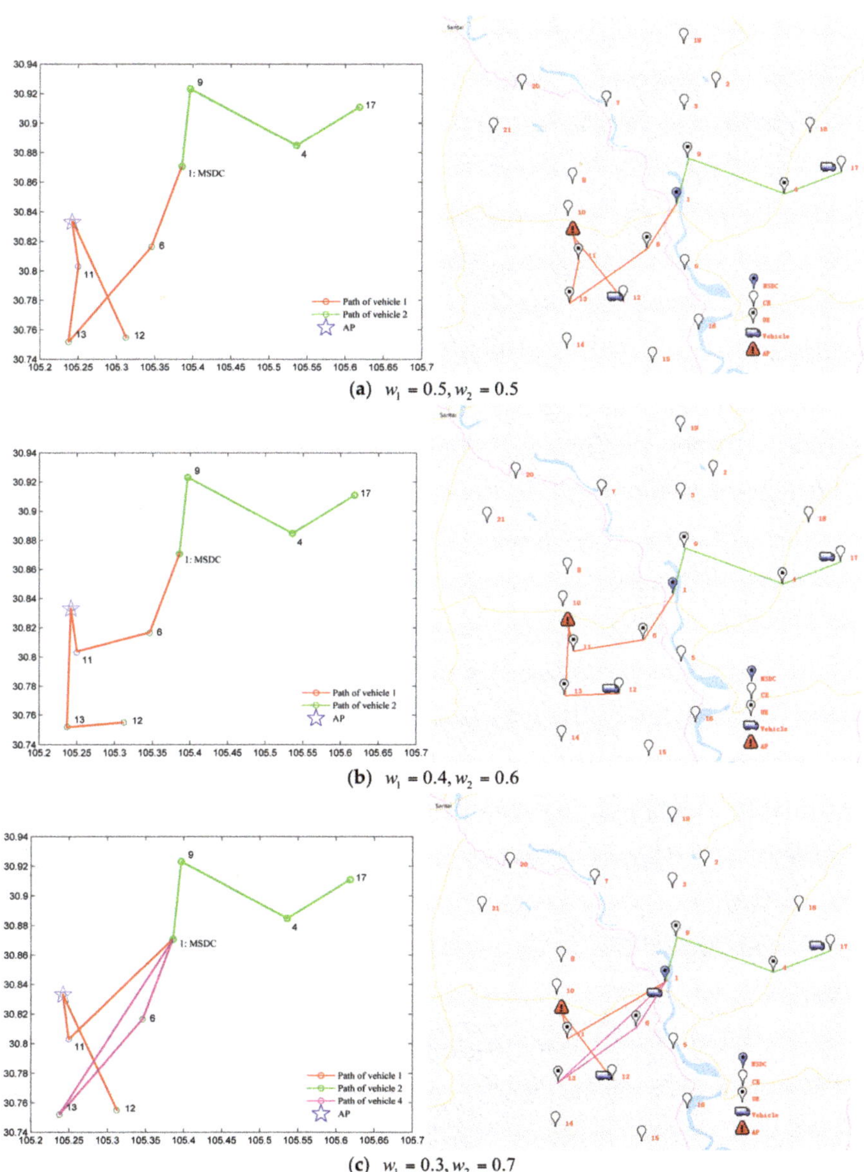

(a) $w_1 = 0.5, w_2 = 0.5$

(b) $w_1 = 0.4, w_2 = 0.6$

(c) $w_1 = 0.3, w_2 = 0.7$

Figure 6. *Cont.*

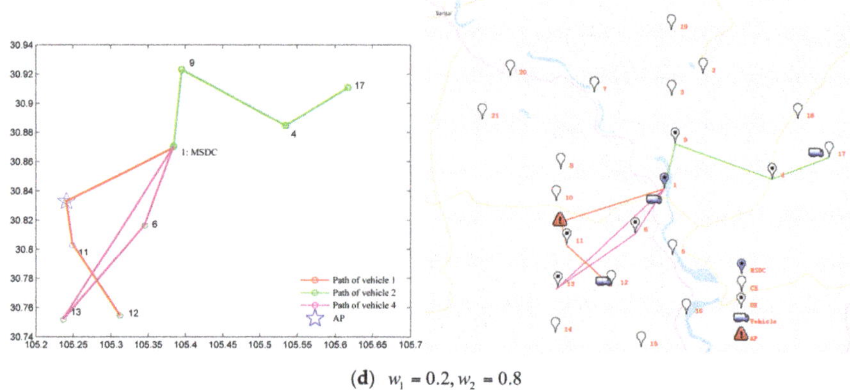

(d) $w_1 = 0.2, w_2 = 0.8$

Figure 6. Distribution schemes under different objective weights.

From the results in Table 6 and Figure 6, we drew the following conclusions:

(1) Different weight coefficients of the objective functions correspond to different disturbance recovery schemes. As shown in Table 6, we set the weight coefficients of the time and cost objective functions to four different sets of numerical values ($w_1 = 0.5, 0.4, 0.3, 0.2$; $w_2 = 0.5, 0.6, 0.7, 0.8$); then, four different disturbance recovery distribution schemes were obtained.

(2) The number of vehicles used in different disturbance recovery distribution schemes is discrepant. As shown in Table 6, there were different numbers of vehicles in the four distribution schemes. The original distribution vehicles continued to be used in the first two distribution schemes; vehicle 1 was dispatched to rescue disturbed vehicle 3 and was responsible for the remaining TMPs that had not been served in the delivery tasks of vehicles 1 and 3 (i.e., the red route in Figure 6a,b). Vehicle 4 was added in the latter two distribution schemes to assist vehicle 1 in completing the service to the remaining TMPs that had not been served in the delivery tasks of vehicles 1 and 3 (i.e., the red route belongs to vehicle 1 and the purple route belongs to vehicle 4 in Figure 6c,d).

(3) For the time disturbance subobjective, the disturbance gradually decreased with an increase in its weight, but the disturbance of the distribution cost gradually increased. As seen from the results in Table 6, $f(x)$ gradually increased with the decrease in w_1, and $g(x)$ continuously decreased with the increase in w_2. In other words, as the weight coefficient of the cost objective function decreased, the cost of the disturbance recovery distribution scheme gradually increased, but the disturbance of the rescue scheme to time gradually decreased.

(4) The different weight coefficient settings of objective functions resulted in the same fitness value. From the results in Table 6, we found that the same value of f could be obtained from different values of w_1, w_2, $f(x)$, $g(x)$ by calculations using Formula (14). This means that the different weight coefficient settings of the objective functions have no influence on the fitness value of the optimal solution, but different values of cost and time disturbance subobjective functions are formed; in addition, different disturbance recovery schemes are obtained at the same time. Therefore, in the face of actual disturbance events, emergency rescue decision makers should set the appropriate weight combination of objective function according to the current disturbance situation.

5.2.2. The Convergence of the Algorithm

During the process of solving the results in Section 5.2.1, the convergence of the HGA under different objective weights is shown in Figure 7.

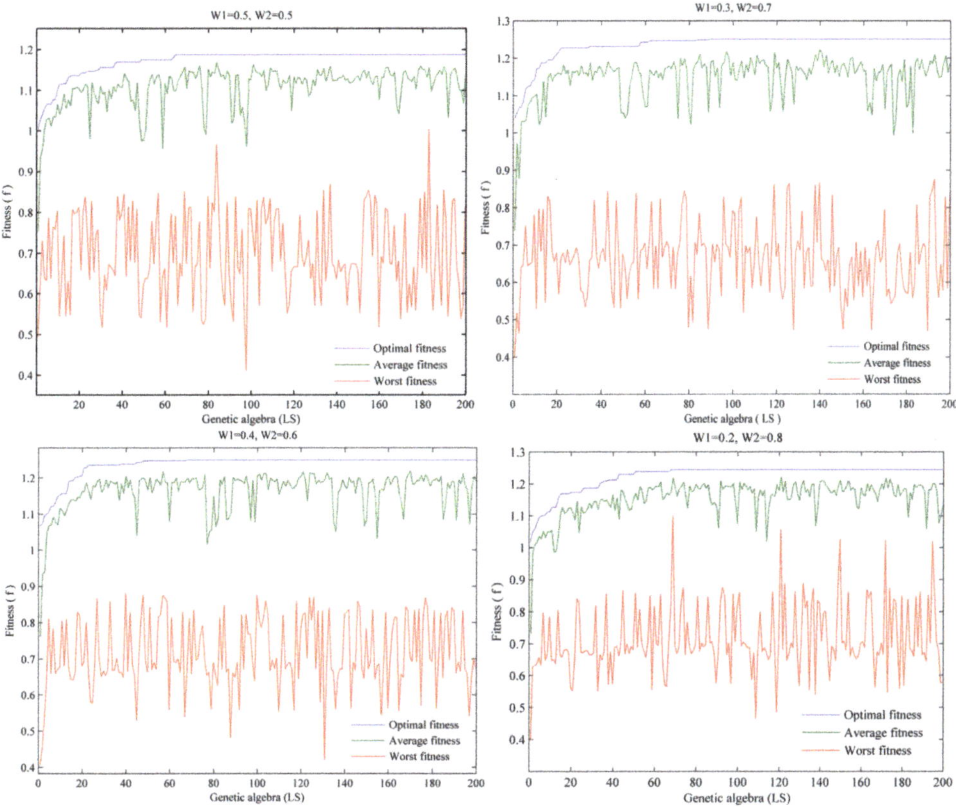

Figure 7. The convergence of the hybrid genetic algorithm (HGA) under different objective weights.

There are many factors that can affect the execution time of the algorithm, such as the size of the problem and the speed at which the computer executes the instructions (running memory, hardware quality, etc.). Therefore, when using different computer solutions, the solution time shown in Table 6 may be different. However, from Figure 7, we can clearly see that when solving the model with different weights, the HGA convergence effect was considerable, and the speed of convergence was fast. The optimal solution was obtained in the 60–80th generation, which proves that the algorithm has high stability.

5.3. Analysis of Experimental Results

Medical supplies are important public health supplies. Based on the concept of disturbance management, the DMMSD model was proposed to make emergency response decisions for disturbance events in the distribution process of these medical supplies. At the same time, we measured the disturbance from the two dimensions of time and cost, thus obtaining disturbance recovery route maps at the different weights to provide a reference for the decision-making of disturbance management scheduling in medical supplies distribution. However, during the actual distribution process, emergency decisionmakers responding to disturbance events need to make reasonable arrangements according to different emergency situations.

After a disturbance event occurs, the rescue decision-makers can weigh the rescue time and cost according to the urgency and scope of the disaster situation. The research results of this paper can be used as a reference for decision makers' scientific decisions. The specific recommendations are shown below.

In an emergency distribution environment with a sudden epidemic situation or a large-scale natural disaster, public health supplies, such as vaccines and blood, need to rapidly be made available to meet the urgent demands of the TMPs. In this case, time is life. The MSDC needs to deliver the medical supplies to the TMPs in the shortest possible time to quickly control the epidemic situation or disease caused by natural disasters. Therefore, keeping the time disturbance of delivering medical supplies to TMPs at a minimum is the main goal. Thus, at this time, the time disturbance subobjective function has a very high weighting, and the cost is second.

However, the distribution of public health medical supplies, such as vaccines, can cause significant costs. Although all costs will be paid during the initial stage of an epidemic situation or large-scale natural disaster, the urgency for the demand of medical supplies will be gradually reduced after the epidemic situation is essentially stabilized or during the general distribution process. Meanwhile, there is a limitation of the actual delivery capacity; thus, what also needs to be considered is the operation costs of the logistics system. At this time, the weighting of the time disturbance is reduced and the weighting of the cost is increased.

6. Conclusions

Special medical supplies, such as blood and vaccines, are the key to reducing the number of casualties and controlling the epidemic after a natural disaster occurs. Therefore, it is obvious that the quality of distribution of medical supplies is important. In order to quickly respond to disturbance events during the distribution of medical supplies, a disturbance management model for medical supplies distribution was proposed in this paper to effectively deal with the interruption of cold-chain logistics caused by disturbance events and to ensure medical supply distribution is safe and effective. In this model, based on the concept of disturbance management, the measurement of disturbance is carried out from two dimensions: time and cost. The objective functions of the model are minimum cost and minimum time disturbance, and a hybrid genetic algorithm was designed to solve the model. Furthermore, disturbance recovery schemes under different weight coefficients were obtained through numerical experiments which provide a reference for the emergency decision makers of disturbance events to reasonably conduct the disturbance management. The validities of the model and algorithm were verified.

In future research, we will consider further optimization of the distribution paths in the case of a combination of disturbances caused by different disturbance events. Meanwhile, real geographic situations should be taken into consideration in the problem of disturbance management.

Author Contributions: Y.S. implemented the experiments with the guidance of Z.H.

Funding: This work was supported by the National Social Science Foundation of China (No. 13CGL127), the Science and Technology Plan Program of Sichuan Province (Grant No.2018ZR0066).

Acknowledgments: Yuhe Shi would specifically like to highlight the ongoing support of Songyi Wang from Chongqing University for his help with the algorithm experiment, and Zhaoxia Guo of Sichuan University for the revision of this manuscript.

Conflicts of Interest: The authors declare no conflict of interest.

References

1. Han, W.; Chen, L.; Jiang, B.; Ma, W.; Zhang, Y. Major natural disasters in China, 1985–2014: Occurrence and damages. *Int. J. Environ. Res. Public Health* **2016**, *13*, 1118. [CrossRef] [PubMed]
2. Chan, E.Y.Y.; Gao, Y.; Griffiths, S.M. Literature review of health impact post-earthquakes in China 1906–2007. *J. Public Health* **2010**, *32*, 52–61. [CrossRef] [PubMed]
3. Chan, E.Y.Y.; Guo, C.; Lee, P.; Liu, S.; Mark, C.K.M. Health emergency and disaster risk management (health-EDRM) in remote ethnic minority areas of rural China: The case of a flood-prone village in Sichuan. *Int. J. Disaster Risk Sci.* **2017**, *8*, 156–163. [CrossRef]

4. Lo, S.T.T.; Chan, E.Y.Y.; Chan, G.K.W.; Murray, V.; Abrahams, J.; Ardalan, A.; Kayano, R.; Yau, J.C.W. Health emergency and disaster risk management (health-EDRM): Developing the research field within the Sendai framework paradigm. *Int. J. Disaster Risk Sci.* **2017**, *8*, 1–5. [CrossRef]
5. Nelson, C.M.; Wibisono, H.; Purwanto, H.; Mansyur, I.; Moniaga, V.; Widjaya, A. Hepatitis B vaccine freezing in the Indonesian cold chain: Evidence and solutions. *Bull. World Health Organ.* **2004**, *82*, 99–105. [PubMed]
6. Haidari, L.A.; Brown, S.T.; Ferguson, M.; Bancroft, E.; Spiker, M.; Wilcox, A.; Ambikapathi, R.; Sampath, V.; Connor, D.L.; Lee, B.Y. The economic and operational value of using drones to transport vaccines. *Vaccine* **2016**, *34*, 4062–4067. [CrossRef] [PubMed]
7. Jozefowiez, N.; Mancel, C.; Mora-Camino, F. A heuristic approach based on shortest path problems for integrated flight, aircraft, and passenger rescheduling under disruptions. *Eur. J. Inf. Syst.* **2013**, *64*, 384–395. [CrossRef]
8. Kohla, N.; Larsenb, A.; Larsenc, J.; Rossd, A.; Tiourinee, S. Airline disruption management—Perspectives, experiences and outlook. *J. Air Transp. Manag.* **2007**, *13*, 149–162. [CrossRef]
9. Ambulkar, S.; Blackhurst, J.; Grawe, S. Firm's resilience to supply chain disruptions: Scale development and empirical examination. *J. Oper. Manag.* **2015**, *33–34*, 111–122. [CrossRef]
10. Revilla, E.; Sáenz, M.J. Supply chain disruption management: Global convergence vs. national specificity. *J. Bus. Res.* **2014**, *67*, 1123–1135. [CrossRef]
11. Yuan, J.; Mu, Y. Rescheduling with release dates to minimize makespan under a limit on the maximum sequence disruption. *Eur. J. Oper. Res.* **2007**, *182*, 936–944. [CrossRef]
12. Wang, K.; Choi, S.H. A decomposition-based approach to flexible flow shop scheduling under machine breakdown. *Int. J. Prod. Res.* **2012**, *50*, 215–234. [CrossRef]
13. Cacchiani, V.; Huisman, D.; Kidd, M.; Kroon, L.; Toth, P.; Veelenturf, L.; Wagenaar, J. An overview of recovery models and algorithms for real-time railway rescheduling. *Transp. Res. B Methodol.* **2014**, *63*, 15–37. [CrossRef]
14. Yu, G.; Qi, X. *Disruption Management: Framework, Models and Applications*; World Scientific: Singapore, 2004.
15. Zeimpekis, V.; Giaglis, G.M.; Minis, I. In A dynamic real-timefleet management system for incident handling in city logistics. In Proceedings of the IEEE Vehicular Technology Conference, Stockholm, Sweden, 30 May–1 June 2005.
16. Potvin, J.Y.; Xu, Y.; Benyahia, I. Vehicle routing and scheduling with dynamic travel times. *Comput. Oper. Res.* **2006**, *33*, 1129–1137. [CrossRef]
17. Taniguchi, E.; Shimamoto, H. Intelligent transportation system based dynamic vehicle routing and scheduling with variable travel times. *Transp. Res. Part C* **2004**, *12*, 235–250. [CrossRef]
18. Ruan, J.; Wang, X. Disruption management of emergency medical supplies intermodal transportation with updated transit centers. *Oper. Res. Manag. Sci.* **2016**, *25*, 114–124.
19. Ding, Q.; Hu, X.; Jiang, Y. A model of disruption management based on prospect theory in logistic distribution. *J. Manag. Sci. China* **2014**, *17*, 1–9.
20. Liu, C.; Zhu, Z.; Liu, L. Disruption management of location-routing problem (LRP) for emergency logistics system in early stage after earthquake. *Comput. Eng. Appl.* **2017**, *53*, 224–230.
21. Ramezanian, R.; Behboodi, Z. Blood supply chain network design under uncertainties in supply and demand considering social aspects. *Transp. Res. Part E* **2017**, *104*, 69–82. [CrossRef]
22. Wang, K.; Ma, Z.; Zhou, Y. A two-phase decision-making approach for emergency blood transferring problem in public emergencies. *J. Transp. Syst. Eng. Inf. Technol.* **2013**, *13*, 169–178.
23. Chen, Y.; Lv, W.; Jiang, J. Research on cold-chain delivery model of multi-vaccines based on time constraint. *Logist. Sci.-Tech.* **2017**, *40*, 24–26.
24. Campbell, A.M.; Vandenbussche, D.; Hermann, W. Routing for relief efforts. *Transp. Sci.* **2008**, *42*, 127–145. [CrossRef]
25. Battini, D.; Peretti, U.; Persona, A.; Sgarbossa, F. Application of humanitarian last mile distribution model. *J. Humanit. Logist. Supply Chain Manag.* **2014**, *4*, 131–148. [CrossRef]
26. Ruan, J.; Wang, X.; Shi, Y. A two-stage approach for medical supplies intermodal transportation in large-scale disaster responses. *Int J. Environ. Res. Public Health* **2014**, *11*, 11081–11109. [CrossRef] [PubMed]
27. Caunhye, A.M.; Nie, X.; Pokharel, S. Optimization models in emergency logistics: A literature review. *Socio-Econ. Plan. Sci.* **2011**, *46*, 4–13. [CrossRef]

28. Galindo, G.; Batta, R. Review of recent developments in or/ms research in disaster operations management. *Eur. J. Oper. Res.* **2013**, *230*, 201–211. [CrossRef]
29. Najafi, M.; Eshghi, K.; Dullaert, W. A multi-objective robust optimization model for logistics planning in the earthquake response phase. *Transp. Res. Part E* **2013**, *49*, 217–249. [CrossRef]
30. Omair, M.; Sarkar, B. Minimum quantity lubrication and carbon footprint: A step towards sustainability. *Sustainability* **2017**, *9*, 714. [CrossRef]
31. Habib, M.S.; Sarkar, B. An integrated location-allocation model for temporary disaster debris management under an uncertain environment. *Sustainability* **2017**, *9*, 716. [CrossRef]
32. Ahmed, W.; Sarkar, B. Impact of carbon emissions in a sustainable supply chain management for a second generation biofuel. *J. Clean. Prod.* **2018**, *186*, 807–820. [CrossRef]
33. Sarkar, B.; Ahmed, W.; Kim, N. Joint effects of variable carbon emission cost and multi-delay-in-payments under single-setup-multiple-delivery policy in a global sustainable supply chain. *J. Clean. Prod.* **2018**, *185*, 421–445. [CrossRef]
34. Sarkar, B. Supply chain coordination with variable backorder, inspections, and discount policy for fixed lifetime products. *Math. Probl. Eng.* **2016**, *2016*, 1–14. [CrossRef]
35. Sarkar, B.; Ganguly, B.; Sarkar, M.; Pareek, S. Effect of variable transportation and carbon emission in a three-echelon supply chain model. *Transp. Res. Part E* **2016**, *91*, 112–128. [CrossRef]
36. Sarkar, B. A production-inventory model with probabilistic deterioration in two-echelon supply chain management. *Appl. Math. Model.* **2013**, *37*, 3138–3151. [CrossRef]
37. Sarkar, B.; Sana, S.S.; Chaudhuri, K. An inventory model with finite replenishment rate, trade credit policy and price-discount offer. *J. Ind. Eng.* **2013**, *2013*, 18. [CrossRef]
38. Moon, I.; Shin, E.; Sarkar, B. Min-max distribution free continuous—Review model with a service level constraint and variable lead time. *Appl. Math. Comput.* **2014**, *229*, 310–315. [CrossRef]
39. Sarkar, B.; Saren, S.; Sinha, D.; Sun, H. Effect of unequal lot sizes, variable setup cost, and carbon emission cost in a supply chain model. *Math. Probl. Eng.* **2015**, *2015*, 1–13. [CrossRef]
40. He, Z.; Chen, P.; Liu, H.; Guo, Z. Performance measurement system and strategies for developing low-carbon logistics: A case study in China. *J. Clean. Prod.* **2017**, *156*, 395–405. [CrossRef]
41. He, Z.; Guo, Z.; Wang, J. Integrated scheduling of production and distribution operations in a global MTO supply chain. *Enterp. Inf. Syst.* **2018**, *19*, 94–122. [CrossRef]
42. Guo, Z.; Zhang, D.; Liu, H.; He, Z.; Shi, L. Green transportation scheduling with pickup time and transport mode selections using a novel multi-objective memetic optimization approach. *Transp. Res. D* **2016**, *60*, 137–152. [CrossRef]
43. Wang, S.; Tao, F.; Shi, Y. In Optimization of air freight network considering the time window of customer, In Proceedings of the IEEE International Conference on Industrial Technology and Management, Oxford, UK, 7–9 May 2018.
44. Wang, X.; Ruan, J.; Zhang, K.; Ma, C. Study on combinational disruption management for vehicle routing problem with fuzzy time windows. *J. Manag. Sci. China* **2011**, *14*, 2–15.
45. Wang, S.; Tao, F.; Shi, Y.; Wen, H. Optimization of vehicle routing problem with time windows for cold chain logistics based on carbon tax. *Sustainability* **2017**, *9*, 694. [CrossRef]
46. Wang, S.; Tao, F.; Shi, Y. Optimization of inventory routing problem in refined oil logistics with the perspective of carbon tax. *Energies* **2018**, *11*, 1437. [CrossRef]
47. Liu, W.Y.; Lin, C.C.; Chiu, C.R.; Tsao, Y.S.; Wang, Q. Minimizing the carbon footprint for the time-dependent heterogeneous-fleet vehicle routing problem with alternative paths. *Sustainability* **2014**, *6*, 4658–4684. [CrossRef]
48. Wang, S.; Tao, F.; Shi, Y. Optimization of location–routing problem for cold chain logistics considering carbon footprint. *Int. J. Environ. Res. Public Health* **2018**, *15*, 86. [CrossRef] [PubMed]

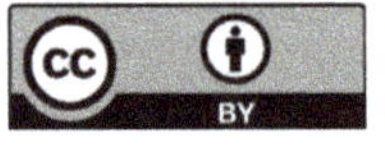

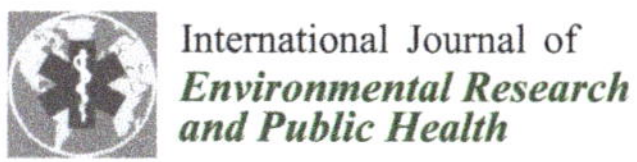

International Journal of
Environmental Research and Public Health

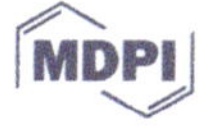

Article

Transmission of Influenza A in a Student Office Based on Realistic Person-to-Person Contact and Surface Touch Behaviour

Nan Zhang and Yuguo Li *

Department of Mechanical Engineering, The University of Hong Kong, Pokfulam Road, Hong Kong, China; zhangnan@hku.hk

* Correspondence: liyg@hku.hk; Tel.: +852-3917-2625

Received: 2 June 2018; Accepted: 7 August 2018; Published: 9 August 2018

Abstract: Influenza A viruses result in the deaths of hundreds of thousands of individuals worldwide each year. In this study, influenza A transmission in a graduate student office is simulated via long-range airborne, fomite, and close contact routes based on real data from more than 3500 person-to-person contacts and 127,000 surface touches obtained by video-camera. The long-range airborne, fomite and close contact routes contribute to 54.3%, 4.2% and 44.5% of influenza A infections, respectively. For the fomite route, 59.8%, 38.1% and 2.1% of viruses are transmitted to the hands of students from private surfaces around the infected students, the students themselves and other susceptible students, respectively. The intranasal dose via fomites of the students' bodies, belongings, computers, desks, chairs and public facilities are 8.0%, 6.8%, 13.2%, 57.8%, 9.3% and 4.9%, respectively. The intranasal dose does not monotonously increase or decrease with the virus transfer rate between hands and surfaces. Mask wearing is much more useful than hand washing for control of influenza A in the tested office setting. Regular cleaning of high-touch surfaces, which can reduce the infection risk by 2.14%, is recommended and is much more efficient than hand-washing.

Keywords: influenza A; airborne; fomite; close contact; infection; surface touch; office; mask; hand-washing

---

1. Introduction

Influenza is a highly contagious respiratory illness that causes 1,250,000 deaths annually worldwide [1]. It is estimated that influenza A viruses result in the deaths of approximately half a million individuals worldwide every year [2]. Influenza A viruses exist on many surfaces in our daily lives, such as towels in homes and medical cart items in hospitals [3].

Despite human beings' vast clinical experience, debate about the transmission of influenza continues [4]. The influenza virus is known to be spread from person to person by at least two mechanisms: direct and indirect transfer of respiratory secretions and contact with large droplets that settle onto fomites [5]. Studies have shown that influenza A may be transmitted by inhalation of small airborne particles [6]. Although some evidence was found of animal-to-animal transmission [7], other evidence of person-to-person transmission was based on observational and epidemiological studies [8]. Influenza can also be transmitted by droplet nuclei [9,10]. In addition, other studies have found that the fomite route could be a potential route of influenza transmission [11]. In general, influenza A can be spread via the airborne, droplet and direct and indirect contact routes.

Many simulations of influenza transmission have been conducted in enclosed spaces such as hospitals [12] and air cabins [13], and in large spaces such as cities [14], and even between cities [15]. Large-scale influenza transmission is usually based on macroscopic factors such as human mobility via airplane and other modes of public transport [15]. Microscopic factors such as how people talk or make contact with each other are ignored because of complexity. Most human behaviour, including person-to-person contact and surface touches, are hypothesised even when all transmission routes are considered. However, human behaviour changes with the environment, and large errors may result if all human behaviour is unknown or randomly set. A simulation of influenza A transmission based on realistic data of human behaviour in a confined space is needed to help understand influenza A transmission and to implement effective measures to prevent and control disease.

In this study, we simulated influenza A transmission in a graduate student office by considering three routes: long-range airborne, fomite and close contact (short-range airborne and droplet spray). All student behaviour, including close contact and surface touches in the office, was recorded by video-camera from 9 a.m. to 9 p.m., from 11 to 15 September 2017. The data included more than 3500 close contacts between students and more than 127,000 surface touches. Influenza A transmission was simulated in the office via three routes based on realistic behaviour obtained from these recorded data. We discovered how influenza A virus is transmitted via air, hands, surfaces, mucous membranes and inhalation. We also analysed the efficacy of various strategies for prevention of influenza A via various transmission routes.

2. Materials and Methods

We simulated influenza A transmission via three routes (long-range airborne, fomite and close contact) in a graduate student office in China. The office measured $12 \times 8.4 \times 2.7$ m and included 39 students. All surfaces were grouped into six categories (primary surfaces): private (i.e., the student [*Std*]; body parts), students' belongings (*Bln*), desks (*Dsk*), chairs (*Chr*), computers (*Cpt*) and public facilities (*Pbf*). These primary surfaces were in turn divided into 31 secondary surfaces consisting of 57 types of sub-surfaces with multiple surfaces for each type, giving a total of 1490 basic surfaces (Supplementary Materials: Table S1).

The data for each student's surface touch behaviour were taken from four video-cameras installed on the office ceiling to monitor student behaviour of close contact and surface touch from 9 a.m. to 9 p.m. on five successive weekdays from 11 to 15 September 2017. All students in the office gave informed consent for inclusion before they participated in the study. Five video image analysis assistants were appointed to process the data second by second, recording all visible touch actions made by every student in the office. A surface touch was defined as any contact between a hand or finger and a solid surface or object lasting for 1 s or longer. The information recorded comprised the onset time, duration, and location of each touch, and details of which student had done the touching, which hand had been used, and which surface had been touched. For quality control during the video image analysis, one author (NZ) verified touch actions at two time points, namely the 15th minute and the 45th minute of each of the 60 h. Verification revealed that 67 out of the 1712 touch actions (3.1%) had been incorrectly recorded by the original video analysers.

In the 5-day study period, 127,052 touches by left and right hands on 1490 coded surfaces were recorded. The surfaces had a total exposure to touch of 1,517,958 person·seconds. The students spent 90.74% of their time in the office touching surfaces [16].

In this paper, we used influenza A as an example. Figure 1 illustrates how influenza A is transmitted via the long-range airborne, fomite and close contact routes. When an infected student breathes, talks, coughs or sneezes, the virus is carried in particles and released into the environment. Small droplets disperse in the air. Some floating particles flow outdoors through the ventilation system, some are inhaled by students, some are deposited on surfaces and those still in the air lose viability over time. Large droplets are rapidly deposited on surfaces near the infected student or are directly sprayed onto the hands of the infected person while covering their mouth and nose while coughing or sneezing. The virus will then be transferred to a surface if it is touched by a contaminated hand. A clean hand can also be contaminated if it touches a contaminated surface. Some large droplets with virus on hands can be transferred to the mucous membranes if the student touches his or her own lips, nose or eyes. Some large droplets are resuspended from surfaces to the air because of human activities such as walking. In addition, viruses on hands and surfaces also lose viability over time. Moreover, when an infected student speaks face-to-face with other students, particles are sprayed from the mouth of the infected student. Some small particles will be directly inhaled via the respiratory tract by students who speak with the infected student, and some large particles might be rapidly deposited on their mucous membranes. The inhalation dose and intranasal dose of susceptible students gradually increase, and each student's infection risk can be calculated based on the dose-response parameters of influenza A.

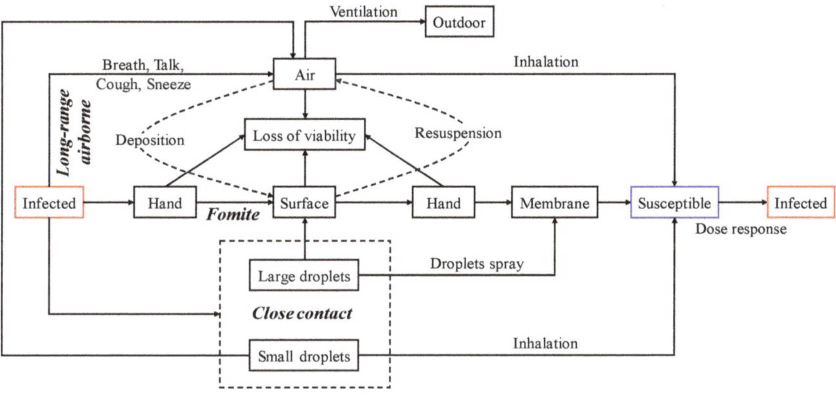

Figure 1. Three routes for influenza A transmission.

All students go to lunch and dinner between 12 a.m. and 1 p.m. and between 5 p.m. and 6 p.m., respectively, every day. In real conditions, all students do not stay in the office all the time. To reduce the randomness caused by their stay duration, all students are assumed to remain in the office from 9 a.m. to 9 p.m. except for lunch and dinner time.

2.1. Parameter Setting

The US Centers for Disease Control and Prevention (CDC) have defined three influenza transmission routes: long-range airborne, fomite (direct and indirect) and close contact (Table 1). Only particles with a diameter of less than 10 μm can penetrate the lungs [17]. Pathogens carried in particles with an aerodynamic diameter (d_a) between 10 and 100 μm are inspired if a person is facing the patient at close range during an expiratory event such as a cough or a talk [18]. More than 99% of the pathogens emitted in a cough are carried by particles with an aerodynamic diameter $d_a > 100$ μm [19], and these particles tend to settle rapidly on surfaces near the point of emission [18].

Table 1. Modes of person-to-person transmission of respiratory viruses [20].

Transmission Route	Definition
Aerosol transmission	Virus is transmitted through the air by aerosols within the inspirable size range or smaller; aerosol particles are small enough to be inhaled into the nasopharynx and distally into the trachea and lung.
Direct transmission	Virus is transferred by contact from an infected person to another person without a contaminated intermediate object (fomite).
Indirect transmission	Virus is transferred by contact with a contaminated intermediate object (fomite).
Droplet spray transmission	Virus is transmitted through the air by droplet sprays (such as those produced by coughing or sneezing); a key feature is deposition of droplets by impaction on exposed mucous membranes.

At the beginning of the simulation, there are 39 students in the office, i.e., one infected student (P_0) and 38 susceptible students (P_1–P_{38}). They touch surfaces and talk with each other based on realistic data on surface touch and interpersonal contacts obtained from the video analysis. In each simulation, all students will select an action, such as with surfaces they touch and with whom they talk, from the database (collected surface touch and close contact data) at each time step (second).

2.2. Long-Range Airborne

Particles of various sizes ae generated by activities such as breathing, talking, coughing and sneezing. We assumed that particles ($d_a < 10$ μm) uniformly floated in the air of the office. The deposition of these small particles is slight because it requires around an hour in a steady environment [21,22]. In an office setting, the deposition rate will be reduced because of frequent walking by the students. We assumed that the deposition rate was 0.1 min^{-1}, which means that 10% of the particles' volume is deposited uniformly on all surfaces per minute.

Because the difference in the association between the size and number of particles from previous researchers is large, we use the average values from previous studies to assess the total virus quantity in small particles. Summarising the previous studies [23–29], the total volume of small particles ($d_a < 10$ μm) by breathing (V'_{vb}), talking (V'_{vt}) (counting from 1 to 100, which takes about 100 s), coughing (V'_{vc}) and sneezing (V'_{vs}) are estimated as 1.02×10^{-10} mL, 1.47×10^{-7} mL, 1.65×10^{-7} mL and 1.27×10^{-6} mL, respectively. The total volume of large particles ($d_a > 10$ μm) generated by breathing (V''_{vb}), talking (V''_{vt}), coughing (V''_{vc}) and sneezing (V''_{vs}) are estimated as 0 mL, 5.15×10^{-3} mL, 6.15×10^{-3} mL and 4.75×10^{-2} mL, respectively. Here, we assumed that the size distribution of particles generated by coughing and sneezing was the same. People take an average of 15 breaths per minute, so a breath takes around 4 s [30]. The average frequencies of coughing and sneezing episodes for an influenza A infected person are 22/h [31] and 5/h [32] respectively. A cough takes 1 s, and a sneeze is assumed to take 3 s. Our recorded data show that students in the office spent an average of 10% of their time talking with others. Therefore, the frequency of breathing (f_b), talking (f_t), coughing (f_c) and sneezing (f_s) of an infected person are 21,600 times, 0.8 h (two students on average share the time during talking), 352 times and 80 times per day (talking, coughing and sneezing during 16 h except 8-h sleep). The total volume of droplets generated by an infected person per day (V_V) is calculated by Equation (1).

$$V_v = V\prime_v + V\prime\prime_v = \sum_{i=1}^{i=4}(V\prime_{vi} + V\prime\prime_{vi})\cdot f_i \approx 6.11 \text{ mL/day} \quad (1)$$

where i = 1 to 4 shows the human activities of breathing, talking, coughing and sneezing, respectively; $V\prime_v$ and $V\prime\prime_v$ are the total volume of small and large droplets generated by an infected person per day, respectively.

We assumed that an infected person's initial viral shedding rate is around 1.5×10^7 TCID50/day [19,24,25,31,33], and it changes with time and the severity of infection. Because the amount of virus in a particle is roughly proportional to the particle's volume [34], we considered the virus concentrations in all particles to be the same. The virus concentration (C_v) in all particles is then obtained ($C_v = 1 \times 10^{6.39}$ TCID50/mL). This value is between the virus concentration in nasopharyngeal fluid (10^2–10^7 TCID50/mL) measured by Douglas [35] and that in saliva (10^4–10^8 TCID50/mL) estimated by Nicas [36].

The ventilation rate (V_{AC}) in offices is usually set to 1 ACH [37]. The respiratory rate (R_R) of a person is around 0.38 m^3/h (0.11 L/s) [38]. The inactivation rate (μ_a) of influenza A in aerosols in the air changes with the relative humidity (RH%) and temperature [39]. We assumed that the relative humidity and temperature in the office were around 50% and 20 °C to 24 °C, respectively; they were not measured. The inactivation rate (μ_a) of influenza A in aerosols in the air is 13.9 day^{-1} [40].

If a susceptible person inhales aerosol that contains influenza A viruses, he or she has a probability of being infected. The infection probability depends on the total inhalation quantity of the virus.

$$IR_I = 1 - \exp(-\alpha_R \times D) \quad (2)$$

where IR_I is the infection risk (probability to be infected), D is the respiratory dose, α_R is the estimated dose-response parameter for exposure to the respiratory tract distal to the head airways from the respirable particle inhalation study, and $\alpha_R = 0.18$ TCID50^{-1} is obtained by influenza A2/Bethesda/10/63 virus aerosol in humans [36].

All values mentioned above are listed in Table 2.

Table 2. Parameters related to long-range airborne.

Parameter	Symbol	Value	Source
Deposition rate	R_D	0.1 min^{-1}	Assumed
Volume of small particles by breathing	V'_{vb}	1.02×10^{-10} mL	[23–29]
Volume of small particles by talking	V'_{vt}	1.47×10^{-7} mL	[23–29]
Volume of small particles by coughing	V'_{vc}	1.65×10^{-7} mL	[23–29]
Volume of small particles by sneezing	V'_{vs}	1.27×10^{-6} mL	[23–29]
Volume of large droplets by breathing	V''_{vb}	0 mL	[23–29]
Volume of large droplets by talking	V''_{vt}	5.15×10^{-3} mL	[23–29]
Volume of large droplets by coughing	V''_{vc}	6.15×10^{-3} mL	[23–29]
Volume of large droplets by sneezing	V''_{vs}	4.75×10^{-2} mL	[23–29]
Frequency of breath	F_b	15 min^{-1}	[30]
Frequency of coughing (infected person)	F_c	22 h^{-1}	[31]
Frequency of sneezing (infected person)	F_s	5 h^{-1}	[32]
Duration per cough	D_c	1 s	Assumed
Duration per sneeze	D_s	3 s	Assumed
Percentage of time on talking with others	P_t	10%	Monitored
Viral shedding rate	R_s	1.5×10^7 TCID50/day	[19,24,25,31,33]
Virus concentration in exhaled particles	C_v	$1 \times 10^{6.39}$ TCID50/mL	Calculated based on [19,23–29,31,33,34]
Ventilation rate in the office	V_{AC}	1 ACH	[37]
Respiratory rate of a person	R_R	0.38 m^3/h	[38]
Inactivation rate of influenza A [1]	μ_a	13.9 day^{-1}	[40]
Dose-response parameter	α_R	0.18 TCID50^{-1}	[36]

[1] The inactivation rate of influenza A in aerosols in the air in the condition of 50% R.H and 20 °C–24 °C.

2.3. Fomite

Large droplets rapidly settle on the ground [41]. In the simulations, we considered that droplets larger than 10 μm ($d_a > 10$ μm) do not remain airborne long enough to become respirable [19]. When an infected student talks, coughs or sneezes, areas 1-m in front of and 0.5-m on both sides of the patient will be contaminated [29]. We assumed that half of the particles are deposited on surfaces that are touched by the infected persons themselves and that the remaining 50% of particles are randomly distributed on the surfaces near the infected persons when they talk, cough and sneeze. If no surface is touched, half of the particles are deposited on the infected student's desktop if he or she sits on his or her own chair; otherwise, half of the particles are deposited on the floor. According to the analysis of human touch behaviour in an office, the touch frequency for each surface is listed in Table 3, and the type and area of each surface are also listed.

Table 3. Detailed information of all sub-surfaces.

Sub-Surf [1]	Surf Type [2]	F [3] (h^{-1})	Area [4] (cm^2)	Hori-Coef [5]	Sub-Surf [1]	Surf Type [2]	F [3] (h^{-1})	Area [4] (cm^2)	Hori-Coef
*Std*H$_1$	S	6.32	469	0.5	*Std*H$_2$	S	19.41	470	0
*Std*H$_3$	S	1.01	470	0	*Std*S$_1$	P	0.28	504	0.5
*Std*S$_2$	P	0.34	504	0.5	*Std*A$_1$	P	1.17	1293	0.5
*Std*A$_2$	P	1.35	1293	0.5	*Std*D$_1$	S	3.76	183	0
*Std*D$_2$	S	3.80	183	0	*Std*B$_1$	P	2.86	2401	0
*Std*B$_2$	P	0.99	940	0	*Std*L$_1$	P	12.64	6592	0
*Bln*B$_1$	P	3.05	2600	0.5	*Bln*C$_1$	N	2.88	500	0
*Bln*E$_1$	N	1.94	10	0.5	*Bln*G$_1$	N	2.71	10	0.5
*Bln*M$_1$	N	15.12	200	0.5	*Bln*O$_1$	P	0.65	7500	0
*Bln*P$_1$	P	0.39	2400	0.5	*Cpt*M$_1$	N	23.61	120	0.5
*Cpt*K$_1$	N	28.98	700	1	*Dsk*T$_1$	N	20.19	6000	1
*Dsk*D$_1$	St	1.04	90	0.25	*Dsk*F$_1$	N	0.08	300	1
*Dsk*F$_2$	N	0.14	180	1	*Dsk*F$_3$	N	0.18	180	1
*Dsk*F$_4$	N	0.06	400	0	*Dsk*F$_5$	N	0.06	400	0
*Chr*A$_1$	N	3.17	200	1	*Chr*A$_2$	N	3.00	200	1
*Chr*C$_1$	P	0.73	1200	1	*Chr*B$_1$	P	1.56	100	1
*Chr*B$_2$	P	0.09	1200	0	*Chr*B$_3$	P	0.23	1200	0
*Chr*B$_4$	P	0.09	80	0	*Chr*B$_5$	P	0.05	80	0
*Pbf*C$_1$	N	0.03	5	0	*Pbf*C$_2$	N	0.01	60	0
*Pbf*P$_1$	N	<0.01	200	1	*Pbf*P$_2$	N	0.28	35	0
*Pbf*P$_3$	N	0.08	100	0	*Pbf*P$_4$	N	0.51	3200	0
*Pbf*P$_5$	N	0.09	660	0	*Pbf*D$_1$	St	0.05	100	0.25
*Pbf*D$_2$	N	0.04	300	0	*Pbf*D$_3$	N	0.01	5000	0
*Pbf*O$_1$	St	<0.01	100	0.25	*Pbf*O$_2$	St	0.01	1600	0
*Pbf*O$_3$	N	<0.01	6000	0	*Pbf*W$_1$	N	0.01	12000	0
*Pbf*W$_2$	N	0.05	2750	0.2	*Pbf*W$_3$	N	0.31	12	1
*Pbf*T$_1$	N	0.18	200	0	*Pbf*R$_1$	N	0.04	400	0
*Pbf*B$_1$	N	0.14	10	0.5	*Pbf*K$_1$	N	0.08	4400	1
*Pbf*H$_1$	N	0.03	4260	0.4					

[1] Sub-surf: sub-surfaces. The codes of 57 sub-surfaces can be found in Table S1. [2] Surf type: type of surfaces including porous (P), non-porous (N), stainless steel (St) and skin (S). No one wears shorts while in the office, so the hands, head, face and neck are regarded as skin, and other body parts are regarded as porous surfaces. [3] Frequency of each sub-surface to be touched (h^{-1}). [4] Data for the human body's skin area were obtained from [42,43]. The area of the hand does not include the back of the hand. Area for other surfaces was measured or estimated. Therefore, the area considered includes only the parts usually touched by hands; for example, the area of a mouse includes only the top and side surfaces because few people will directly touch its bottom surface. [5] Horizontal coefficient of area. It means that the portion of the area that is horizontal can gather particles caused by deposition. For example, a horizontal coefficient of 1 means that all surface areas are horizontal and are totally exposed to particle deposition (e.g., *Dsk*T1: desktop).

When a hand touches a surface, the total quantity of virus (TCID50) on the hand and on the surface can be calculated based on Equations (3) and (4).

$$\frac{\mathrm{d}V_h(t)}{\mathrm{d}t} = R_{sh} \cdot A_C \cdot \frac{V_s}{A_S} - R_{hs} \cdot A_C \cdot \frac{V_h}{A_h}, \tag{3}$$

$$\frac{\mathrm{d}V_s(t)}{\mathrm{d}t} = R_{hs} \cdot A_C \cdot \frac{V_h}{A_h} - R_{sh} \cdot A_C \cdot \frac{V_s}{A_S}, \tag{4}$$

where $V_h(t)$ and $V_s(t)$ are the total quantity of virus ($TCID_{50}$) on a hand and a surface at time t caused by surface touch, respectively; R_{sh} and R_{hs} are the virus transfer rates from surfaces to hands and from hands to surfaces, respectively; A_s, A_h and A_C represent the area of the surface, the hand (palm) and the parts of the hand and the surface that make contact.

The transfer rate between hands and various surfaces directly determines the amount of influenza A that is transmitted via the fomite route. Table 4 lists some values for the transfer rate between hands and surfaces with various materials.

Table 4. [1] Virus transfer rate between hands and surfaces.

Donor	Recipient	Transfer Rate	Donor	Recipient	Transfer Rate
Porous	Hand	3% [44]	Hand	Porous	80% [45]
Non-porous	Hand	7% [46]	Hand	Non-porous	12% [47]
Stainless steel	Hand	7.9% [48]	Hand	Stainless steel	16.1% [49]
Hand	Hand	25.5% [50]			

[1] All surfaces in the office are regarded as composed by materials shown in the Table. In addition, many factors influence the transfer rate, including temperature, humidity, touch duration and dry/wet hand, thus causing some errors here.

Virus can reach the mucous membranes if a student touches his or her mouth, nasopharynx and eyes with a contaminated hand. Studies have shown that the mean rate of all finger contacts with the lips, nostrils and eyes ranges from 0.7 h^{-1} to 15 h^{-1} [36,51]. In this study, we assumed that the frequency of mucous membrane touching is 5 h^{-1}. Therefore, from Table 1, one of four hand-face contacts are hand-mucous membrane contacts. The virus transfer rate from the fingertip to the mucous membranes is set to 35% [52]. The dose-response parameter based on intranasal inoculation of humans $\alpha_I = 5.7 \times 10^{-5}\ TCID_{50}^{-1}$.

Resuspension of microorganisms from the floor, clothing and furniture acts as a secondary source [53]. Resuspended dust comprises up to 60% of the total particulate matter in indoor air [54,55]. The resuspension rate depends on many factors, such as the room height, the relative humidity and the particle size. To simplify the resuspension, we assumed that resuspension rate in the office is $10^{-4}\ h^{-1}$ [56]. Only resuspension between surfaces and the air is considered, while that between skin and the air is ignored because skin is usually moist.

Influenza A virus loses viability on surfaces over time. Porous and non-porous surfaces are both considered because the death rate of the virus differs significantly between the two surfaces [31]. According to a previous study [48], the inactivation rate of influenza A virus on a porous surface such as pyjamas (μ_p) is $1.6 \times 10^{-2}\ min^{-1}$, that on a non-porous surface such as stainless steel (μ_s) is $2.0 \times 10^{-3}\ min^{-1}$ and that on the hand (μ_h) is 1.2 min^{-1}. Inactivation on mucous membranes is not considered here.

Based on the balance between virus generation and disappearance (flew out of the room, lost viability or inhaled by people), the virus quantity in the air and on the surfaces can be calculated (Equations (5) and (6)).

$$\frac{\mathrm{d}V_{Air}(t)}{\mathrm{d}t} = V_{Ps} + R_{SA} - D_{AS} - \frac{V_{Air}}{V_R} \cdot V_{AC} - \left(1 - e^{-V_{Da}}\right) \cdot V_{Air} - V_I, \tag{5}$$

$$\frac{dV_{Sf}(t)}{dt} = V_{Pl} + D_{AS} - R_{SA} - \left(1 - e^{-V_{Ds}}\right) \cdot V_{sf}(t) + V_{HS} - V_{SH}, \tag{6}$$

where V_{Air} and V_{Sf} are the quantity of virus (TCID$_{50}$) in the air and on surfaces in the office; V_{Ps} and V_{Pl} are the virus generation velocity in small droplets and large droplets, respectively, generated by breathing, talking, coughing and sneezing by the infected student; D_{AS} and R_{SA} are the particle deposition velocity from the air to surfaces and the resuspension velocity from surfaces to the air, respectively; V_R is the room's total volume; V_{AC} is the air change rate; V_{Da} and V_{Ds} are the inactivation rate of virus in the air and on surfaces, respectively; V_{HS} and V_{SH} are the quantity of virus (TCID$_{50}$) transferred from the hands to surfaces and from surfaces to the hands at each step, respectively; and V_I is the inhalation velocity of each student.

2.4. Close Contact

Close contact is usually defined as being within 3 ft (~1 m) of the infector [36]. When two or more students talk, small and large droplets will be sprayed from the infected student's mouth. Large droplets are likely deposited on the mucous membranes of susceptible students, some small droplets are directly inhaled by the students who are talking with the infected student and some of the remaining small droplets are inhaled by others via the long-range airborne route. In this study, a close contact was counted when a face to face contact occurs between any two students who are within 3 ft (~1m). The quantity of virus (TCID$_{50}$) changes via inhalation and deposition on mucous membranes according to factors such as relative height, distance and direction in which the two students were facing and the room's airflow. Here we assumed that 50% of small droplets [18,19] are inhaled by the student who is talking with the infected student and 30% of large droplets are deposited on that student's face (10% of droplets on the face are deposited directly on the mucous membranes). Other small droplets diffuse into the air, and large droplets are deposited on surfaces nearby.

We observed 3526 close contacts between students in an office over the course of 5 days. Figure 2 shows the association between the duration of close contact and percentage of contacts. The frequency of close contact per person is 9.64 h^{-1} per student, including active and passive contacts. Each student spent an average of 9.86% of their time in close contact. The average duration and the mean duration of close contact were 53.8 s and 17 s, respectively.

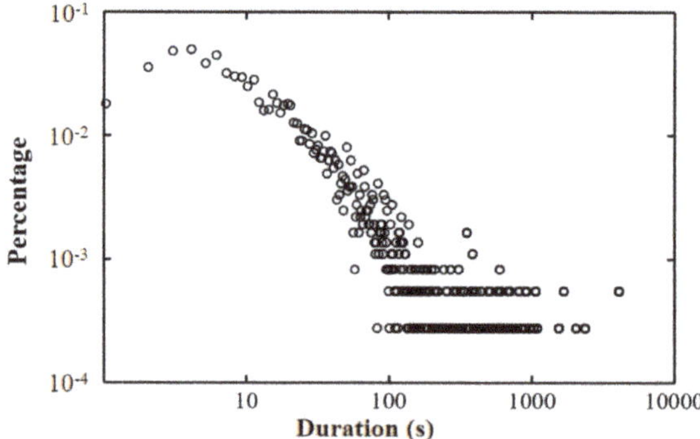

Figure 2. Association between the duration of close contact and the percentage of contacts.

3. Results

3.1. Spatio-Temporal Virus Distribution

Students move, make contact with other students, and touch surfaces in the office. Influenza A virus will be transferred between the hands and surfaces over time. From Figure 3a, the virus on the hands of the infected student increases rapidly and reaches a balance because limited numbers of his or her private surfaces share the virus. The hands of other students (susceptible) will be gradually contaminated, and virus on the hands of susceptible students almost reach a balance after 3 h (12 a.m.). The private surfaces of infected students are highly contaminated, and the quantity of virus ($TCID_{50}$) on the private surfaces of the infected student is almost three orders of magnitude of that on the private surfaces of susceptible students. Public surfaces are dirtier than the private surfaces of susceptible students, and they also play important roles in the spread of infection like hubs in the surface touch network. The cumulative quantity of virus ($TCID_{50}$) on the mucous membranes of susceptible students expresses each student's intranasal dose and gradually increases over time.

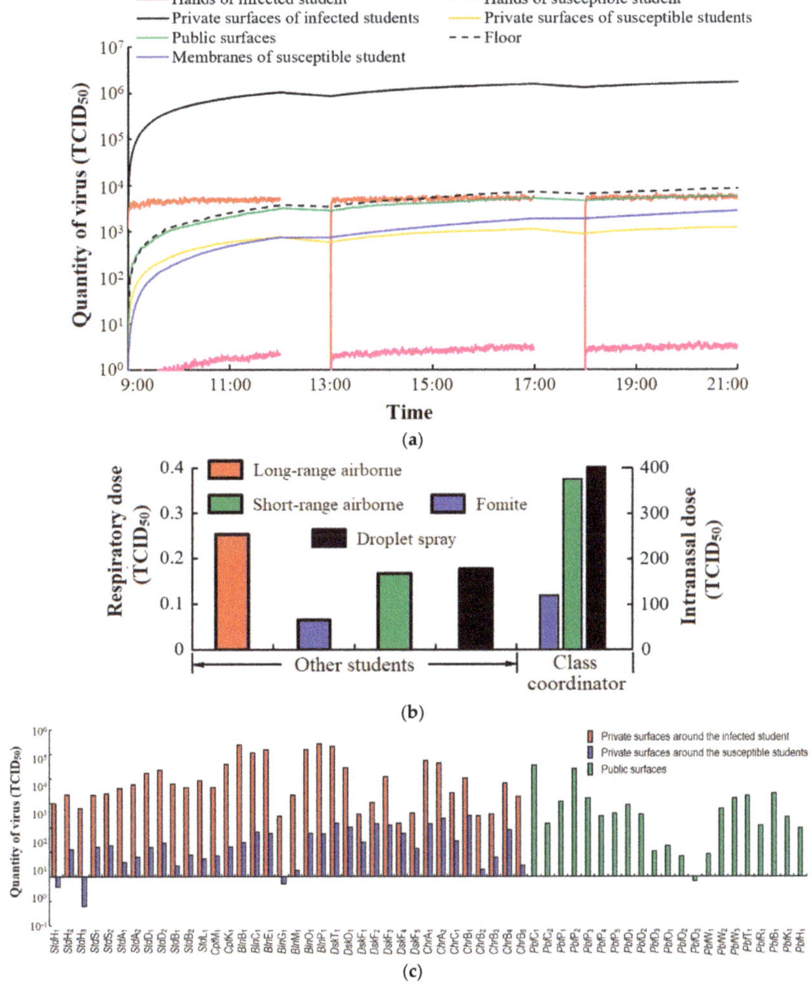

Figure 3. Quantity of virus ($TCID_{50}$) (**a**) on different types of surface [1]; (**b**) absorbed by the class coordinator and other students via various transmission routes (close contact includes both short-range airborne and droplet spray); (**c**) on different types of sub-surfaces after a whole day ($TCID_{50}$ per surface).[1] Quantity of virus ($TCID_{50}$) on private surfaces, hands and mucous membranes of susceptible students are the average value of each student rather than a summation of all susceptible students.

The quantity of virus ($TCID_{50}$) on the floor is relatively low because we assumed that most large droplets generated by talking, coughing and sneezing are deposited on the top surfaces of the desk, if the infected student is sitting in his or her own seat. In a 1-day simulation, we found that the respiratory dose per day of each susceptible student from the long-range and short-range airborne routes are 0.25 and 0.17 $TCID_{50}$, respectively, and the intranasal dose per day from the fomite and droplet spray routes are 63.81 and 185.24 $TCID_{50}$ (Figure 3b). All results are average values from 1000 simulations. Based upon the dose-response parameters from two routes, the total infection risk for each susceptible student during 1 day in the office is 8.75%, of which 54.31%, 4.23% and 44.46% are contributed by the long-range airborne, fomite and close contact routes. The class coordinator usually has more frequent interaction with other students, and we assumed that the probability of the class coordinator touching others' desks and chairs and talking with others is twice that of the other students. The infection risk of the monitor is 13.79% (Figure 3b). The virus distribution on the surfaces of the desks and chairs of the class coordinator and the other students is shown in Figure S1 (Supplementary Materials). The class coordinator has a higher infection risk than the other students. There are 57 types of sub-surfaces, and the final quantity of virus ($TCID_{50}$) on each type of sub-surface ($TCID_{50}$ per surface) is shown in Figure 3c. The quantity of virus ($TCID_{50}$) is much higher on the private surfaces around the infected student (approaching 800 times) than around susceptible students. Keyboards, headphones, desktops, mice and mobile phones are the five most-contaminated private surfaces around the infected student. The top of the seat back, the right chair arm, the desktop, the left chair arm and the top of the left desk's fence are the five most-contaminated private surfaces around the susceptible students. Air conditioning (AC) controllers, printer touch screens, cabinet handles, tissue dispensers and the printer drawer are the dirtiest of all public surfaces. Surfaces with small areas, such as headphones and the buttons on the AC controller usually have a high virus concentration.

3.2. Infection Spread via the Fomite Route

The spread of infection can be controlled only after the route of virus transmission is known. Figure 4 shows that 95.1% of virus is transmitted via private surfaces, while only 4.9% is transmitted via public surfaces. In all private surfaces, 59.8% of virus is transmitted via the private surfaces around the infected student, 38.1% of virus is transmitted via the private surfaces around the self and only 2.1% of virus is transmitted via the private surfaces of other susceptible students. The percentage of intranasal doses of susceptible students from the fomites of six primary surfaces—students, their belongings, computers, desks, chairs and public facilities—are 8.0%, 6.8%, 13.2%, 57.8%, 9.3% and 4.9%, respectively. Most virus absorbed by susceptible students comes from desktops, mice, mobile phones, faces, chair arms, keyboards, hands, printer touch screens and the button of the water dispenser. In addition, most virus absorbed by students comes from the private surfaces of infected students and the student himself or herself. The face is dirty, because some large droplets are deposited upon it when two students speak. Few students touch the faces of other students; therefore, the main sources of virus on the face are from the student himself or herself. During disinfection, the red and orange surfaces labelled in Figure 4 should receive more attention because of the high rate of virus transmission through them.

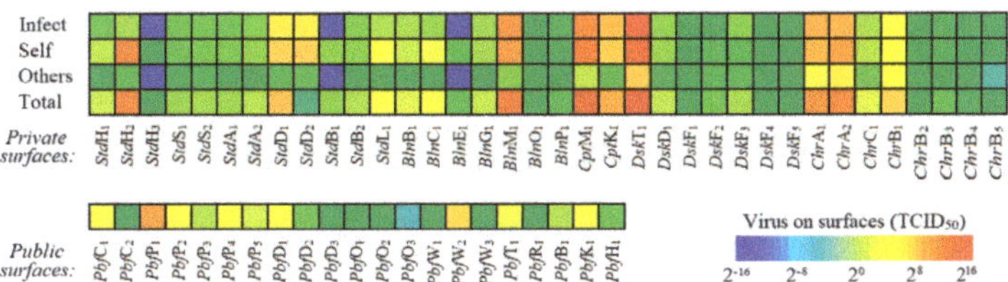

Figure 4. Quantity of virus ($TCID_{50}$) transmitted from various types of sub-surfaces from the private surfaces of the infected student, the student's own private surfaces, the private surfaces of other susceptible students and public surfaces to the hands ($TCID_{50}$).

Many factors influence effectiveness of virus transmission via fomites such as virus inactivation on surfaces and the virus transfer rate between hands and surfaces. With decreasing R_{sh} and increasing R_{hs}, the respiratory dose per student per day gradually increases (Figure 5a). When $R_{sh} > 0.1$, the intranasal dose increases as R_{hs} increases, while when $R_{sh} < 0.1$, the intranasal dose is negative in proportion with R_{hs} (Figure 5b). When R_{sh} is high, the quantity of virus ($TCID_{50}$) on surfaces increases as R_{hs} increases because more viruses are transferred from the hands of the infected student. When susceptible students touch the surfaces, more virus will be transferred from the surfaces to their hands. The intranasal dose of the susceptible students increases. When R_{sh} is very low, it is difficult for the virus to transfer from surfaces to the hands. Although the virus from the hands of the infected student to surfaces increases as R_{hs} increases, the transmission of virus from surfaces to the hands of susceptible students is limited because of small R_{sh}. As R_{hs} increases, more virus is transmitted from the hands of susceptible students to surfaces than from the surfaces to their hands, and the intranasal dose of the susceptible students decreases. In reality, adjustment of R_{sh} and R_{hs} to a specific value can efficiently limit virus transmission via fomites, thus reducing the infection risk, especially in infectious diseases that are transmitted mainly via fomites such as norovirus. From Figure 5c,d, the respiratory dose gradually decreases as R_{sh} increases and as R_{hs} decreases. In contrast, the intranasal dose gradually increases, thus the total quantity of virus ($TCID_{50}$) on surfaces decreases. The amount of virus aerosol in the air as a result of resuspension decreases. Therefore, in most cases, the respiratory dose decreases as intranasal dose increases.

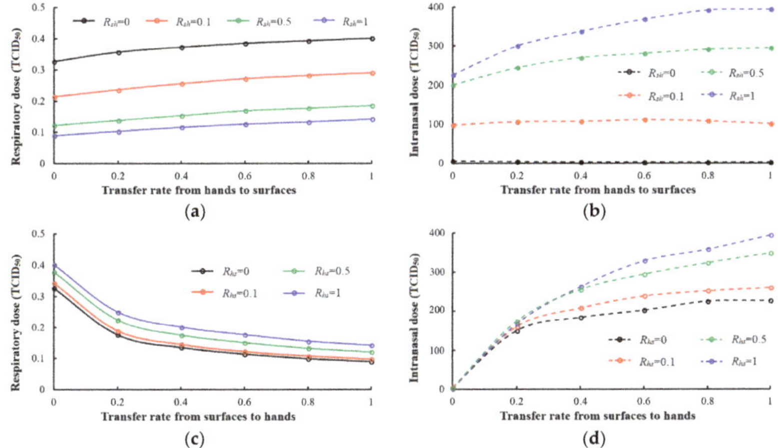

Figure 5. Different transfer rate between surfaces and hands (R_{hs} & R_{sh}). (**a**) Respiratory dose changes with R_{sh}; (**b**) intranasal dose changes with R_{sh}; (**c**) respiratory dose changes with R_{hs}; (**d**) intranasal dose changes with R_{hs}.

3.3. Strategies for Influenza A Prevention

3.3.1. Mask Wearing

Masks have various filtrating resolutions and efficacies. Surgical masks can only prevent large droplets, and N95 masks can prevent both large and small droplets. We hypothesised that 95% of both large and small droplets can be blocked by a tightly worn N95 mask. The particle block efficiency reduces if the mask is not tightly worn. Figure 6a,b show the respiratory and intranasal dose absorbed by susceptible students with different large and small droplets blocking efficiency and mask wearing strategies (the infected or the susceptible students wearing masks). When the blocking efficiency for large droplets (E_{BL}) is reduced from 100% to 30%, the respiratory dose of susceptible students from the long-range airborne route increases from 0.04 to 0.19 $TCID_{50}$. The intranasal dose via fomites and droplet spray increase from 0.01 to 42.53 $TCID_{50}$ and from 0 to 131.79 $TCID_{50}$, respectively (Figure 6b). When $E_{BL} = 100\%$, the intranasal dose comes only from the deposition of small aerosol in the air. Therefore, comparing no mask with wearing mask with 100% E_{BL}, each susceptible student's average infection risk is reduced from 8.75% to 3.82%. When an N95 mask is worn, small droplets can also be filtered. By increasing the mask's blocking efficiency for small droplets (E_{BS}), the respiratory dose via both long-range and short airborne routes decreases (Figure 6a). However, the intranasal dose via the fomite and droplet spray routes remain nearly the same if E_{BS} increases (Figure 6b). When 95% of both small and large droplets are blocked ($E_{BL} = E_{BS} = 95\%$), the infected student's total risk of infection will be reduced from 8.75% to 0.45%.

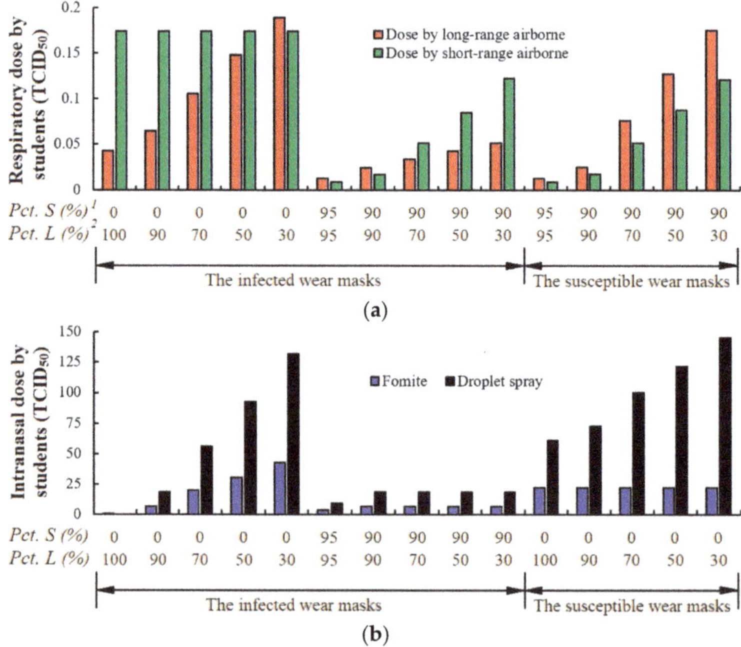

Figure 6. Dose of influenza A virus by susceptible students under different mask wearing strategies and efficiencies. (**a**) Long-range and short-range airborne routes; (**b**) fomite and droplet spray routes.[1] Pct.S (%): Percentage of small particles blocked by masks.[2] Pct.L (%): Percentage of large droplets blocked by masks.

If only susceptible students wear the mask rather than the infected student, the infection risk changes. The respiratory dose via the long-range and short-range airborne routes decreases with increasing E_{BS}. When 95% of both small and large droplets are blocked, the respiratory dose from the airborne route is reduced to 0.02 $TCID_{50}$ (Figure 6a). A mask can block the virus from the hands to the nose and lips because the mask isolates them. When all susceptible students wear masks with high E_{BL}, intranasal dose through fomites can hardly be further reduced. This case differs when only the infected student wears the high-E_{BL} mask. The intranasal dose caused by droplet spray decreases as E_{BL} increases (Figure 6b). The total infection risk will be reduced to 0.87% if all susceptible students tightly wear N95 masks.

3.3.2. Ventilation

It is well known that ventilation can efficiently reduce the risk of infection via the long-range airborne route. It is determined by natural and mechanical ventilation, which are influenced by many factors such as open doors, open windows and AC systems. When the ventilation rate changes from 1 ACH to 4 ACH, the respiratory dose via the long-range airborne route will be reduced from 0.26 to 0.19 $TCID_{50}$, and the general infection risk will be reduced by 1.2% (Figure 7). If the ventilation rate increases to 10 ACH, the infection risk via the long-range airborne route will be less than half under only 1 ACH. With no ventilation, all virus in the air moves out only through inactivation and deposition, and the virus concentration in the air is much higher.

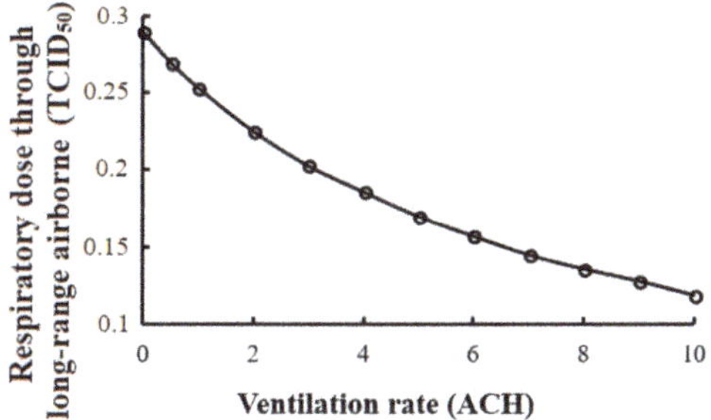

Figure 7. Respiratory dose via the long-range airborne route at various ventilation rates.

3.3.3. Hand Washing

Figure 8 shows how hand washing by the infected student and susceptible students influences the respiratory and intranasal dose. In the simulation, we hypothesised that hands become completely clean (no virus) after hand washing. The infected student's hands usually possess a large quantity of virus ($TCID_{50}$), which will then be transmitted to surfaces and resuspended in the air. As shown in blue and red lines in Figure 8, when the infected student's hand washing frequency is less than 6 times per hour, the decrease in the respiratory and intranasal doses for susceptible students is obvious. If susceptible students wash their hands, rather than the infected student, the infection risk reduction via fomites is slightly higher. If the hand washing frequency is less than 6 times per hour, the intranasal dose reduction via fomites will be obviously limited. Moreover, hand washing by susceptible students hardly reduces the respiratory dose. In general, focusing on the influenza A virus, if the frequency of hand washing is more than twice per hour, very little further improvement can be made in the efficacy for infection risk reduction.

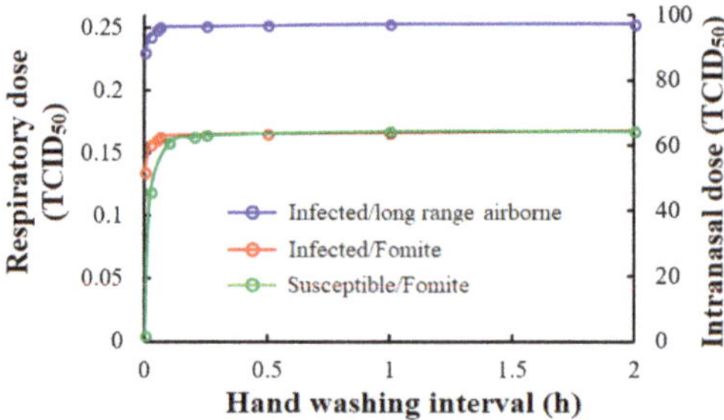

Figure 8. Infection risk reduction by hand washing (Blue and red lines show the respiratory and intranasal doses of the susceptible students when only the infected student washes his or her hands; the green line shows the intranasal dose from susceptible students when only they wash hands).

3.3.4. Surface Cleaning

In the simulation, we hypothesised that surfaces become completely clean (no virus) after surface cleaning. Figure 9a shows how respiratory and intranasal doses change with various strategies of surface cleaning with frequency of 0.5 h^{-1}. No student touches the floor, and a clean floor can only reduce the resuspension of aerosol. Regular desktop cleaning can reduce the respiratory and intranasal dose from 0.26 to 0.14 $TCID_{50}$ and from 65.87 to 35.10 TCID50, respectively (the general infection risk ranges from 8.75% to 6.71%). The cleaning of more surfaces, such as the top five high-touch surfaces and all private surfaces, can slightly reduce the infection risk from 6.71% to 6.61%, and to 6.17%, respectively.

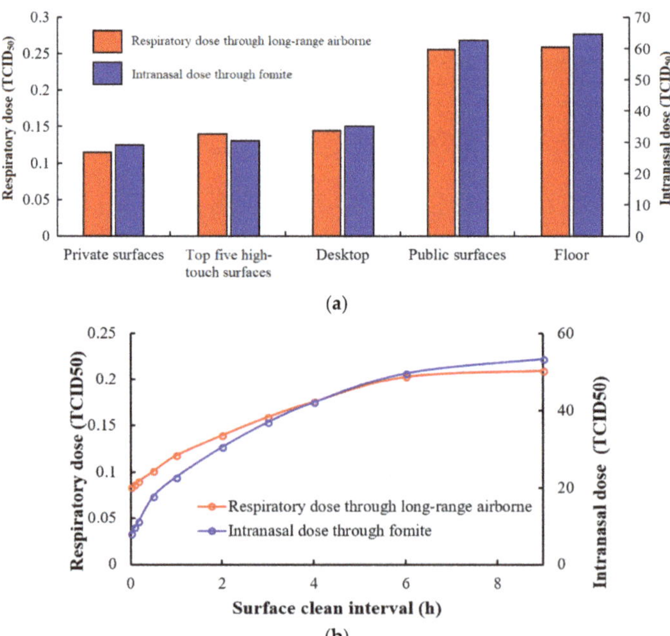

Figure 9. Surface cleaning. (**a**) Various types of surfaces with a cleaning frequency of 0.5 h−1; (**b**) different clean interval for top five high-touch surfaces [1]. [1] Top five high-touch surfaces: desktop, mouse, mobile phone, keyboard and chair arms.

Figure 9b shows that the respiratory and intranasal dose grows logarithmically as the interval at which high-touch surfaces are cleaned increases. If only a regular high-touch surface cleaning is conducted at 3 p.m. each day, the respiratory dose via long-range airborne and the intranasal dose via fomites are 0.16 and 36.97 $TCID_{50}$ (infection risk = 6.97%), respectively. However, if the frequency of surface cleaning is increased to once per hour (surface clean interval = 1 h), the infection risk is reduced to 6.19%. With a continuous decrease in the clean frequency when it is lower than once per hour, the infection risk will be reduced quickly, but the workload is huge.

4. Discussion

In this paper, we studied how influenza A transmits in a graduate student office in one day from 9 a.m. to 9 p.m. through long-range airborne, fomite and close contact (short-range airborne and droplets spray) routes based on real recorded data of contacts between students and surfaces touch. Most parameters set in the simulation are from real recorded data and existing studies.

We found that each susceptible student's average infection risk during a day in the office is 8.75%, of which 54.31%, 4.23%, 33.24% and 11.22% are contributed by the long-range airborne, fomite, short-range airborne and droplet spray routes. However, in an air cabin, focusing on influenza A H1N1, the contributions via the airborne, close contact and fomite routes are 34.30%, 64.98% and 0.72% [13]. In the air cabin, close contact is more frequent because of the high density of passengers. Fomites contribute less due to the low probability of direct touch between the infected and susceptible passengers. The long-range airborne route is less frequent because a high ventilation rate (25 ACH) is set in the air cabin even though the population density is high. Focusing on virus on surfaces, the private surfaces around the infected student had the most virus, because most contaminated droplets are deposited on surfaces around the infected person, and nearby surfaces are also easily touched [18]. The quantity of virus ($TCID_{50}$) on all surfaces stops its rapid increase after 3 h. Virus on the hands of susceptible students always remains at a lower level because the inactivation rate of influenza A on the hands is high. The quantity of virus ($TCID_{50}$) on public surfaces is higher than on private surfaces around the susceptible students. Moreover, some active students such as the class coordinator have more contacts and a higher probability of touching other's private surfaces. We found that the class coordinator's infection risk is almost 1.6 times that of other students.

Approximately 4.2% of the influenza A infection risk comes from fomites. However, for other infectious diseases such as norovirus, which makes more than 85% of the contribution to infection risk [13], and fomite plays an important role. In the office, 95.1% of viruses were transmitted via private surfaces and only 4.9% via public surfaces. The desk is the dirtiest of all private surfaces. In this study, we hypothesised that most contaminated droplets generated by talking, coughing and sneezing are deposited on desks. Desktops, mice, mobile phones and keyboards transmit virus easily. This result accords with previous studies on microbiome [57,58]. Public surfaces are the hubs of the surface touch network [16]. AC controller buttons, printer touch screens and public cabinet handles are highly contaminated. The button of the water dispenser is frequently touched. However, the infected students usually touched the chair arms, cups and seatbacks of other students before getting a cup of water. The virus on hands is diluted, and the total quantity of virus ($TCID_{50}$) on the water dispenser is limited. These high-risk surfaces should be given more attention in infectious disease transmission, especially on some diseases that are highly dependent on fomite, such as norovirus. If we can design an anti-virus material to build all high-touch surfaces, we could efficiently control virus transmission via fomites.

From a virus transfer rate perspective, if we can create a surface that can block virus transmission from surfaces to hands ($R_{sh} = 0$), the virus from fomites could be efficiently controlled. Indeed, the transfer rate between surfaces and hands cannot reach 0 or 1. A material with low R_{sh} can limit virus transmission from surfaces to hands, such as porous materials [44]. Surfaces made with material with a high R_{hs} can absorb more virus from hands of both the infected student and susceptible students. Therefore, the means by which to adjust the virus transfer rate between surfaces and hands by using materials with different R_{sh} and R_{hs} is very helpful to prevent virus transmission via fomites. We found that when $R_{sh} > 0.1$, the intranasal dose increases as R_{hs} increases, while when $R_{sh} < 0.1$, it decreases with R_{hs} in an office setting.

Many strategies, such as mask wearing [59], ventilation [4], hand washing [11] and surface cleaning [60], can limit the spread of influenza A in a confined room. Wearing a mask can control the spread of disease via the long-range airborne, fomite and close contact routes. A high ventilation rate helps to dilute the virus concentration in the air, and the respiratory dose from the long-range airborne route will be obviously reduced. Hand washing can reduce the infection risk directly via fomites and indirectly via the long-range airborne route because of the lower rate of resuspension from surfaces to the air. The same effects are brought by surface cleaning. Mask wearing is much more efficient than hand washing because influenza A is transmitted mainly via the airborne and close contact routes. Mask wearing by the infected student has greater efficiency at reducing the infection risk than simply having the susceptible students wear masks (infection risk of 0.87% vs. 0.45% when an N95 mask is tightly sealed). According to the test in hospitals, tightly sealing a mask to the face can block the entry of 94.5% of total virus and 94.8% of infectious virus [59]. We found that 94.9% of the infection risk can be reduced if an N95 mask is tightly sealed on the infected student, which is very useful in influenza A transmission control. The airborne route is the main route of influenza A virus spread. In a norovirus outbreak, the efficiency of mask-wearing should be reassessed.

Hands play a very important role in the surface touch network, because hands can be contaminated by covering the mouth and nose when coughing and sneezing or by touching contaminated surfaces, and thus can also contaminate surfaces. Some previous studies have shown that hand washing can cut the risk of respiratory infection by 16% [61]. We found that only hand washing is limited to reduce infection risk. When the hand washing frequency is greater than six times per hour, the infection risk can be obviously reduced. However, in the hospital, when all doctors and nurses wear masks, hand washing is more efficient because hands are one of the main ways to spread virus from hospital workers to susceptible people. We also found that if the susceptible students wash their hands (rather than the infected student), the efficiency of infection risk reduction is slightly higher.

Students spent more than 90% of their time in the office touching surfaces. The intranasal dose due to contact between hands and mucous membranes depends on the quantity of viable pathogens on the office's surfaces, the frequency of contact between hands and contaminated surfaces, contact between hands and mucous membranes and the efficiency of pathogen transfer to and from hands-on contact [18]. Regular surface cleaning can reduce the infection risk. Public surfaces are frequently touched, so viruses on public surfaces are diluted by many touches by susceptible students. Public surface cleaning every 2 h is not very efficient because there are few public surfaces in the office. Desktops are among the most contaminated surfaces in the office because the students spent most of their time at their desks. Contaminated droplets are deposited on the desktop when an infected student talks, coughs or sneezes. Students often touch the desktops of other students, because of the high frequency of discussions between students in the office. Cleaning of all private surfaces can reach a better condition (infection risk reduced by 2.56%), but the workload is too large. Therefore, regular cleaning of desktops or high-touch surfaces is suggested if the virus is very severe. In addition, cleaning of high-touch surfaces is much more efficient than hand-washing because high-touch surfaces gathered more virus and because the inactivation rate on surfaces is much lower than on the hands. The results of influenza A simulation based on real data of human behaviour in a confined space is very helpful to help understand the real characteristics of influenza A transmission and to make effective plans to prevent and control diseases.

This work perhaps lacks a direct and strong connection to Health-EDRM (health-related emergency disaster risk management). However, the model that we built and suggestions that we put forward are useful in for controlling infectious diseases transmission, and major outbreaks if infectious diseases can be itself a health-related disaster. Moreover, natural and complex disasters such as floods, tsunamis, and earthquakes can dramatically increase the risk of infectious diseases outbreak including malaria, measles, viral hepatitis, etc. [62,63]. After a serious disaster, many people who have been affected by the disaster will be gathered in an emergency shelter. Risk of infectious disease transmission through different routes can be calculated based on our model, and suggestions we obtained also can guide disaster managers in making efficient emergency plans for infectious disease control and prevention after disasters.

This study has various limitations. All students are assumed to stay in the office at all times except at lunch and dinner time, virus generation is overestimated, and a higher infection risk of susceptible students is calculated. The virus transfer rate between surfaces and hands is influenced by many factors, such as force, area and touch duration. We assumed that each touch between a specific surface and a hand has the same transfer rate. Most particles are deposited on the desktop when the infected student talks, coughs or sneezes, and we did not consider that some private things such as mice, keyboards and cups share the virus on the desk. Therefore, the quantity of virus ($TCID_{50}$) on the desk is overestimated. Moreover, in our simulation, some parameters such as transfer rate between hand and various surfaces are not based on influenza virus due to data unavailability. Heterogeneity exists in the study, and it may result in some errors. The differences in human behaviour by gender are ignored, and relative positions, heights and angles between two students during close contact are not considered. A future study should collect some samples in the office if any students are infected with influenza A. We can then compare the real virus distribution data with our simulation data to verify the accuracy of our model.

5. Conclusions

Influenza A transmission in a graduate student office is simulated via long-range airborne, fomite, and close contact routes based on realistic data of human behaviours. The long-range airborne, fomite and close contact routes contribute to 54.3%, 4.2% and 44.5% of influenza A infections, respectively. For the fomite route, 59.8%, 38.1% and 2.1% of viruses are transmitted to the hands of students from private surfaces around the infected students, the students themselves and other susceptible students, respectively. The private surfaces of infected students are highly contaminated. The quantity of virus ($TCID_{50}$) is much higher on the private surfaces around the infected student (approaching 800 times) than around susceptible students. Keyboards, headphones, desktops, mice and mobile phones are the five most-contaminated private surfaces around the infected student. Public surfaces are dirtier than the private surfaces of susceptible students. The intranasal dose via fomites of the students' bodies, belongings, computers, desks, chairs and public facilities are 8.0%, 6.8%, 13.2%, 57.8%, 9.3% and 4.9%, respectively. The intranasal dose does not monotonously increase or decrease with the virus transfer rate between hands and surfaces, and a specific value setting can optimally limit influenza A virus transmission via fomites Mask wearing is much more useful than hand washing for control of influenza A in the tested office setting, and the total risk can be reduced from 8.75% to 0.45% if an N95 mask is tightly sealed by infected students. Regular cleaning of high-touch surfaces, which can reduce the infection risk by 2.14%, is recommended and is much more efficient than hand-washing.

Supplementary Materials: The following are available online at http://www.mdpi.com/1660-4601/15/8/1699/s1, Figure S1: Surfaces contamination around the class coordinator and other students, Table S1: Types of surfaces in student office.

Author Contributions: Conceptualization, N.Z. and Y.L; Data curation, N.Z.; Formal analysis, N.Z.; Funding acquisition, Y.L.; Investigation, N.Z.; Methodology, N.Z.; Software, N.Z.; Supervision, Y.L.; Writing—original draft, N.Z.; Writing—review & editing, Y.L.

Funding: This research was funded by a Collaborative Research Fund provided by the Research Grants Council of Hong Kong [grant number C7025-16G].

Conflicts of Interest: The authors declare no conflict of interest.

References

1. Monto, A.S.; Whitley, R.J. Seasonal and pandemic influenza: A 2007 update on challenges and solutions. *Clin. Infect. Dis.* **2008**, *46*, 1024–1031. [CrossRef] [PubMed]
2. Englund, J.A. Antiviral therapy of influenza. *Semin. Pediatr. Infect. Dis.* **2002**, *13*, 120–128. [CrossRef] [PubMed]
3. Morens, D.M.; Rash, V.M. Lessons from a nursing home outbreak of influenza A. *Infect. Control Hosp. Epidemiol.* **1995**, *16*, 275–280. [CrossRef] [PubMed]
4. Brankston, G.; Gitterman, L.; Hirji, Z.; Lemieux, C.; Gardam, D.M. Transmission of influenza A in human beings. *Lancet Infect. Dis.* **2007**, *7*, 257–265. [CrossRef]
5. Weinstein, R.A.; Bridges, C.B.; Kuehnert, M.J.; Hall, C.B. Transmission of influenza: Implications for control in health care settings. *Clin. Infect. Dis.* **2003**, *37*, 1094–1101. [CrossRef] [PubMed]
6. Tellier, R. Review of aerosol transmission of influenza A virus. *Emerg. Infect. Dis.* **2006**, *12*, 1657–1662. [CrossRef] [PubMed]
7. Lowen, A.C.; Mubareka, S.; Tumpey, T.M.; García-Sastre, A.; Palese, P. The guinea pig as a transmission model for human influenza viruses. *Proc. Natl. Acad. Sci. USA* **2006**, *103*, 9988–9992. [CrossRef] [PubMed]
8. Moser, M.R.; Bender, T.R.; Margolis, H.S.; Noble, G.R.; Kendal, A.P.; Ritter, D.G. An outbreak of influenza aboard a commercial airliner. *Am. J. Epidemiol.* **1979**, *110*, 1–6. [CrossRef] [PubMed]
9. McLean, R.L. General discussion. *Am. Rev. Respir. Dis.* **1961**, *83*, 36–38.
10. Schulman, J.L.; Kilbourne, E.D. Airborne transmission of influenza virus infection in mice. *Nature* **1962**, *195*, 1129. [CrossRef] [PubMed]
11. Hertzberg, V.S.; Weiss, H.; Elon, L.; Si, W.P.; Norris, S.L. the FlyHealthy Research Team. Behaviors, movement, and transmission of droplet-mediated respiratory diseases during transcontinental airline flights. *Proc. Natl. Acad. Sci. USA* **2018**. [CrossRef] [PubMed]
12. Gilardi, F.; Castelli, G.G.; Vinci, M.R.; Ciofi, D.A.M.; Santilli, V.; Brugaletta, R.; Santoro, A.; Montanaro, R.; Lavorato, L.; Raponi, M.; et al. Seasonal influenza vaccination in health care workers. A pre-post intervention study in an Italian paediatric sospital. *Int. J. Environ. Res. Public Health* **2018**, *15*, 841. [CrossRef] [PubMed]
13. Lei, H.; Li, Y.; Xiao, S.; Lin, C.H.; Norris, S.L.; Wei, D.; Hu, Z.; Ji, S. Routes of transmission of influenza A H1N1, SARS CoV, and norovirus in air cabin: Comparative analyses. *Indoor Air* **2017**, *28*, 394–403. [CrossRef] [PubMed]
14. Chong, K.C.; Goggins, W.; Zee, B.C.Y.; Wang, M.H. Identifying meteorological drivers for the seasonal variations of influenza infections in a subtropical city—Hong Kong. *Int. J. Environ. Res. Public Health* **2015**, *12*, 1560–1576. [CrossRef] [PubMed]
15. Charu, V.; Zeger, S.; Gog, J.; Bjørnstad, O.N.; Kissler, S.; Simonsen, L.; Grenfell, B.T.; Viboud, C. Human mobility and the spatial transmission of influenza in the United States. *PLoS Comput. Biol.* **2017**, *13*, e1005382. [CrossRef] [PubMed]
16. Zhang, N.; Li, Y.G.; Huang, H. Surface touch and its network growth in a graduate student office. *Indoor Air*, under review.
17. Bolashikov, Z.D.; Melikov, A.K. Methods for air cleaning and protection of building occupants from airborne pathogens. *Build. Environ.* **2009**, *44*, 1378–1385. [CrossRef]
18. Nicas, M.; Sun, G. An integrated model of infection risk in a health-care environment. *Risk Anal.* **2006**, *26*, 1085–1096. [CrossRef] [PubMed]
19. Nicas, M.; Nazaroff, W.W.; Hubbard, A. Toward understanding the risk of secondary airborne infection: Emission of respirable pathogens. *J. Occup. Environ. Hyg.* **2005**, *2*, 143–154. [CrossRef] [PubMed]
20. Approaches to Better Understand Human Influenza Transmission (CDC). Available online: https://www.cdc.gov/influenzatransmissionworkshop2010/ (accessed on 1 May 2018).
21. Yang, W.; Elankumaran, S.; Marr, L.C. Concentrations and size distributions of airborne influenza A viruses measured indoors at a health centre, a day-care centre and on aeroplanes. *J. R. Soc. Interface* **2011**, *8*, 1176. [CrossRef] [PubMed]
22. Drossinos, Y.; Housiadas, C. Aerosol flows. In *Multiphase Flow Handbook*; Crowe, C.T., Ed.; CRC Press: Boca Raton, FL, USA, 2006; pp. 6-1–6-58.
23. Duguid, J.P. The size and the duration of air-carriage of respiratory droplets and droplet-nuclei. *Epidemiol. Infect.* **1946**, *44*, 471–479. [CrossRef]

24. Loudon, R.G.; Roberts, R.M. Relation between the airborne diameters of respiratory droplets and the diameter of the stains left after recovery. *Nature* **1967**, *213*, 95–96. [CrossRef]
25. Hayden, F.G.; Fritz, R.; Lobo, M.C.; Alvord, W.; Strober, W.; Straus, S.E. Local and systemic cytokine responses during experimental human influenza A virus infection. Relation to symptom formation and host defense. *J. Clin. Investig.* **1998**, *101*, 643–649. [CrossRef] [PubMed]
26. Zhu, S.; Kato, S.; Yang, J.H. Study on transport characteristics of saliva droplets produced by coughing in a calm indoor environment. *Build. Environ.* **2006**, *41*, 1691–1702. [CrossRef]
27. Fabian, P.; McDevitt, J.J.; DeHaan, W.H.; Fung, R.O.P.; Cowling, B.J.; Chan, K.H.; Leung, G.M.; Milton, D.K. Influenza virus in human exhaled breath: An observational study. *PLoS ONE* **2008**, *3*, e2691. [CrossRef] [PubMed]
28. Chao, C.Y.H.; Wan, M.P.; Morawska, L.; Johnson, G.R.; Ristovski, Z.D.; Hargreaves, M.; Mengersen, K.; Corbett, S.; Li, Y.; Xie, X.; et al. Characterization of expiration air jets and droplet size distributions immediately at the mouth opening. *J. Aerosol Sci.* **2009**, *40*, 122–133. [CrossRef]
29. Xie, X.; Li, Y.; Sun, H.; Liu, L. Exhaled droplets due to talking and coughing. *J. R. Soc. Interface* **2009**, *6*, S703. [CrossRef] [PubMed]
30. Sinnreich, R.; Kark, J.D.; Friedlander, Y.; Sapoznikov, D.; Luria, M.H. Five minute recordings of heart rate variability for population studies: Repeatability and age–sex characteristics. *Heart* **1998**, *80*, 156–162. [CrossRef] [PubMed]
31. Atkinson, M.P.; Wein, L.M. Quantifying the routes of transmission for pandemic influenza. *Bull. Math. Biol.* **2008**, *70*, 820–867. [CrossRef] [PubMed]
32. Chen, S.C.; Liao, C.M. Probabilistic indoor transmission modeling for influenza (sub) type viruses. *J. Infect.* **2010**, *60*, 26–35. [CrossRef] [PubMed]
33. Knight, V.; Fedson, D.; Baldini, J.; Douglas, R.G.; Couch, R.B. Amantadine therapy of epidemic influenza A2 (Hong Kong). *Infect. Immun.* **1970**, *1*, 200–204. [PubMed]
34. Couch, R.B.; Gerone, P.J.; Cate, T.R.; Griffith, W.R.; Alling, D.W.; Knight, V. Preparation and properties of a small-particle aerosol of coxsackie A21. *Proc. Soc. Exp. Biol. Med.* **1965**, *118*, 818–822. [CrossRef] [PubMed]
35. Douglas, R. Influenza in man. In *fluenza Virus and Influenza: Kilbourne*; Academic Press, Inc.: New York, NY, USA, 1975; pp. 395–445.
36. Nicas, M.; Jones, R.M. Relative contributions of four exposure pathways to influenza infection risk. *Risk Anal.* **2009**, *29*, 1292–1303. [CrossRef] [PubMed]
37. Zhang, N.; Huang, H.; Su, B.; Ma, X.; Li, Y. A human behavior integrated hierarchical model of airborne disease transmission in a large city. *Build. Environ.* **2018**, *127*, 211–220. [CrossRef]
38. Chen, S.C.; Chang, C.F.; Liao, C.M. Predictive models of control strategies involved in containing indoor airborne infections. *Indoor Air* **2006**, *16*, 469–481. [CrossRef] [PubMed]
39. Weber, T.P.; Stilianakis, N.I. Inactivation of influenza A viruses in the environment and modes of transmission: A critical review. *J. Infect.* **2008**, *57*, 361–373. [CrossRef] [PubMed]
40. Harper, G.J. Airborne micro-organisms: Survival tests with four viruses. *Epidemiol. Infect.* **1961**, *59*, 479–486. [CrossRef]
41. Blachere, F.M.; Lindsley, W.G.; Pearce, T.A.; Anderson, S.E.; Fisher, M.; Khakoo, R.; Meade, B.J.; Lander, O.; Davis, S.; Thewlis, R.E.; et al. Measurement of airborne influenza virus in a hospital emergency department. *Clin. Infect. Dis.* **2009**, *48*, 438. [CrossRef] [PubMed]
42. Yang, J. Numerical and Experimental Study on Physiological Responses in Hot Environments Based on Human-Clothing-Environment System. Ph.D. Thesis, Tsinghua University, Beijing, China, 2015. (in Chinese).
43. Wester, R.C.; Maibach, H.I. Regional variation in percutaneous absorption. *Drugs Pharm. Sci.* **1999**, *97*, 107–116.
44. Sattar, S.A.; Jacobsen, H.; Springthorpe, V.S.; Cusack, T.M.; Rubino, R. Chemical disinfection to interrupt transfer of rhinovirus type 14 from environmental surfaces to hands. *Appl. Environ. Microbiol.* **1993**, *59*, 1579–1585. [PubMed]
45. Mackintosh, C.A.; Hoffman, P.N. An extended model for transfer of micro-organisms via the hands: Differences between organisms and the effect of alcohol disinfection. *Epidemiol. Infect.* **1984**, *92*, 345–355. [CrossRef]
46. Mokhtari, A.; Jaykus, L.A. Quantitative exposure model for the transmission of norovirus in retail food preparation. *Int. J. Food Microbiol.* **2009**, *133*, 38–47. [CrossRef] [PubMed]

47. Lopez, G.U.; Gerba, C.P.; Tamimi, A.H.; Kitajima, M.; Maxwell, S.L.; Rose, J.B. Transfer efficiency of bacteria and viruses from porous and nonporous fomites to fingers under different relative humidity conditions. *Appl. Environ. Microbiol.* **2013**, *79*, 5728–5734. [CrossRef] [PubMed]
48. Bean, B.; Moore, B.M.; Sterner, B.; Peterson, L.R.; Gerding, D.N.; Balfour, H.H. Survival of influenza viruses on environmental surfaces. *J. Infect. Dis.* **1982**, *146*, 47–51. [CrossRef] [PubMed]
49. Ansari, S.A.; Sattar, S.A.; Springthorpe, V.S.; Wells, G.A.; Tostowaryk, W. Rotavirus survival on human hands and transfer of infectious virus to animate and nonporous inanimate surfaces. *J. Clin. Microbiol.* **1988**, *26*, 1513–1518. [PubMed]
50. Pancic, F.; Carpentier, D.C.; Came, P.E. Role of infectious secretions in the transmission of rhinovirus. *J. Clin. Microbiol.* **1980**, *12*, 567–571. [PubMed]
51. Hendley, J.O.; Wenzel, R.P.; Gwaltney, J.M., Jr. Transmission of rhinovirus colds by self-inoculation. *N. Eng. J. Med.* **1973**, *288*, 1361–1364. [CrossRef] [PubMed]
52. Rusin, P.; Maxwell, S.; Gerba, C. Comparative surface-to-hand and fingertip-to-mouth transfer efficiency of gram-positive bacteria, gram-negative bacteria, and phage. *J. Appl. Microbiol.* **2002**, *93*, 585–592. [CrossRef] [PubMed]
53. Prussin, A.J.; Marr, L.C. Sources of airborne microorganisms in the built environment. *Microbiome* **2015**, *3*, 78. [CrossRef] [PubMed]
54. Alshitawi, M.S.; Awbi, H.B. Measurement and prediction of the effect of students' activities on airborne particulate concentration in a classroom. *HVAC&R Res.* **2011**, *17*, 446–464.
55. Ocak, Y.; Kılıçvuran, A.; Eren, A.B.; Sofuoglu, A.; Sofuoglu, S.C. Exposure to particulate matter in a mosque. *Atmos. Environ.* **2012**, *56*, 169–176. [CrossRef]
56. Qian, J.; Ferro, A.R. Resuspension of dust particles in a chamber and associated environmental factors. *Aerosol Sci. Technol.* **2008**, *42*, 566–578. [CrossRef]
57. Fierer, N.; Lauber, C.L.; Zhou, N.; McDonald, D.; Costello, E.K.; Knight, R. Forensic identification using skin bacterial communities. *Proc. Natl. Acad. Sci. USA* **2010**, *107*, 6477–6481. [CrossRef] [PubMed]
58. Meadow, J.F.; Altrichter, A.E.; Green, J.L. Mobile phones carry the personal microbiome of their owners. *PeerJ* **2014**, *2*, e447. [CrossRef] [PubMed]
59. Noti, J.D.; Lindsley, W.G.; Blachere, F.M.; Cao, G.; Kashon, M.L.; Thewlis, R.E.; McMillen, C.M.; King, W.P.; Szalajda, J.V.; Beezhold, D.H. Detection of infectious influenza virus in cough aerosols generated in a simulated patient examination room. *Clin. Infect. Dis.* **2012**, *54*, 1569. [CrossRef] [PubMed]
60. Kramer, A.; Schwebke, I.; Kampf, G. How long do nosocomial pathogens persist on inanimate surfaces? A systematic review. *BMC Infect. Dis.* **2006**, *6*, 130. [CrossRef] [PubMed]
61. Rabie, T.; Curtis, V. Handwashing and risk of respiratory infections: A quantitative systematic review. *Trop. Med. Int. Health* **2006**, *11*, 258–267. [CrossRef] [PubMed]
62. Jafari, N.; Shahsanai, A.; Memarzadeh, M.; Loghmani, A. Prevention of communicable diseases after disaster: A review. *J. Res. Med. Sci.* **2011**, *16*, 956–962. [PubMed]
63. Kouadio, I.K.; Aljunid, S.; Kamigaki, T.; Hammad, K.; Oshitani, H. Infectious diseases following natural disasters: Prevention and control measures. *Expert Rev. Anti-Infect. Ther.* **2012**, *10*, 95–104. [CrossRef] [PubMed]

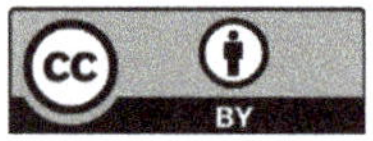

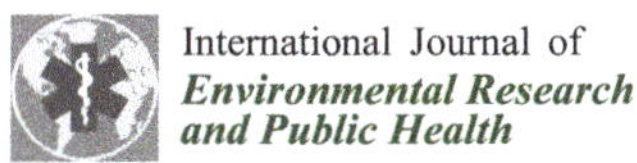
International Journal of
Environmental Research and Public Health

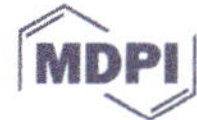

Article

Reducing the Future Risk of Trauma: On the Integration of Global Disaster Policy within Specific Health Domains and Established Fields of Practice

Lennart Reifels [1,2]

[1] Centre for Mental Health, Melbourne School of Population and Global Health, The University of Melbourne, Melbourne, VIC 3010, Australia; l.reifels@unimelb.edu.au; Tel.: +61-3-8344-0667

[2] Disaster Research Unit, Department of Political and Social Sciences, Free University of Berlin, 12165 Berlin, Germany

Received: 2 August 2018; Accepted: 3 September 2018; Published: 5 September 2018

Abstract: The global increase in the frequency and severity of natural hazards and extreme climatic events necessitates more efficient global and national strategies to reduce the likelihood and impact of traumatic consequences for disaster-affected populations. The recent inclusion of mental health in the Sendai Framework for Disaster Risk Reduction marks a pivotal point in the recognition of the significant burden of disasters on mental health, and a global commitment to reducing its impacts. Nevertheless, effective agreement implementation and efforts to reduce disaster mental health risks are facing significant challenges. These include a lack of clarity about the conceptual interlinkages and place of disaster risk reduction principles within the field of disaster mental health, which is traditionally marked by a prevailing recovery orientation, and the need for effective translation into disaster mental health policy and practice. Therefore, this study drew on data from interviews with European disaster mental health and risk reduction experts in order to appraise the merit and implications of a global disaster risk reduction policy for advancing population mental health in the context of disaster. Study findings outline existing opportunities, challenges, and key strategies for the integration of disaster risk reduction within disaster mental health policy and practice.

Keywords: disaster; disaster risk reduction; Sendai framework; mental health

---

1. Introduction

At the global level, human mental health and wellbeing is being increasingly jeopardised through rising trends in population exposure to severe natural hazards and extreme climatic events [1,2]. Despite the often remarkable resilience of communities to the onslaught of such events, decades of disaster mental health research have demonstrated the significant burden that mass-traumatic events can inflict on the mental health of affected populations [3]. This mental health impact can vary in intensity, course, and duration, and find expression in temporary distress reactions among a large majority, ongoing mental health problems of mild to moderate severity, as well as more severe mental health issues (such as post-traumatic stress disorder or depression) among a significant minority of those affected by disaster [4]. Apart from constituting an important outcome domain in its own right, population mental health also plays a key role in facilitating effective rebuilding and recovery efforts and in terms of broader social, socio-economic, and societal functioning [5].

International recognition of the need to better manage the varied risks associated with disaster exposure has resulted in seminal intergovernmental agreements and policy frameworks to guide global and societal disaster risk reduction [6,7]. The Sendai Framework for Disaster Risk Reduction 2015–2030, which was adopted by 187 United Nations (UN) member states in March 2015, reflects an important conceptual shift in global disaster policy—away from managing disaster impacts and consequences, toward a proactive approach to managing and reducing disaster risks. Although this relatively subtle shift in global disaster policy may be unbeknownst to many outside of the field, it is likely to have important practical ramifications for concerted societal efforts to address disaster risks across varied sectors and practice domains over the next 15 years. It further requires a thorough understanding of both existing and newly emerging disaster risks facing societies today and the adoption of proactive and effective strategies to manage and reduce these risks in future.

The Sendai Framework is structured around the key elements of a global goal and expected outcome, operationalised through seven global targets primarily aimed at reducing: disaster mortality, the number of people affected, economic losses, damage to infrastructure, and disruption of basic (e.g., health) services. In addition, four cross-cutting priority areas for global action highlight the critical importance of: (1) understanding disaster risk, (2) strengthening disaster risk governance, (3) investing in disaster risk reduction, and (4) enhancing disaster preparedness for effective response and to 'build back better'. As part of a concerted implementation effort, the Sendai Framework also outlines local, national, and regional level stakeholder roles and responsibilities.

One of the cornerstones of the Sendai Framework is its strong emphasis on human health. This is particularly evident in 35 direct references to health, the explicit inclusion of health in the expected Sendai outcome ("the substantial reduction of disaster risk and losses in lives, livelihoods, and health and in the economic, physical, social, cultural, and environmental assets of persons, businesses, communities, and countries"), and direct links to health in four of the framework's seven global targets [8,9]. Within the context of this strong health emphasis, the explicit inclusion of mental health in the Sendai Framework marks a pivotal point in the recognition of the significant burden of disasters on the mental health of affected populations, and a simultaneous global commitment to reducing its impacts [10]. Mental health features, perhaps most prominently, as a national and local level responsibility under Sendai's priority action area (4) in terms of the aim to "enhance recovery schemes to provide psychosocial support and mental health services for all people in need" (paragraph 33o); whereas other key action areas underpin the critical importance of a better understanding of disaster risks across varied societal sectors and domains.

However, despite the formal inclusion and recognition of the importance of population mental health, significant challenges remain to the effective Sendai agreement implementation and associated efforts to reduce disaster mental health risks and consequences. These include a lack of clarity about the conceptual interlinkages and place of disaster risk reduction principles within the field of disaster mental health, which is traditionally marked by a prevailing recovery orientation, and the need for translation into disaster mental health policy and practice.

Conversely, key aspects relevant to disaster mental health have thus far received relatively little systematic attention in the context of disaster risk reduction frameworks. This, however, is in stark contrast to more general and public health domains, which are increasingly being considered in disaster risk reduction contexts [8,9,11,12]. As a direct consequence, the Sendai Framework currently provides little conceptual elaboration of the nature of disaster mental health risks or necessary guidance for future societal strategies to reduce and manage associated mental health risks and consequences of extreme climatic events and disasters. In view of the inevitable limits of global disaster treaties to provide health domain-specific guidance, there is therefore an urgent need to carefully consider the implications of the Sendai Framework for specific health domains, and to facilitate its integration within established fields of practice [13].

For brevity, this article adopts an inclusive definition of disaster mental health (DMH) as a scientific discipline and field of practice that is concerned with understanding, preventing, and addressing mental health problems and promoting psychosocial wellbeing and resilience in disaster and emergency contexts. Thus understood, DMH is not merely limited to efforts that seek to better understand or address psychiatric phenomena via therapeutic interventions, but rather includes recognition of the vital importance of a broader range of psycho-social factors, outcomes, and support strategies in disaster and emergency contexts. Emerging from traditions, such as trauma and stress studies, and incorporating related humanitarian practice fields, such as Mental Health and Psychosocial Support, DMH has amassed a considerable body of knowledge about the potential spectrum of disaster mental health outcomes and relevant intervention and support strategies over time [14,15]. Yet, traditionally, the primary focus of DMH strategies has been on facilitating recovery in the wake of disaster, whereas the field has remained fairly oblivious to broader developments in global disaster policy. In view of this circumstance, the current shift in disaster policy in the context of the Sendai Framework—from managing disaster impacts to reducing disaster risks—provides a pertinent and timely opportunity to examine the intersection of these two fields in more depth, and to explore the DMH field through a disaster risk reduction (DRR) lens.

This study therefore drew on data from interviews with European disaster mental health and risk reduction experts in order to appraise the merit and implications of global disaster risk reduction policy for advancing population mental health in the context of disaster. More specifically, this study examined the conceptual nature of disaster mental health risks, as well as concrete opportunities, current challenges, and key strategies for the integration of disaster risk reduction within disaster mental health policy and practice.

2. Materials and Methods

This study drew on data from interviews with 17 European key informants (including 14 DMH and 3 DRR experts), which were conducted between May and September 2016, as part of a larger research project that examined the early implementation of the Sendai Framework in Europe. In view of the relatively small pool of key informants in this area, this exploratory study adopted a purposive sampling frame informed by prior stakeholder mapping to recruit eminent DMH and DRR experts at the European regional and national levels (in the UK, the Netherlands, and Germany) for participation in semi-structured interviews. Participating DRR experts represented three of the 17 DRR experts recruited for the larger study who were both directly involved in the Sendai implementation and in a position to complete an interview schedule focused on disaster mental health. Key informants (10 men, 7 women) were typically affiliated with scientific institutions and national DMH or DRR advisory bodies across the UK, the Netherlands, and Germany, or European-based advisory bodies with a broader international mandate.

Semi-structured interviews were conducted on the basis of an interview schedule. The schedule included 15 questions that explored the intersection of DRR and DMH by eliciting information on: principal mental health risks in disaster contexts, DMH strategies to address these risks, and existing opportunities, current challenges, and key strategies for the integration of disaster risk reduction and disaster mental health. A copy of the full interview schedule is available from the author upon request. The interviews, which lasted between 40 and 95 minutes, were conducted either in person or remotely (via telephone or Skype), audio-recorded, and analysed thematically using NVivo11 (QSR International Pty Ltd., Melbourne, Australia). All key informants provided consent for study participation. The study protocol was approved by the Human Research Ethics Committee at the University of Melbourne (ID: 1646655.1).

3. Results

Key themes resulting from the expert interviews are summarised in the following, with the study's thematic coding framework and illustrative participant quotes outlined in Table S1.

3.1. Principal Disaster Mental Health Risks

Key informants were asked about what they would regard as the principal mental health risks in disaster contexts. The principal mental health risks identified by the experts fell into five broad thematic categories. The first two of these highlighted commonly established risk factors for adverse mental health outcomes, as well as newly emerging risks that were contextually bound to the unfolding European refugee/migration crisis. The three remaining categories were focused on risks associated with the conduct of appropriate disaster mental health responses and intervention strategies, e.g., in relation to the adequate recognition and detection of complex mental health impacts, the provision of appropriate mental health support, and overarching disaster response communication and coordination.

3.1.1. Common Risk Factors

Key informants frequently identified established risk factors for adverse mental health outcomes. These factors included, amongst others, the nature of the hazard, exposure level, peri-traumatic and post-event reactions, various forms of loss (of persons, resources, livelihoods), lack of (received or perceived) social support, distress impacting on normal functioning, the decay of the recovery environment, and secondary stressors in the disaster aftermath (related to damaged infrastructure, lacking health support, social conflict, and uncertainties about the future). Vulnerable population groups identified to be at particular risk and warranting special attention included those with pre-existing difficulties or severe mental illness, children, the elderly, socially isolated individuals, and people with disabilities.

3.1.2. Emerging Risks (European Migration Crisis)

A second set of emerging mental health risks revolved around the unfolding refugee and migration crisis in Europe, with many experts indicating involvement in this crisis either inside or outside of Europe. Principal mental health risks identified in this context were often reflective of underpinning social and physical determinants of health. These highlighted the role of displacement as a major mental health risk factor given the loss of continuity of care, the impact of family separation (on anxiety, depression, identity loss), as well as frequent occurrences of unresolved missing person situations (which provided no opportunity for closure or appropriate mourning). Mental health risks specific to younger generations were posed by: disrupted education and development paths for youth (during an already challenging and critical developmental stage); the impact of disrupted schooling and language barriers on cognitive development; as well as lacking access to normal peers, play, and structure for children; and the impacts of malnutrition on the mother-child bond, routine lactation, and cognitive/physical development of infants.

3.1.3. Recognition of Complex Mental Health Impacts

Failure to recognise the complexity and diversity of mental health impacts in disaster-affected populations was identified as a pivotal risk in the design and conduct of appropriate disaster mental health responses. Importantly, this included the risk of failing to detect those individuals who proceed to develop more persistent or severe mental health problems, distinct from those who initially experience common transitory distress responses. The shortcomings of a reductionist view were highlighted in terms of the failure to differentiate varying mental health risks of specific population groups (e.g., those affected directly or indirectly, or first responders), and in terms of a sole focus on specific signature disorders (such as post-traumatic stress disorder), rather than the relevant broader spectrum of disaster mental health outcomes and psychosocial consequences. Over-pathologisation on the part of disaster response planners further entails the risk of mismanaging normal human distress reactions to abnormal or disastrous circumstances. However, under-pathologisation may run the risk of failing to identify or reach those with significant mental health problems who may not otherwise readily access or seek support. Varied mental health risks posed by different disaster types and contexts, and interactions with pre-existing problems in disaster-affected communities, further compound the challenge of recognising complex disaster impacts in the design of appropriate mental health responses.

3.1.4. Provision of Appropriate Mental Health Support

Specific risks associated with the provision of appropriate mental health support to disaster-affected populations include the potential use of ineffective early interventions (such as debriefing), the lack of timely psychosocial care, the absence of clear and timely community information, and the lack of recognition of longer-term mental health provisions that needed to be put in place. In view of diverse emerging mental health problems and known barriers in the access to mental healthcare, the need was highlighted for a delicate balance between an emphasis on proactive support intervention and a stance of watchful waiting. This balance would help optimally align support efforts with the stage of recovery and nature of presenting problems, and not alienate affected individuals and communities in the process.

3.1.5. Disaster Response Communication and Coordination

Broader mental health risks were also identified in the context of disaster response communication and coordination. Non-consultative and top-down approaches of disaster response authorities can create mental health risks for affected communities further down the track. Politician behavior in disaster contexts can also be informed by and affecting public sentiment, whereas public perception of the way in which presenting health problems are handled or addressed by responsible authorities may pose a political risk for decision makers. Inherent risks of public disaster response communication included a general lack of communication, the uncertainty of (intended) outcomes, and possibility of unintended consequences. Moreover, disaster-poor countries can face challenges in communicating disaster risks to the wider public with a view to motivate self-protective action, which may lead to a stronger reliance on public authorities and experts in disaster contexts. Hierarchically organised civil protection systems, which are not traditionally citizen-centric, have therefore often failed to recognise existing community agency, resources, and self-help potential, or have struggled to translate a prevailing rhetoric of citizen engagement into effective practice. Conversely, the lack of public risk awareness, proper citizen engagement, and overarching stakeholder coordination and cooperation also increases the risk of adverse disaster outcomes and consequences.

3.2. *Current DMH Strategies to Address Risks*

When asked about key strategies through which the DMH field was addressing these principal disaster mental health risks, experts identified strategies within four main areas.

3.2.1. Development of Guidelines and Response Plans

The development of overarching psychosocial disaster guidelines and response plans was seen as pivotal to the design and conduct of effective disaster responses and to addressing mental health risks in disaster contexts. Specifically, organisations with routine involvement in disaster responses will need to have psychosocial disaster plans in place. Although generic plans may never be specific enough to capture unique disaster circumstances, these nevertheless provide an important planning framework that can be adapted to concrete scenarios.

3.2.2. Mechanisms to Identify and Direct People to Appropriate Support

Key mechanisms to detect and direct disaster-affected individuals to appropriate mental health support included the establishment of on-scene information and advice centres, the implementation of psychological screen and treat programs, and the establishment of disaster health registers. The role of public mental health awareness and wellbeing campaigns was raised in this context, as was the newly-developed concept of health passports for refugees and migrants, which may assist in providing greater continuity of care and access to vital medications across national boundaries.

3.2.3. Psychosocial and Mental Health Support Strategies

Designated mental health support strategies emphasised the need to provide screening, effective early intervention, and psychosocial support within the broader context of practical assistance. The need for basic psychosocial support strategies that could be provided by lay people and volunteer-based disaster relief agencies was highlighted. Specific psychosocial support strategies identified included the creation of safe spaces for vulnerable groups (in terms of child-friendly spaces, non-formal schooling, or breast-feeding tents), as well as the provision of parental support, livelihood skill building, general information, or legal advice. Awareness raising for the specific situation and issues affecting (and advocating the protection of) vulnerable groups was considered particularly critical in the context of violence against women and for residents of psychiatric institutions. The integration of mental health support within primary care and ceasing of opportunities to strengthen existing mental health systems and 'build back better' after disaster were equally highlighted as key avenues to address systemic mental health risks in disaster contexts.

3.2.4. Disaster Preparedness Planning

Other strategies and avenues to reduce disaster mental health risks were identified in the context of disaster preparedness planning. These included the provision of dedicated first responder training, the establishment of organisational support systems, mechanisms to facilitate multiagency networking, cooperation and joint planning, and the mapping of existing services. The importance of prior vulnerability and needs assessments (including geographical mapping of vulnerable groups) was highlighted, as was the need to involve these groups and the broader public in disaster preparedness planning. The resulting need to adapt existing alert systems, evacuation plans, and risk/crisis communication to the needs of vulnerable groups was emphasised, as was the potential to adopt a stronger focus on resilience-building activities throughout the whole cycle of disaster prevention, preparedness, response, and recovery planning.

3.3. *Challenges to DMH/DRR Integration*

Several questions explored the intersection of DMH and DRR in more depth, including existing challenges and opportunities for the integration of the two fields. Key integration challenges highlighted DMH and DRR as rather separate fields of practice, marked by practitioners from different professional backgrounds and a mutual lack of awareness. The use of technical jargon on either side was seen as an impediment to effective integration, as was the lack of DMH stakeholder involvement in the Sendai implementation process. The relative vagueness of the Sendai Framework, which does not specify key mental health risks to be addressed, along with its broad aims were seen to harbor the potential to lead to mental health initiatives that are not necessarily the most beneficial. Key challenges to greater recognition and use of existing DMH strategies within DRR included the lack of an empirical evidence base for specific psychosocial support strategies (which science requires to inform policy), and challenges in effective targeting of more preventative resilience-building initiatives before disaster strikes. Conversely, it was recognised that the Sendai implementation process did not necessarily follow a uniform international pattern but rather required unique integration within national systems and structures. Potential professional role and resource implications of the integration of the two fields were raised in terms of the necessary willingness of professionals to step outside of their brief, the perception that extra work or resources may be required, or that a stronger focus on community empowerment within DMH could result in less funding for traditional clinical or other core work. Other integration challenges included the limited sustainability of project-based initiatives, and lacking recognition of the vital role of DMH stakeholders in joint pre-disaster planning (beyond common ad-hoc involvement in response and recovery).

3.4. DMH/DRR Integration Opportunities

Notwithstanding these challenges, experts identified wide ranging opportunities for the stronger integration of the two fields. Key integration avenues involved the use of inter-sectoral platforms, joint stakeholder meetings, and preparedness summits, as well as disaster-related information and referral websites, and mobile phone applications. Joint DRR-DMH fact sheets and DRR primers for DMH staff may facilitate mutual practitioner understanding. Building on existing European projects and networks, the development of a shared European position was regarded as useful. In this context, major disaster events were also seen as progress catalysts that can provide opportunities to explore new solutions and trial different ways of operating.

DMH experts and practitioners can facilitate DMH/DRR integration by advocating the recognition of mental health issues in disaster prevention and response planning, integrating mental health knowledge at higher strategy and local planning levels, providing guidance on where mental health funding and efforts are best spent, and by continuing to build the underpinning DMH evidence base. Simultaneously, it was recognised that DMH must become better at providing clear and understandable messages and at marketing DMH knowledge, so that it can be more readily used by local authorities and stakeholders. Other DMH contributions to foster integration included psychosocial capacity analysis at the municipal level, prior vulnerability mapping, and knowledge and skill building in vulnerable groups to enhance self-help capacity and psychosocial stress management.

Integration can also be facilitated by expanding the prevailing DRR mandate to include mental health, such as by addressing psychological stressors in public crisis communication, including mental health messaging in non-formal education, as well as through professional selection and equipment of first responders with the vital skills to handle common stress reactions.

Promising conceptual interlinkages that facilitate future DMH/DRR integration efforts revolved around a shared focus on resilience building, the use of health promotion strategies, community-based and self-help approaches, and community mobilisation concepts that are already embedded in international guidelines for psychosocial emergency response. Other interlinkages exist between health and disaster literacy approaches, and between healthy cities and urban resilience frameworks.

Formal integration steps highlighted the benefits of incorporating DMH guidelines as an appendix to the Sendai Framework, the need to operationalise DMH/DRR linkages and interventions to support broader application and effectiveness testing, devote project funding to integration efforts, and mandate stronger interdisciplinary and interagency work, such as in joint disaster planning.

4. Discussion

The findings of this exploratory study provide a first look at the DMH field through a DRR lens, and a vital perspective on the intersection of these two fields that can facilitate future integration efforts. Study findings indicate that it is clearly early days in terms of the formal integration of the fields, and that Sendai disaster policy awareness within the mental health field may be limited. Yet, the impending application of DRR concepts and approaches across varied societal sectors and health domains in the context of the Sendai implementation provides a pertinent and timely opportunity to examine its conceptual and practical implications for DMH and other established fields of practice.

4.1. Conceptualising DMH Risks: The Place of Risk Within DMH

Application of the Sendai objective of understanding disaster risk within the context of a specific health domain and field of practice (such as DMH) inevitably involves the task of fleshing out an otherwise generic (or content-neutral) notion of disaster risk, with domain-specifically relevant content that is consistent with the broader Sendai notion. A better understanding of pre-existing notions of disaster risk held among practitioners within a given health domain therefore constitutes an important preliminary step in developing a shared conceptual understanding and joint future integration and work agenda.

In appraising the nature of principal DMH risks identified by the experts, and the place of risk within the DMH field more broadly, it is evident that DMH has developed an existing risk vocabulary (and associated evidence base) that is primarily centered on established risk factors for adverse disaster mental health outcomes. Such risk factors include a wide range of predisposing factors (such as age, gender, socio-economic status, or pre-existing difficulties), as well as factors related to disaster exposure and secondary stressors, all of which have been well established in the literature [3].

Nevertheless, beyond the primacy of this risk factor-driven understanding, the broad scope of identified principal DMH risks also spanned newly emerging mental health risks (contextually bound to the European migration crisis) and risks associated with the design and delivery of adequate support interventions (such as the recognition of complex disaster mental health impacts, the provision of appropriate mental health support, and broader disaster response communication and coordination). As a whole, these principal DMH risks are reflective of the developmental stage, existing sophistication, and key challenges of the field. Moreover, all these DMH risk notions (either directly or indirectly) have a shared concern with the potential for adverse disaster mental health outcomes.

Specific DMH risk factors identified in this study are structurally different from the broader (probabilistic) notion of disaster risk, elaborated and defined in the Sendai Framework as "The potential loss of life, injury, or destroyed or damaged assets which could occur to a system, society, or a community in a specific period of time, determined probabilistically as a function of hazard, exposure, vulnerability, and capacity" [16]. DMH risk factors are perhaps more akin to various elements of this definition, such as the key concepts of vulnerability, exposure, and (as in the case of the latter DMH risks) capacity.

When DMH risks are classified in terms of the specific nature of adverse disaster outcomes considered, it becomes possible to distinguish at least three different types of DMH risk, and to conceive of DMH risk more generally, as the likelihood and severity of:

(1) Newly emerging or exacerbated mental health issues among disaster-affected populations (Type A)
(2) Adverse impacts on existing mental health support systems (Type B), for example, in terms of client/staff safety and wellbeing, infrastructure damage, service disruption, surge capacity, evacuation, and business continuity
(3) Secondary effects of A and B on individual, community, business, and societal functioning (Type C)

Beyond these principal DMH risk types, it is also possible to identify more intermediate DMH risks, such as:

(4) Lack of DMH preparedness or capacity (Type D)
(5) Poor quality, lacking efficiency, efficacy, and coordination of DMH responses (Type E)

Nevertheless, although these latter intermediate risks may constitute ongoing key challenges of the field, these can also generally be regarded subordinate to principal DMH risks of Types A and B. In considering the nature of domain-specific DMH risks of Types A–C, it is again helpful to draw upon the broader Sendai notion of disaster risk. This notion calls us to move beyond the mere consideration of adverse outcomes, and to adopt a comprehensive understanding of disaster risk as determined by the key aspects of hazard, exposure, and existing vulnerabilities and capacities [16].

4.2. Current Focus of DMH (Risk Reduction) Strategies

In view of the nature of identified mental health risks in disaster contexts, much of the existing arsenal of DMH strategies has traditionally been focused on addressing these risks during disaster response and recovery phases. As such, these strategies could be seen to require the prior occurrence of disaster event exposure in order to become relevant or applicable. Yet, interview data also suggested an increasing trend toward the exploration of more proactive, preventative, and resilience building initiatives within DMH, which, while still fledging in terms of an empirical evidence base [17], would also be well aligned with broader developments in disaster policy and the move toward the promotion of disaster resilient communities, health systems, and societies [18,19].

4.3. Sendai's Dual Challenge for DMH

In this context, it is interesting to note that the principal reference to mental health in the Sendai Framework (Priority 4, paragraph 33o; see Introduction) encapsulates an implicit understanding of DMH that firmly locates the role of the field within disaster recovery and building back better phases. As such, this conceptual understanding also reinforces the traditional DMH focus and self-understanding. It is also in this narrow sense that the genuine conceptual challenge posed by the Sendai Framework for DMH policy may be considered comparatively negligible, notwithstanding substantial variability in the existing capacity of countries to effectively apply DMH policy and know-how in practice [20]. Put differently, the implications of this narrowly conceived Sendai challenge for DMH may be less about the aim of finding new and innovative ways of doing things, but rather about becoming more professional at those activities in which the field at large is already engaged; perhaps resulting in a greater need for capacity building or upscaling (particularly in resource-poor countries), rather than broader reorientation or reinvention.

Yet, while undoubtedly more work must be done in terms of strengthening the existing capacity, effectiveness, integration, and sustainability of DMH systems [21], Sendai's conceptual challenge for DMH policy and practice (in a broader sense) goes further. When Sendai's underpinning philosophy of understanding and reducing disaster risk is taken to heart, it becomes possible to look beyond DMH's established role as post-disaster savior, and to explore the potential role that the DMH field (via existing or future strategies) may be able to assume in reducing disaster risks and in averting adverse disaster mental health consequences, before these occur. The implications of this broader Sendai challenge for DMH may thus require a potential shift in conceptual emphasis—away from the current focus on downstream interventions and toward the exploration of more proactive upstream strategies that are effective at reducing DMH risks [13].

4.4. Sendai Implementation Requirements

Global Sendai Framework implementation between 2015 and 2030 will be monitored on the basis of national progress reporting across UN member states against agreed targets and indicators [16]. The ability of member states to demonstrate progress in terms of not only the existence but outcomes of effective DRR strategies has direct implications for societal sectors and health domains, and for the field of DMH. Key Sendai progress indicators of relevance to health include quantifiable reductions in the number of deaths (A-2), missing persons (A-3), injured or ill people (B-2), each per 100,000 population; as well as in the number of destroyed or damaged health facilities (D-2), and disruptions to health services (D-7) attributable to disasters [16,22].

When these health-related Sendai implementation requirements are viewed through the lens of the above DMH risk typology, these would primarily call for a better understanding and the reduction of principal DMH risks of Type A (in alignment with Sendai indicator B-2) and Type B (in alignment with indicators D-2 and D-7), whereas wider societal benefits of monitoring, enumerating, and reducing secondary, or more intermediate DMH risks of Types C–E, are also evident.

In this context, the Bangkok Principles, in support of the implementation of the health aspects of the Sendai Framework [23] and related UN guidance directives, also specifically highlight the importance of incorporating relevant (mental) health indicator data within comprehensive national disaster risk assessments [24], associated disaster loss databases [25], and multi-hazard early warning systems. Future monitoring of Sendai implementation progress in terms of the reduction of principal DMH risks is therefore critically dependent on the systematic identification, collection, and incorporation of mental health indicator data within these planning and reporting processes to ascertain reduced disaster impacts at population and service system levels over time.

4.5. Study Limitations

As the first study explicitly focussing on the nexus of DMH and DRR, this study adopted an open-exploratory and not theoretically-driven approach to examining DMH risks, strategies, and conceptual interlinkages of these fields from the perspective of European DMH and DRR experts. In view of the social construction of disaster risk [26], it is conceivable that exploration of these issues with other stakeholder groups (such as lay people or professionals from other regions) may have resulted in different conceptualisations of risk or priority strategies to address these. Specific DMH risks identified in this study may also, at least in part, be socio-historically contingent upon major events unfolding in the study region at the time. Although interview participants in this exploratory study represented eminent DMH and DRR experts at each of the targeted European regional and national levels, the purposive study sampling frame and relatively small sample size may have limited the representativeness and generalisability of study findings. The broader project policy focus on the Sendai Framework implementation across Europe placed restrictions on the extent to which its implications could be examined for more specific national or local DMH practice traditions.

4.6. Implications and Future Directions

DMH is in a favorable position to tackle the Sendai challenge to both inform DRR, and in turn, be informed by DRR. Expert identification of mental health risks and strategies does not necessarily imply that these risks are generally well understood or that such strategies are already widely in place across countries. The inclusion of mental health in the Sendai Framework is laudable, yet its general formulation does not reflect the existing key challenges and sophistication of the DMH field. DMH therefore needs to guide DRR on the relevant mental health risks and aspects of disasters and on the choice of effective strategies to address these. In turn, a shift in DMH orientation and further steps will be required to effectively translate DRR principles and concepts into DMH policy and practice.

This study outlined several strategies and conceptual interlinkages that can facilitate future DMH/DRR integration efforts and provided valuable insights and lessons for the integration of global disaster policy in other health domains and established fields of practice.

Future efforts to integrate global DRR policy within a given health domain need to address several interrelated levels. At a conceptual level, key DRR concepts and principles, such as disaster risk and risk reduction, need to be examined in terms of their compatibility with and implications for prevailing doctrines and practice approaches [27]. The application of a DRR approach within a given health domain, such as DMH, thus first and foremost requires completing a rather abstract notion of disaster risk with health domain-specifically relevant content and meaning. Whereas the Sendai Framework provides broad parameters and agreed-upon definitions of key DRR concepts, it is essential that we turn to practitioners and experts within these fields to better understand principal disaster risks and existing strengths and limitations of key strategies to address these risks at present.

At a policy level, integration can be facilitated through systematic mapping of the Sendai Framework against existing policies and practice guidelines to identify key areas of overlap, existing gaps, inform strategic future planning, and focus areas for further development. Insightful examples of comprehensive Sendai mapping exercises already exist in regard to EU policies [28], and the U.K.'s existing doctrine of integrated emergency management [29]. Future efforts to integrate DRR within DMH would thus benefit from systematically mapping the Sendai Framework against DMH policies and guidelines at varied entity levels including international, national, sub-national, and agency levels.

At a translational level, results of these foundational exercises can inform the shape and focus of key activities to operationalize existing linkages between these fields. These include the identification of promising bridging approaches or innovative case studies—at policy, service, or practical intervention levels—that can be applied more broadly and tested for effectiveness. Capitalizing upon and further developing existing avenues for joint cooperation between DMH and DRR sectors will become increasingly important, as is ensuring adequate DMH and health sector representation at all levels of the Sendai implementation process. In this respect, it is critical that mental health specific indicators be developed that align with broader Sendai indicators to facilitate ongoing monitoring and reporting of Sendai progress in terms of reduced mental health impacts at population and service system levels over time. One of the key strengths of the Sendai Framework is that it combines an ambitious and timely global policy program with broad multinational buy-in and clear guidance to facilitate its implementation at global, regional, national, and local levels.

Health domain-specific DRR integration efforts can complement broad-based, whole-society DRR approaches by highlighting the relevance of DRR policy and implications of key DRR concepts, addressing existing translation barriers, and helping to unlock the unique DRR potential within established fields of practice. Notably, designated DMH interventions constitute one key element in the broader arsenal of DRR strategies that can reduce future risk of disaster exposure, associated traumatic impacts, and adverse mental health consequences. Therefore, effective disaster mental health risk reduction requires the application and integration of effective DMH strategies in the context of broad-based DRR strategies [13]. To further strengthen its unique role and contribution in the Sendai implementation process, the DMH field needs to intensify its efforts to establish a sound evidence base to support the choice of effective interventions, to sustainably build its disaster preparedness and response capacity, and to actively explore the merit of more preventative upstream strategies. The recently established World Health Organization (WHO) Thematic Platform for Health Emergency and Disaster Risk Management Research [30,31] provides a promising overarching context in which to further examine principal disaster mental health risks (Types A–E) and more effective strategies to reduce these risks in future.

5. Conclusions

Successful Sendai Framework implementation and efforts to reduce disaster mental health risks critically hinge upon the application of both concerted broad-based DRR and effective DMH strategies, and on the effective integration of DRR principles within existing health domains and established fields of practice.

Supplementary Materials: The following are available online at http://www.mdpi.com/1660-4601/15/9/1932/s1, Table S1: Thematic Coding Framework.

Funding: This work was supported through a EU Residency Scholarship from the European Union Centre on Shared Complex Challenges, which was co-funded by the European Commission and The University of Melbourne.

Acknowledgments: Some of the central ideas expressed in this paper were originally presented at the UNISDR Science and Technology Conference in Geneva, Switzerland in January 2016 and at the 32nd Annual Meeting of the International Society for Traumatic Stress Studies in Dallas, TX, USA in November 2016.

Conflicts of Interest: The author declares no conflict of interest. The funders had no role in the design of the study; in the collection, analyses, or interpretation of data; in the writing of the manuscript, and in the decision to publish the results.

References

1. The Human Cost of Weather-related Disasters 1995–2015. Available online: https://www.unisdr.org/files/46796_cop21weatherdisastersreport2015.pdf (accessed on 4 September 2018).
2. Berry, H.L.; Bowen, K.; Kjellstrom, T. Climate change and mental health: A causal pathways framework. *Int. J. Public Health* **2010**, *55*, 123–132. [CrossRef] [PubMed]
3. Norris, F.H.; Friedman, M.J.; Watson, P.J.; Byrne, C.M.; Diaz, E.; Kaniasty, K. 60,000 disaster victims speak: Part I. An empirical review of the empirical literature, 1981–2001. *Psychiatry* **2002**, *65*, 207–239. [CrossRef] [PubMed]
4. Neria, Y.; Nandi, A.; Galea, S. Post-traumatic stress disorder following disasters: A systematic review. *Psychol. Med.* **2008**, *38*, 467–480. [CrossRef] [PubMed]
5. The Economic Cost of the Social Impact of Natural Disasters. Available online: http://australianbusinessroundtable.com.au/our-research/social-costs-report (accessed on 4 September 2018).

6. Sendai Framework for Disaster Risk Reduction 2015–2030. Available online: https://www.preventionweb.net/files/43291_sendaiframeworkfordrren.pdf (accessed on 4 September 2018).
7. Hyogo Framework for Action 2005–2015: Building the Resilience of Nations and Communities to Disasters. Available online: https://www.unisdr.org/files/1037_hyogoframeworkforactionenglish.pdf (accessed on 4 September 2018).
8. Murray, V.; Aitsi-Selmi, A.; Blanchard, K. The role of public health within the United Nations post-2015 framework for disaster risk reduction. *Int. J. Disaster Risk Sci.* **2015**, *6*, 28–37. [CrossRef]
9. Aitsi-Selmi, A.; Murray, V. The Sendai framework: Disaster risk reduction through a health lens. *Bull. World Health Organ.* **2015**, *93*, 362. [CrossRef] [PubMed]
10. Tsutsumi, A.; Izutsu, T.; Ito, A.; Thornicroft, G.; Patel, V.; Minas, H. Mental health mainstreamed in new UN disaster framework. *Lancet Psychiatry* **2015**, *2*, 679–680. [CrossRef]
11. Murray, V. Disaster Risk Reduction, Health, and the Post-2015 United Nations Landmark Agreements. *Disaster Med. Public Health Prep.* **2014**, *8*, 283–287. [CrossRef] [PubMed]
12. Dar, O.; Buckley, E.J.; Rokadiya, S.; Huda, Q.; Abrahams, J. Integrating health into disaster risk reduction strategies: Key considerations for success. *Am. J. Public Health* **2014**, *104*, 1811–1816. [CrossRef] [PubMed]
13. Reifels, L. Disaster Mental Health Risk Reduction: An Upstream Paradigm Shift for Disaster Mental Health. In Proceedings of the UNISDR Science and Technology Conference on the Implementation of the Sendai Framework for Disaster Risk Reduction 2015–2030, Geneva, Switzerland, 27–29 January 2016.
14. Halpern, J.; Tramontin, M. A history of disaster mental health. In *Disaster Mental Health: Theory and Practice*; Thomson: Belmont, CA, USA, 2007; pp. 46–79.
15. Watson, P.J.; Brymer, M.J.; Bonanno, G.A. Postdisaster psychological intervention since 9/11. *Am. Psychol.* **2011**, *66*, 482–494. [CrossRef] [PubMed]
16. Report of the Open-Ended Intergovernmental Expert Working Group on Indicators and Terminology Relating to Disaster Risk Reduction. Available online: https://www.preventionweb.net/files/50683_oiewgreportenglish.pdf (accessed on 4 September 2018).
17. Joyce, S.; Shand, F.; Tighe, J.; Laurent, S.J.; Bryant, R.A.; Harvey, S.B. Road to resilience: A systematic review and meta-analysis of resilience training programmes and interventions. *BMJ Open* **2018**, *8*, e017858. [CrossRef] [PubMed]
18. Beerlage, I. Community resilience. In *Atlas of Vulnerability and Resilience—Pilot Version for Germany, Austria, Liechtenstein and Switzerland*; Fekete, A., Hufschmidt, G., Eds.; Cologne: Bonn, Germany, 2016; pp. 32–33, ISBN 978-3-946573-12-8.
19. World Health Organization. *Operational Framework for Building Climate Resilient Health Systems*; World Health Organization: Geneva, Switzerland, 2015; ISBN 978 92 4 156507 3.
20. Te Brake, H.; Dückers, M. Early psychosocial interventions after disasters, terrorism and other shocking events: Is there a gap between norms and practice in Europe? *Eur. J. Psychotraumatol.* **2013**, *4*, 19093. [CrossRef] [PubMed]
21. Reifels, L.; Pietrantoni, L.; Prati, G.; Kim, Y.; Kilpatrick, D.G.; Dyb, G.; Halpern, J.; Olff, M.; Brewin, C.R.; O'Donnell, M. Lessons learned about psychosocial responses to disaster and mass trauma: An international perspective. *Eur. J. Psychotraumatol.* **2013**, *4*. [CrossRef] [PubMed]
22. Maini, R.; Clarke, L.; Blanchard, K.; Murray, V. The Sendai Framework for Disaster Risk Reduction and Its Indicators—Where Does Health Fit in? *Int. J. Disaster Risk Sci.* **2017**, *8*, 150–155. [CrossRef]
23. Bangkok Principles for the Implementation of the Health Aspects of the Sendai Framework for Disaster Risk Reduction 2015–2030. Available online: http://www.who.int/hac/events/2016/Bangkok_Principles.pdf (accessed on 4 September 2018).
24. Words into Action Guidelines: National Disaster Risk Assessment. Governance System, Methodologies, and Use of Results (Consultative Version). Available online: https://www.unisdr.org/files/52828_nationaldisasterriskassessmentwiagu.pdf (accessed on 4 September 2018).
25. Disaster Loss Data in Monitoring the Implementation of the Sendai Framework. Available online: https://council.science/cms/2017/05/DRR-policy-brief-2-data.pdf (accessed on 4 September 2018).
26. Chipangura, P.; Van Niekerk, D.; Van Der Waldt, G. An exploration of objectivism and social constructivism within the context of disaster risk. *Disaster Prev. Manag.* **2016**, *25*, 261–274. [CrossRef]

27. Phibbs, S.; Kenney, C.; Severinsen, C.; Mitchell, J.; Hughes, R. Synergising Public Health Concepts with the Sendai Framework for Disaster Risk Reduction: A Conceptual Glossary. *Int. J. Environ. Res. Public Health* **2016**, *13*, 1241. [CrossRef] [PubMed]
28. Action Plan on the Sendai Framework for Disaster Risk Reduction 2015–2030. A Disaster Risk-Informed Approach for All EU Policies. Available online: http://ec.europa.eu/echo/sites/echo-site/files/1_en_document_travail_service_part1_v2.pdf (accessed on 4 September 2018).
29. Disaster Risk Reduction and the Sendai Framework. What Does it Mean for UK resilience practitioners? Available online: https://www.epcresilience.com/EPC/media/Images/Knowledge%20Centre/Occasionals/OP21-Disaster-Risk-Reduction-Jun-2017.pdf (accessed on 4 September 2018).
30. Lo, S.T.T.; Chan, E.Y.Y.; Chan, G.K.W.; Murray, V.; Abrahams, J.; Ardalan, A.; Kayano, R.; Yau, J.C.W. Health Emergency and Disaster Risk Management (Health-EDRM): Developing the Research Field within the Sendai Framework Paradigm. *Int. J. Disaster Risk Sci.* **2017**, *8*, 145–149. [CrossRef]
31. Health Emergency and Disaster Risk Management: Mental Health and Psychosocial Support Factsheet. Available online: http://www.who.int/hac/techguidance/preparedness/risk-management-mental-health-december2017.pdf (accessed on 4 September 2018).

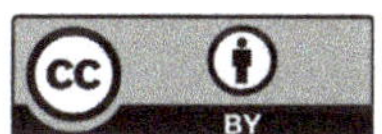

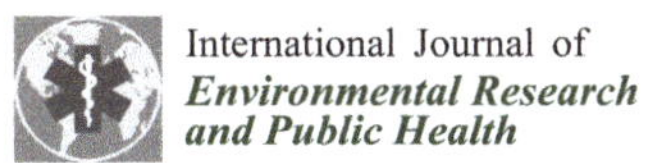
International Journal of
Environmental Research and Public Health

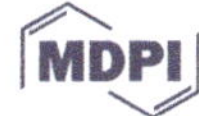

Article

Spatio-Temporal Distribution of Negative Emotions in New York City After a Natural Disaster as Seen in Social Media

Oliver Gruebner [1,2,*], Sarah R. Lowe [3], Martin Sykora [4], Ketan Shankardass [5], SV Subramanian [6] and Sandro Galea [7]

1 Department of Geography, Humboldt-Universität zu Berlin, Berlin 10099, Germany
2 Epidemiology, Biostatistics, and Prevention Institute (EBPI), University of Zurich, 8001 Zurich, Switzerland
3 Department of Psychology, Montclair State University, Montclair, NJ 07043, USA; lowes@mail.montclair.edu
4 Centre for Information Management (CIM), School of Business and Economics (SBE), Loughborough University, Loughborough LE11 3TU, UK; M.D.Sykora@lboro.ac.uk
5 Department of Health Sciences, Wilfrid Laurier University, Waterloo, ON M5B 1W8, Canada; ketan.shankardass@gmail.com
6 Department of Social and Behavioral Sciences, Harvard T.H. Chan School of Public Health, Boston, MA 02115, USA; svsubram@hsph.harvard.edu
7 School of Public Health, Boston University, Boston, MA 02118, USA; sgalea@bu.edu
* Correspondence: oliver.gruebner@geo.hu-berlin.de; Tel.: +49-30-2093-6905

Received: 7 September 2018; Accepted: 12 October 2018; Published: 17 October 2018

Abstract: Disasters have substantial consequences for population mental health. We used Twitter to (1) extract negative emotions indicating discomfort in New York City (NYC) before, during, and after Superstorm Sandy in 2012. We further aimed to (2) identify whether pre- or peri-disaster discomfort were associated with peri- or post-disaster discomfort, respectively, and to (3) assess geographic variation in discomfort across NYC census tracts over time. Our sample consisted of 1,018,140 geo-located tweets that were analyzed with an advanced sentiment analysis called "Extracting the Meaning Of Terse Information in a Visualization of Emotion" (EMOTIVE). We calculated discomfort rates for 2137 NYC census tracts, applied spatial regimes regression to find associations of discomfort, and used Moran's I for spatial cluster detection across NYC boroughs over time. We found increased discomfort, that is, bundled negative emotions after the storm as compared to during the storm. Furthermore, pre- and peri-disaster discomfort was positively associated with post-disaster discomfort; however, this association was different across boroughs, with significant associations only in Manhattan, the Bronx, and Queens. In addition, rates were most prominently spatially clustered in Staten Island lasting pre- to post-disaster. This is the first study that determined significant associations of negative emotional responses found in social media posts over space and time in the context of a natural disaster, which may guide us in identifying those areas and populations mostly in need for care.

Keywords: advanced sentiment analysis; digital epidemiology; geographic information system; geo-social media; hotspots; post-disaster mental health; psychogeography; spatial epidemiology; spatial regimes regression; Twitter data

---

1. Introduction

Large-scale natural disasters are observed worldwide [1–3] and can have substantial consequences for population mental health [4–7]. Although research to date has documented a great deal of mental health resilience in the aftermath of disasters, elevated rates of mental health consequences, including depression and post-traumatic stress, have been observed [7–10]. One of the key risk factors for adverse post-disaster mental health outcomes is experiencing overwhelming emotions in the context of disaster, which may be caused by the event itself, such as by exposure to trauma (i.e., actual or threatened death, serious injury, or sexual violence) [9]. These emotions may also be influenced by non-traumatic *stressors* either in the short or long term, such as loss of financial property, personal belongings, and/or one's home [4,7,9–11]. For example, emotions may convey information about how people evaluate what is happening and how they cope with it when they experience stress [11]. Sadness is usually related to experiencing an irreversible loss, and fright related to perception of immediate, concrete, and overwhelming physical danger [11]. Many studies have shown such negative emotional responses during a disaster being predictive of mental health problems in the aftermath of disaster [4], which may reflect the impact of disaster in terms of experienced stress. It is, however, important to differentiate "normal responses to abnormal events" from a lack of mental health resilience because the majority of people who report negative emotional reactions during a disaster do not develop mental health problems in the aftermath [7,10]. Nevertheless, we might expect the spatial and temporal distribution of emotional responses to follow the location and timing of disaster impacts, with implications for the burden of related adverse mental health problems.

The majority of studies on disaster mental health to date have relied solely on post-disaster data. Post-disaster studies are prone to possible recall bias, with the consequence that we are potentially missing important information on the time before the event. Some notable studies to date have included pre-event data [12–14]. Although these studies have brought a much better understanding of changes in mental health from pre- to post-disaster, research on this topic would further benefit from information that is gathered both prior to and during the event. Such information could, for example, demonstrate multiple dimensions of emotional reactions over time in the context of a disaster that could increase the precision of data relevant to mental health responses. Specifically, investigating multiple specific emotions, as defined by Ekman [15], such as fear, anger or disgust, or a combination thereof, could inform about the quality and strength of emotions as they are experienced during the disaster and could inform about risk for possible post-disaster mental health outcomes [16–23].

Research to date has provided little insight into geographic variability in where emotions are excessively expressed during or in the aftermath of large-scale disasters. Geographic concentrations of emotional expression would be indicative of some form of stress that is jointly experienced in specific populations within areas at specific times. Information on the concentration of specific emotional responses may exhibit people's alertness, and geographically mapping those places could reveal the spatial extent of areas in which possible issues arise guiding early intervention to minimize adverse mental health consequences. Better knowledge about the location and timing of specific emotional concentrations could provide important information about how to more efficiently roll out emergency public health interventions in the aftermath of disasters and other mass traumatic events.

Social media data, such as from Twitter, may help to fill these gaps, as they are largely and publicly available, have been successfully applied to disaster research, and provide pre-, peri-, and post-disaster information [23–25]. For example, specific emotions, such as fear or sadness, can be detected from Twitter streams through advanced sentiment analysis [26,27] and can be related to periods before, during, and after disasters. Furthermore, such data provide the opportunity for the geographic assessment of single posts. Hence, ecological momentary assessment of emotional reactions—that is, ongoing evaluation of in-the-moment experiences—becomes possible [26]. For example, in a study on emotional responses in the greater New York City area during Superstorm Sandy, Gruebner et al. [21] used Twitter data and found specific negative emotions clustered over space and time. However, this previous study used a relatively narrow time frame during the disaster.

We set out to explore the spatial distribution of *discomfort* in the population before, during, and after Superstorm Sandy that formed over the Caribbean on 22 October, hit the New York City (NYC) area on 29 October, and disappeared on 2 November 2012 [28]. The storm caused 43 deaths and about US$ 19 billion in damages within NYC alone making it the most costly and destructive disaster to impact public housing in the history of this city [29]. Specifically, we aimed to (1) identify a composite of negative emotions (i.e., discomfort) as expressed by the population that posted geo-located Twitter tweets in NYC over three time periods, each of approximately two weeks, representative of the pre-disaster period, the peri-disaster period, and the post-disaster period. We further aimed to (2) assess whether pre- or peri-disaster discomfort were associated with peri- or post-disaster discomfort, and to (3) investigate whether there was geographic variation in discomfort risk across NYC boroughs over time.

2. Materials and Methods

We used Twitter for this study because it is a publicly available resource that can be widely used for research purposes. Furthermore, tweets were geo-referenced facilitating spatial analysis informing our research questions. In addition, Twitter has already been used in other studies in that context [21,30–32].

About 45 million social media users that were mostly under the age of 50 in the United States were monthly active on Twitter by the end of 2012 [33–35]. Approximately three percent of them potentially used geolocation services producing geo-located Twitter data [36]. We used geo-located Twitter data published within NYC for the time frame of 10 October to 18 November 2012. Our sample was composed of 1,018,140 tweets that were suitable for our analysis, i.e., had information about geographic locations from where the tweets had been issued and were in English (see Table 1). We used tweets that were geo-located within those NYC census tracts that shared a border in order to facilitate spatial analyses at the census tract level. Thereby, 399,089 tweets were within the pre-disaster period (8 October to 21 October), 235,423 tweets were within the peri-disaster period (22 October to 4 November), and 383,628 tweets were within the post-disaster period (5 November to 18 November). Our level of analysis was the census tract (N = 2137). The dataset was available from the Harvard Center for Geographic Analysis Geo-tweet Archive (CGA) [37], the institution that collected the data. For transparency in research, the Tweet IDs used in this study can be made available for interested researchers, according to Twitter's sharing policy. Harvard provides a rehydration app to facilitate conversions of TweetIDs back to full tweets [38].

Table 1. Descriptive figures for aggregated Tweets at the census tract level over the entire study period in New York City from 10 October–18 November 2012. For example, the range of tweet population (or individual emotions) indicates the minimum and maximum number of all tweets, or of tweets with a specific emotion, found in census tracts. Note that discomfort is a combination of the negative emotions anger, confusion, disgust, fear, sadness, and shame. Tweets were coded as discomfort when they were indicative of any of these emotions at the individual level. Therefore, the numbers do not sum up at the census tract level when single emotions are compared to discomfort at that level.

Variable	Range	1st/3rd Quintile	Median	Mean	Sum
Tweet population	1–6507	24/149	59	158.8	1,018,140
Discomfort	0–158	0/5	2	5.03	32,254
Anger	0–119	0/1	0	0.77	4918
Confusion	0–8	0/0	0	0.25	1620
Disgust	0–45	0/1	0	1.11	7126
Fear	0–34	0/1	0	0.59	3841
Sadness	0–77	0/3	1	2.24	14,333
Shame	0–23	0/0	0	0.17	1079

We first analyzed the raw data with the advanced sentiment detection program "Extracting the Meaning Of Terse Information in a Visualization of Emotion" (EMOTIVE) [25,39]. While standard sentiment analysis tools only separate the mood as identified from social media texts into negative, positive, or neutral, EMOTIVE is able to detect basic emotions as defined by Ekman [40], such as *anger, disgust, fear, happiness, sadness, surprise,* and also *shame* and *confusion,* thereby preserving the original tweet texts and timestamps. We combined six of these emotions that are typically considered as negative emotions, i.e., *anger, confusion, disgust, fear, sadness*, and *shame* into one single emotion which we named *discomfort* to maximize statistical power. We coded each tweet dichotomously for the presence (case = 1) or absence (no case = 0) of discomfort. We then separated the dataset into three sets of two weeks each, representative of the pre-disaster period (8 October to 21 October), the peri-disaster period (22 October to 4 November), and the post-disaster period (5 November to 18 November). We then noted all discomfort cases at the census tract level and calculated smoothed spatial empirical Bayes (SEB) rates using the percentage of tweets that were indicative of discomfort out of all tweets (tweet population) for each census tract during each time period. This method was used to adjust for heterogeneity of variances of the rates [41] that evolved due to varying population sizes in the total tweets across NYC's census tracts. Empirical Bayes rates were calculated in GeoDa (Center for Spatial Data Science, Chicago, IL, USA) [41]. In addition, we checked whether SEB rates were significantly different across pre-, peri-, and post-disaster with paired t-tests in R (The R Foundation, Vienna, Austria) [42].

Second, we assessed associations between pre- and peri-disaster discomfort and between pre- as well as peri- and post-disaster discomfort rates at the census tract level initially with Ordinary Least Squares (OLS) regression models. Because OLS residuals exhibited spatial autocorrelation indicated by a Lagrange multiplier test, with the lag model performing well over the spatial error model, we chose a spatial lag model (Spatial Two Stage Least Squares regression (S2SLS)) as suggested in Anselin and Rey [43]. This model explicitly included a spatial lag variable on the right-hand side of the regression equation to account for the spatial structure found in the data stemming from non-independence of discomfort SEB rates in neighboring census tracts.

Third, we investigated spatial clusters of above average SEB (discomfort) across the census tracts at each time period by applying spatial autocorrelation analyses (Global and local Moran's I) in GeoDa [41]. We then ran a series of spatial regimes regression models (S2SLS) to further account for structural instability [43], that is, geographic variation in the associations between pre- and peri-disaster discomfort and post-disaster discomfort across NYC boroughs, i.e., the regimes. Furthermore, a Chow test [44] was applied for regime diagnostics. Regression analysis was applied in GeoDaSpace (Center for Spatial Data Science, Chicago, IL, USA) [45].

3. Results

3.1. Rates of Discomfort in Twitter Data

We extracted and combined six negative emotions from the Twitter activity of users in the given area and time frames in a single index that we termed *discomfort*. We identified 2649 cases (i.e., tweets) (0.66%) indicative of discomfort pre-disaster, 1641 cases (0.70%) peri-disaster, and 2845 cases (0.74%) post-disaster. We noted that compared to pre-disaster, overall discomfort rates were significantly different peri-disaster with $t(2136) = -6.65$, $p < 0.001$ and a mean of difference of -0.003. Post-disaster rates were also significantly different from pre-disaster rates $t(2136) = -3.06$, $p = 0.002$ (mean of difference = -0.001) and from peri-disaster rates $t(2136) = 4.76$, $p < 0.001$ (mean of difference -0.002). In addition, we noted that median rates of discomfort were different across boroughs and time periods, with the highest rates across all time periods in Staten Island as compared to the other boroughs, and Brooklyn having the lowest rates across all time periods compared to the other boroughs (Figure 1).

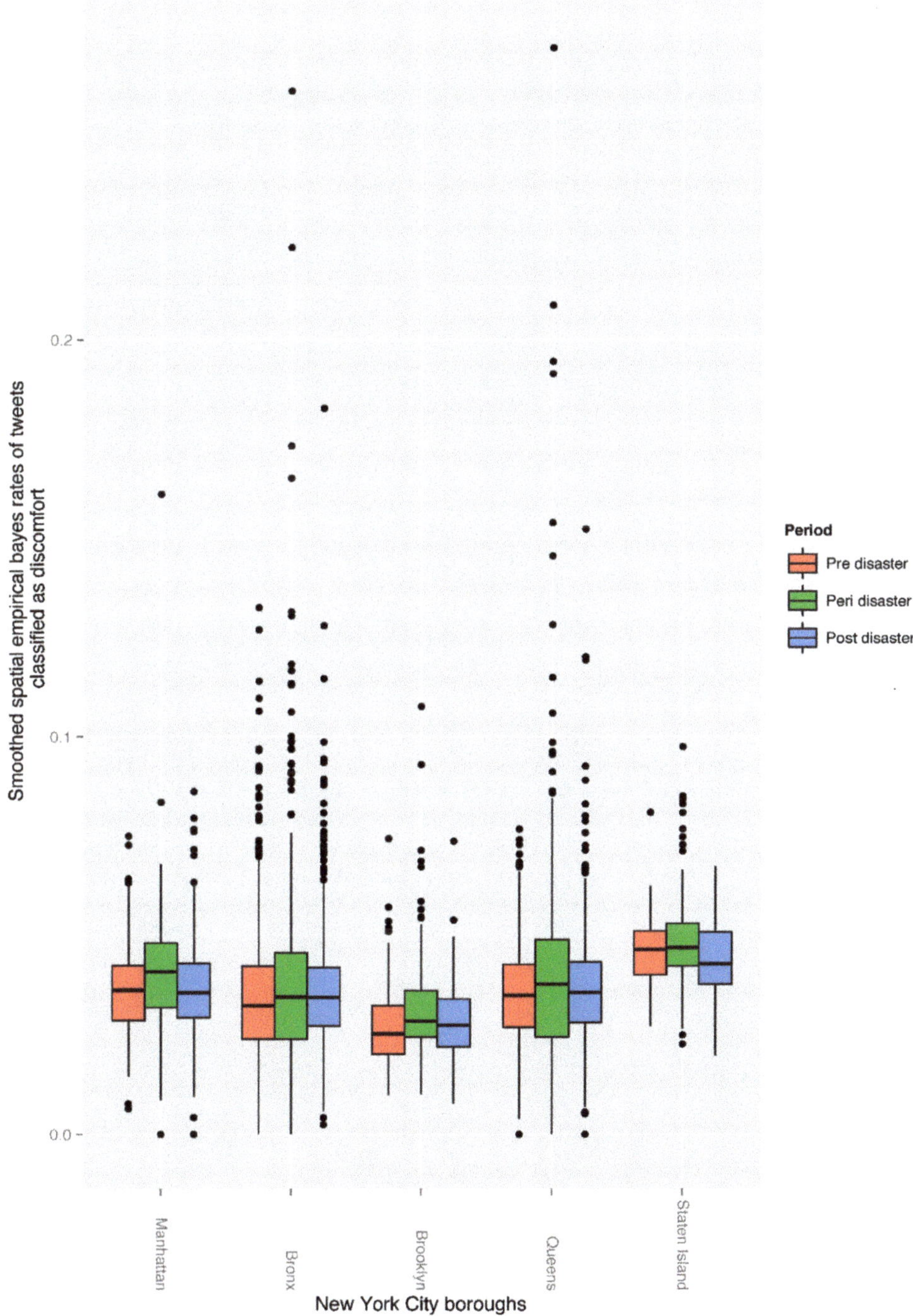

Figure 1. Spatial Empirical Bayes smoothed rates of tweets classified as discomfort for each NYC borough across time periods.

3.2. Associations of Discomfort Over Time

In multivariable regression models, we found a significant association between pre-disaster discomfort and post-disaster discomfort (Beta = 0.11, $p < 0.001$) as well as between peri-disaster discomfort and post-disaster discomfort (Beta = 0.10, $p < 0.001$) (see Table 2). Pre-disaster discomfort and peri-disaster discomfort were, however, not significantly associated. Additionally, both peri- (Beta = 0.68, $p < 0.001$) and post-disaster discomfort (Beta = 0.61, $p < 0.001$) were spatially interdependent across neighboring census tracts, that is, peri- and post-disaster levels of discomfort in one census tract were significantly associated with those in adjacent census tracts.

Table 2. Spatial regression results. Model 1 is a spatial lag regression model.

Variable	Peri-Disaster Discomfort		Post-Disaster Discomfort	
	Coef.	S.E.	Coef.	S.E.
Model 1: New York City				
NYC Intercept	0.00	0.01	0.01 **	0.00
Pre-disaster discomfort	0.03	0.04	0.11 ***	0.02
Peri-disaster discomfort	/		0.10 ***	0.01
Spatial lag of peri-disaster discomfort	0.68 ***	0.18	/	
Spatial lag of post-disaster discomfort	/		0.61 ***	0.07
Model diagnostic				
Pseudo R-squared	0.33		0.47	
Spatial Pseudo R-squared	0.03		0.13	
Anselin-Kelejian Test	1.99		2.67	

Coef. = Coefficient estimate; S.E. = Standard Error; Significance level: *** <0.001, ** <0.01.

3.3. Spatial Variation in Discomfort Risk

We found significant spatial clusters of above average rates of discomfort in all time frames, i.e., pre-, peri-, and post-disaster (Figure 2). The most prominent cluster of discomfort in terms of size was located in Staten Island and was persistent at all time periods, albeit with a varying number of census tracts that were included in the cluster. Although Chow tests did not reveal significant structural instability across the boroughs with spatial regimes regression, we noted that pre-disaster discomfort was significantly and positively associated with post-disaster discomfort in Manhattan (Beta = 0.18, $p < 0.01$), the Bronx (Beta = 0.22, $p < 0.001$), and Queens (Beta = 0.09, $p < 0.01$) (Table 3). Furthermore, peri-disaster discomfort was also significantly and positively associated with post-disaster discomfort in Manhattan (Beta = 0.13, $p < 0.01$) and Queens (Beta = 0.10, $p < 0.05$). In addition, peri- (Beta = 0.91, $p < 0.001$) and post-disaster discomfort (Beta = 0.64, $p < 0.001$) remained spatially interdependent across neighboring census tracts.

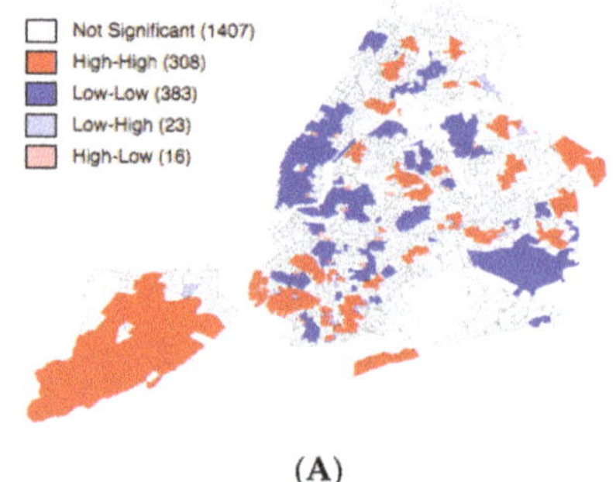

(A)

Figure 2. *Cont.*

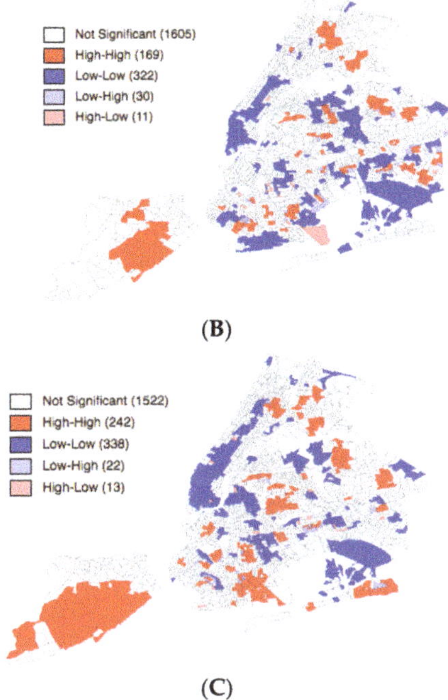

Figure 2. Local clusters of above average discomfort rates (shaded in red) in NYC geo-located Twitter tweets for the three periods before (**A**), during (**B**) and after (**C**) Superstorm Sandy, indicating that high rates were found next to other high rates (High-High). Rates were smoothed with the spatial empirical Bayes smoother prior to the cluster analysis. Notably, the statistic also calculates below average rates (low rates next to other low rates) and outliers (high rates next to low rates and vice versa) that are not considered in this study.

Table 3. Spatial regression results. Model 2 is a spatial lag regression model with regimes, i.e., the boroughs.

Variable	Peri-Disaster Discomfort		Post-Disaster Discomfort	
	Coef.	S.E.	Coef.	S.E.
Model 2: New York City boroughs				
Manhattan Intercept	0.00	0.01	0.00	0.00
Pre-disaster discomfort	0.09	0.12	0.18 **	0.06
Peri-disaster discomfort	/		0.13 **	0.04
Bronx Intercept	0.00	0.01	0.00	0.00
Pre-disaster discomfort	0.07	0.07	0.22 ***	0.07
Peri-disaster discomfort	/		0.05	0.04
Brooklyn Intercept	0.00	0.01	0.01	0.00
Pre-disaster discomfort	0.01	0.06	0.07.	0.04
Peri-disaster discomfort	/		0.10	0.06
Queens Intercept	0.00	0.01	0.01	0.00
Pre-disaster discomfort	0.03	0.08	0.09 **	0.04
Peri-disaster discomfort	/		0.10 *	0.05
Staten Island Intercept	0.01	0.01	0.01 *	0.01
Pre-disaster discomfort	−0.03	0.09	0.07	0.09
Peri-disaster discomfort	/		0.04	0.04

Table 3. *Cont.*

Variable	Peri-Disaster Discomfort		Post-Disaster Discomfort	
	Coef.	**S.E.**	**Coef.**	**S.E.**
Global spatial lag of peri-disaster discomfort	0.91 ***	0.25	/	
Global spatial lag of post-disaster discomfort	/		0.64 ***	0.14
Model diagnostic				
Pseudo R-squared	0.33		0.47	
Spatial Pseudo R-squared	0.03		0.14	
Chow test for intercept	1.84		9.09	
Chow test for pre-disaster discomfort	1.97		6.99	
Chow test for peri-disaster discomfort	/		4.01	
Global Chow test	2.36		18.06	
Anselin-Kelejian Test	1.93		1.04	

Coef. = Coefficient estimate, S.E. = Standard Error, Significance level: *** <0.001, ** <0.01, * <0.1.

4. Discussion

We found negative emotional reactions that we combined in one variable, which we called discomfort. Overall, discomfort rates were significantly different after the disaster as compared to before or during the pre-disaster period across boroughs. Further, we showed that pre- and peri-disaster discomfort were significantly associated with post-disaster discomfort rates. Moreover, discomfort rates were spatially clustered across NYC census tracts and associations of discomfort rates over time were different across boroughs with significant associations only in Manhattan, the Bronx, and Queens.

The Twitter activity of users can exhibit perceived and real risk as experienced by users [21,31]. Our results show that there were higher rates of discomfort expressed in Tweets during the post-disaster period as compared to during the peri-disaster period, likely corresponding to the time period in which residents had to deal with the greatest stressors (e.g., losses) after the storm. Staten Island had the highest median rates of discomfort among all boroughs and across all time frames, which was consistent with what one might expect based on the variability of Sandy's impact across NYC. Staten Island was one of the boroughs that was hit the hardest by Superstorm Sandy due to a combination of the storm's arrival and high tide leading to high levels of inundations and crucial service outage after the storm [46]. All the above might explain why we see highest rates of discomfort in Staten Island.

Taking into account all census tracts in a global regression model, we found that higher volumes of specific negative emotions at pre- or during the disaster were associated with negative emotions also after the disaster. From studies that compared mental health symptoms from before with after the disaster we know that pre-disaster conditions are one of the strongest predictors for post-disaster conditions [12–14]. This may also be true for emotional responses as expressed on Twitter and other social media platforms.

We further investigated geographic concentrations in discomfort rates across NYC regions (i.e., census tracts) within and across the boroughs and found significant spatial clustering of above average discomfort rates in all boroughs except Manhattan, with biggest clusters across census tracts in Staten Island. Spatial clusters may occur due to spatial dependence of rates across census tracts. Our analysis did not investigate the possible causes of small-area variation in discomfort over time; however, we have at least three possible explanations for spatial dependence causing the clusters. First, there were environmental issues, such as flooding and houses affected by the storm with some of them being totally destroyed [47]. Further, reported power shortages, falling trees, or strong winds spanning across census tracts may have affected a wider population in several neighboring census tracts simultaneously. This might have been particularly true across several neighboring census tracts in Staten Island, where considerable flooding and destroyed houses have been reported by the Federal Emergency and Management Agency (FEMA) [47,48]. While people collectively experienced these environmental issues, they may have processed feelings in the affected areas leading to these spatial patterns of negative emotions. There has also been more localized environmental damage, such as floods and affected houses in parts of other boroughs, for example in the Queens areas spanning from Averne to the Far Rockaway, where we found clusters, too [47,48].

Second, daily interaction of, for example, residents of one census tract with facilities of other census tracts (e.g., coffee shop, work place, shelter, drop-off location for receiving aid and goods) while tweeting might have produced spatial patterns of emotions spanning across several adjacent census tracts.

Third, people may have perceived environmental issues differently depending on their socio-demographic characteristics or socio-ecological context in which they live, for example with people living in better structural quality of housing worrying less about strong winds. Socio-demographic characteristics or socio-ecological contexts vary substantially across NYC boroughs (with some neighborhoods being highly segregated across census tracts), which may have further contributed to the clusters. Future studies should include neighborhood level socio-demographic and socio-ecologic variables to further understand these patterns.

We also found that clusters of above average discomfort rates in several census tracts were persistent over time from peri- to post-disaster. The most prominent clusters at all time periods spanning across the largest number of census tracts were also located in Staten Island. These clusters and those elsewhere may exhibit areas of increased risk for mental health needs due to, e.g., increased environmental issues, mobility (or displacement) of tweeters, different perceptions among tweeters, or a combination of the three.

In addition, we investigated the spatial variability of associations of discomfort rates over time. We found that pre-disaster discomfort was significantly associated with post-disaster discomfort only in Manhattan, the Bronx, and Queens, while peri-disaster discomfort was significantly associated with post-disaster discomfort only in Manhattan and Queens. We may expect other factors being more important predictors for post-disaster discomfort in the other boroughs, such as neighborhood-level socio-ecological factors (e.g., socio-economic status, physical exposure to the storm). With regard to the boroughs in which we found significant positive associations of discomfort rates across the time periods, our results may indicate that the associations were place dependent with socio-ecological factors specific to local census tracts and boroughs. Our results may also indicate that those areas with higher discomfort rates during the storm—presumably due to issues such as service outfalls or strong winds—may be more likely to exhibit discomfort also after the storm, when neighborhoods were flooded or houses seriously affected by the storm. Since early emotional reactions predict post-disaster mental health problems [4], this should be investigated in more depth in future studies.

Our study had several limitations. First, we used geo-located English tweets from Twitter. Future studies may also include non-geo referenced data including further languages or data sources. Second, due to likely service shortages during and in the immediate aftermath of the storm, the three time frames under investigation had different number of tweets with the lowest number of tweets during the disaster, which should be kept in mind when interpreting the findings. For example, it is possible that Twitter users were unable to charge their phones, that they were trying to conserve battery life, or that they were restricted in their cell phone usage due to interrupted cell phone services, hence limiting the activity of Twitter users during that time. Third, we only used tweets from NYC census tracts that shared a border with another NYC census tract to facilitate spatial analysis. This excluded tweets that were published in census tracts not directly connected to other census tracts (e.g., Ellis Island) or that were posted while travelling on water. Fourth, since tweeters were assumingly using mobile devices while tweeting, it is possible that tweets were not always sent from the same location but rather while on the daily commute, at home, at work, or in a shelter before or during the storm. After the storm, some of the Twitter population may have been displaced and would be tweeting from other locations as before or during the storm. Finally, we have worked at the ecological level, that is, census tracts in which tweets have been posted rather than at the individual Twitter user level. Use of individual Twitter identifiers would permit the application and testing of more traditional paradigms of stress response variation during a trauma as predicting post-trauma distress.

5. Conclusions

This is the first study that identified emotions representative of discomfort in social media along with their concentration in space and time. Discomfort, i.e., negative emotional responses including amongst others fear, anger, and sadness, were concentrated in some neighborhoods across NYC and were persistent over time, most prominently so in Staten Island. These concentrations may provide knowledge about areas and communities with mental health need.

High discomfort rates pre-disaster were associated with high rates during and after the disaster. The association of pre-, peri-, and post-disaster discomfort over time was place dependent, suggesting different socio-ecological factors responsible for discomfort across the five boroughs.

Since early emotional reactions may predict longer-term mental health needs, this approach could further assist in the long-term allocation of services. EMOTIVE is currently being extended to also evaluate stress responses that in conjunction with a spatially explicit approach, as it has been applied here may help to estimate the development of symptoms indicative of depression and PTSD [49,50]. Given that social media use has dramatically increased worldwide since 2012, these data provide enormous potential for mental health research to study e.g., the functional relationship between socio-ecological factors and mental health. For example, working at the individual social media user level might inform about individual people's exposure in addition to weather-related damage and flooding, such as loss of resources and restricted access to services in real time. In addition, this level of analysis could also capture other community-level risk factors such as geographic variation in pre-existing mental health conditions or social support. In countries with limited formal surveillance infrastructure, the approach may also have potential for the identification of areas and populations in need for care.

Author Contributions: Conceptualization, O.G. and S.R.L.; Methodology, M.S. and O.G.; Software, M.S.; Formal Analysis, M.S. and O.G. Data Curation, M.S. and O.G. Writing-Original Draft Preparation, O.G. and S.R.L.; Writing-Review & Editing, O.G., S.R.L. and K.S.; Visualization, O.G.; Supervision, S.G. and S.V.S.

Funding: This research received no external funding.

Acknowledgments: We thank Suzanne Elayan for her help with data preparation for EMOTIVE. We acknowledge support by the German Research Foundation (DFG) and the Open Access Publication Fund of Humboldt-Universität zu Berlin.

Conflicts of Interest: The authors declare no conflict of interest.

References

1. International Federation of Red Cross and Red Crescent Societies World disasters report: Focus on Culture and Risk. Available online: http://www.ifrc.org/Global/Documents/Secretariat/201410/WDR%2014.pdf (accessed on 12 October 2018).
2. Hoeppe, P. Trends in weather related disasters—Consequences for insurers and society. *Weather Clim. Extrem.* **2015**. [CrossRef]
3. NOAA National Centers for Environmental Information, N. O. and A. A. Billion-Dollar Weather and Climate Disasters: Summary Stats. Available online: http://www.ncdc.noaa.gov/billions/summary-stats (accessed on 12 October 2018).
4. Norris, F.H.; Friedman, M.J.; Watson, P.J.; Byrne, C.M.; Diaz, E.; Kaniasty, K. 60,000 disaster victims speak: Part I. An empirical review of the empirical literature, 1981–2001. *Psychiatry-Interpers. Biol. Process.* **2002**, *65*, 207–239. [CrossRef]
5. Neria, Y.; Galea, S. *Mental Health and Disasters*; Cambridge University Press: Cambridge, UK, 2009; ISBN 0521883873.
6. Neria, Y.; Nandi, A.; Galea, S. Post-traumatic stress disorder following disasters: A systematic review. *Psychol. Med.* **2008**, *38*, 467–480. [CrossRef] [PubMed]

7. Goldmann, E.; Galea, S. Mental health consequences of disasters. *Annu. Rev. Public Health* **2014**, *35*, 169–183. [CrossRef] [PubMed]
8. Dückers, M.L.A. A multilayered psychosocial resilience framework and its implications for community-focused crisis management. *J. Contingencies Crisis Manag.* **2017**, *25*, 182–187. [CrossRef]
9. North, C.S.; Pfefferbaum, B. Mental health response to community disasters. *JAMA* **2013**, *310*, 507. [CrossRef] [PubMed]
10. North, C.S. Disaster mental health epidemiology: Methodological review and interpretation of research findings. *Psychiatry* **2016**, *79*, 130–146. [CrossRef] [PubMed]
11. Lazarus, R.S. *Stress and Emotion A New Synthesis*; SPRINGER: New York, NY, USA, 2006; ISBN 9780826102614.
12. Lowe, S.R.; Chan, C.S.; Rhodes, J.E. Pre-hurricane perceived social support protects against psychological distress: A longitudinal analysis of low-income mothers. *J. Consult. Clin. Psychol.* **2010**, *78*, 551–560. [CrossRef] [PubMed]
13. Weems, C.F.; Pina, A.A.; Costa, N.M.; Watts, S.E.; Taylor, L.K.; Cannon, M.F. Predisaster trait anxiety and negative affect predict posttraumatic stress in youths after Hurricane Katrina. *J. Consult. Clin. Psychol.* **2007**, *75*, 154–159. [CrossRef] [PubMed]
14. La Greca, A.M.; Silverman, W.K.; Wasserstein, S.B. Children's predisaster functioning as a predictor of posttraumatic stress following Hurricane Andrew. *J. Consult. Clin. Psychol.* **1998**, *66*, 883–892. [CrossRef] [PubMed]
15. Ekman, P. Basic emotions. In *Handbook of Cognition and Emotion*; John Wiley&Sons, Ltd.: Chichester, UK, 2005; pp. 45–60. ISBN 9780471978367.
16. Sutton, J.; Gibson, C.B.; Phillips, N.E.; Spiro, E.S.; League, C.; Johnson, B.; Fitzhugh, S.M.; Butts, C.T. A cross-hazard analysis of terse message retransmission on Twitter. *Proc. Natl. Acad. Sci. USA* **2015**, *112*, 14793–14798. [CrossRef] [PubMed]
17. Houston, J.B.; Hawthorne, J.; Perreault, M.F.; Park, E.H.; Goldstein Hode, M.; Halliwell, M.R.; Turner McGowen, S.E.; Davis, R.; Vaid, S.; McElderry, J.A.; et al. Social media and disasters: A functional framework for social media use in disaster planning, response, and research. *Disasters* **2015**, *39*, 1–22. [CrossRef] [PubMed]
18. Glass, K.; Colbaugh, R. Estimating the sentiment of social media content for security informatics applications. *Secur. Inform.* **2012**, *1*, 3. [CrossRef]
19. Johansson, F.; Brynielsson, J.; Quijano, M.N. Estimating Citizen Alertness in Crises Using Social Media Monitoring and Analysis. In Proceedings of the 2012 European Intelligence and Security Informatics Conference, Odense, Denmark, 22–24 August 2012. [CrossRef]
20. Kumar, S.; Barbier, G.; Abbasi, M.A.; Liu, H. Tweet Tracker: An Analysis Tool for Humanitarian and Disaster Relief. In Proceedings of the Fifth International AAAI Conference on Weblogs and Social Media, Barcelona, Spain, 17–21 July 2011.
21. Gruebner, O.; Lowe, S.R.; Sykora, M.; Shankardass, K.; Subramanian, S.V.; Galea, S. A novel surveillance approach for disaster mental health. *PLoS ONE* **2017**, *12*, e0181233. [CrossRef] [PubMed]
22. Gruebner, O.; Sykora, M.; Lowe, S.R.; Shankardass, K.; Trinquart, L.; Jackson, T.; Subramanian, S.V.; Galea, S. Mental health surveillance after the terrorist attacks in Paris. *Lancet* **2016**, *387*, 2195–2196. [CrossRef]
23. Gruebner, O.; Sykora, M.; Lowe, S.R.; Shankardass, K.; Galea, S.; Subramanian, S.V. Big data opportunities for social behavioral and mental health research. *Soc. Sci. Med.* **2017**, *2012*, 2016–2018. [CrossRef] [PubMed]
24. Hirschberg, J.; Manning, C.D. Advances in natural language processing. *Science* **2015**, *349*, 261–266. [CrossRef] [PubMed]
25. Sykora, M.D.; Jackson, T.W.; OBrien, A.; Elayan, S. Emotive Ontology: Extracting Fine-Grained Emotions from Terse, Informal Messages. In Proceedings of the IADIS International Conference Intelligent Systems and Agents 2013, Prague, Czech Republic, 22–24 July 2013.
26. Shaughnessy, K.; Reyes, R.; Shankardass, K.; Sykora, M.; Feick, R.; Lawrence, H.; Robertson, C. Using geolocated social media for ecological momentary assessments of emotion: Innovative opportunities in psychology science and practice. *Can. Psychol. Can.* **2017**. [CrossRef]
27. Hofmann, W.; Patel, P.V. Survey signal. *Soc. Sci. Comput. Rev.* **2015**, *33*, 235–253. [CrossRef]
28. National Oceanic and Atmospheric Administration Hurricane Sandy. Available online: https://www.weather.gov/okx/HurricaneSandy (accessed on 28 July 2018).
29. NYC Housing Authority Sandy Recovery and Progress. Available online: https://www1.nyc.gov/site/nycha/about/recovery-history.page (accessed on 28 July 2018).

30. Shelton, T.; Poorthuis, A.; Graham, M.; Zook, M. Mapping the data shadows of Hurricane Sandy: Uncovering the sociospatial dimensions of 'big data'. *Geoforum* **2014**, *52*, 167–179. [CrossRef]
31. Kryvasheyeu, Y.; Chen, H.; Obradovich, N.; Moro, E.; Van Hentenryck, P.; Fowler, J.; Cebrian, M. Rapid assessment of disaster damage using social media activity. *Sci. Adv.* **2016**, *2*, e1500779. [CrossRef] [PubMed]
32. Takayasu, M.; Sato, K.; Sano, Y.; Yamada, K.; Miura, W.; Takayasu, H. Rumor diffusion and convergence during the 3.11 Earthquake: A twitter case study. *PLoS ONE* **2015**, *10*, e0121443. [CrossRef] [PubMed]
33. Statista Number of Monthly Active Twitter Users in the United States from 1st Quarter 2010 to 2nd Quarter 2018 (In Millions). Available online: https://www.statista.com/statistics/274564/monthly-active-twitter-users-in-the-united-states/ (accessed on 12 October 2018).
34. Pew Research Center Social Media Fact Sheet. Available online: http://www.pewinternet.org/fact-sheet/social-media/ (accessed on 16 October 2018).
35. Pew Research Center Demographics of Key Social Networking Platforms. Available online: http://www.pewinternet.org/2015/01/09/demographics-of-key-social-networking-platforms-2/ (accessed on 16 October 2018).
36. Sloan, L.; Morgan, J. Who tweets with their location? Understanding the relationship between demographic characteristics and the use of geoservices and geotagging on twitter. *PLoS ONE* **2015**, *10*, e0142209. [CrossRef] [PubMed]
37. Harvard Center for Geographic Analysis Geo-tweet Archive. Available online: http://www.gis.harvard.edu (accessed on 16 October 2018).
38. Harvard Center for Geographic Analysis Twitter Rehydration Script. Available online: https://github.com/cga-harvard/hhypermap-bop/tree/master/BOP-utilities/Twitter_Rehydration (accessed on 16 October 2018).
39. Sykora, M.D.; Jackson, T.W.; OBrien, A.; Elayan, S. National security and social media monitoring: A presentation of the EMOTIVE and related systems. In Proceedings of the 2013 European Intelligence and Security Informatics Conference, Uppsala, Sweden, 12–14 August 2013; pp. 172–175.
40. Ekman, P. Are there basic emotions? *Psychol. Rev.* **1992**, *99*, 550–553. [CrossRef] [PubMed]
41. Anselin, L.; Syabri, I.; Kho, Y. GeoDa: An introduction to spatial data analysis. *Geogr. Anal.* **2006**, *38*, 5–22. [CrossRef]
42. R Development Core Team. *R: A Language and Environment for Statistical Computing*; R Foundation for Statistical Computing: Vienna, Austria, 2013; ISBN 3-900051-07-0.
43. Anselin, L.; Rey, S.J. *Modern Spatial Econometrics in Practice: A Guide to GeoDa, GeoDaSpace and PySAL*; GeoDa Press LLC: Chicago, IL, USA, 2014.
44. Chow, G.C. Tests of equality between sets of coefficients in two linear regressions. *Econometrica* **1960**, *28*, 591. [CrossRef]
45. GeoDa Center for Geospatial Analysis and Computation GeoDaSpace 2013. Available online: https://geodacenter.asu.edu/software (accessed on 16 October 2018).
46. Gammon, C. Why Hurricane Sandy Hit Staten Island So Hard/New York City Hurricanes. Available online: http://www.livescience.com/24616-hurricane-sandy-staten-island-effects.html (accessed on 12 October 2018).
47. Federal Emergency and Management Agency FEMA MOTF Hurricane Sandy Impact Analysis. Available online: http://fema.maps.arcgis.com/home/item.html?id=307dd522499d4a44a33d7296a5da5ea0 (accessed on 10 October 2015).
48. Bloch, M.; Fessenden, F.; McLean, A.; Tse, A. Derek Watkins Surveying the destruction Caused by Hurricane Sandy. Available online: http://www.nytimes.com/newsgraphics/2012/1120-sandy/survey-of-the-flooding-in-new-york-after-the-hurricane.html (accessed on 28 July 2018).
49. Sykora, M.D.; Robertson, C.; Shankardass, K.; Feick, R. Stresscapes: Validating Linkages Between Place and Stress Expression on Social Media. In Proceedings of the 2nd International Workshop on Mining Urban Data, Lille, France, 11 July 2015.
50. Chen, X.; Sykora, M.D.; Jackson, T.W.; Elayan, S. Tweeting Your Mental Health: Exploration of Different Classifiers and Features with Emotional Signals in Identifying Mental Health Conditions. In Proceedings of the 51st Hawaii International Conference on System Sciences, Waikoloa Village, HI, USA, 3–6 January 2018.

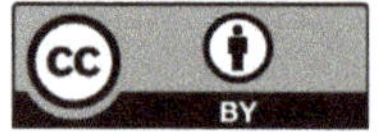

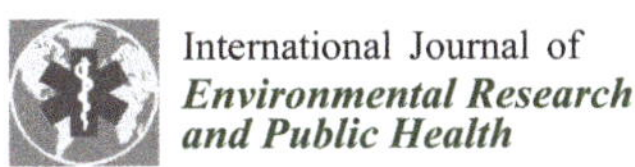
International Journal of
Environmental Research and Public Health

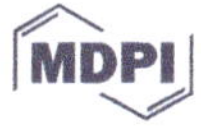

Review

Resilience to Climate-Induced Disasters and Its Overall Relationship to Well-Being in Southern Africa: A Mixed-Methods Systematic Review

Joseph K. Kamara [1,*], Blessing J. Akombi [1], Kingsley Agho [2] and Andre M. N. Renzaho [1]

1 School of Social Sciences and Psychology, Western Sydney University, Sydney, Locked Bag 1797, Penrith, NSW 2751, Australia; B.Akombi@westernsydney.edu.au (B.J.A.); Andre.Renzaho@westernsydney.edu.au (A.M.N.R.)
2 School of Sciences and Health, Western Sydney University, Locked Bag 1797, Penrith, NSW 2751, Australia; k.agho@westernsydney.edu.au
* Correspondence: j.kamara@westernsydney.edu.au; Tel.: +61-481-005-279

Received: 29 August 2018; Accepted: 23 October 2018; Published: 26 October 2018

Abstract: The available literature suggests that natural disasters, especially droughts and floods, were occurring in southern Africa in the early 1900s. However, their frequency and intensity increased during the 1980s. The aim of this systematic review was to assess the relationship between resilience to droughts and people's well-being in southern Africa. A combination of keywords was used to search the following 13 electronic bibliographic databases: Africa Journal Online (AJOL), MEDLINE, Academic Search Complete, Environment Complete, Humanities International Complete, Psychology and Behavioral Sciences Collection, PsycINFO, Embase, Scopus, Web of Science, Applied Social Science Index and Abstracts, ProQuest Central, and CINAHL. Relevant websites were also searched and potential studies for inclusion were downloaded in an EndNote database and screened for eligibility using pre-determined criteria. Quality assessment of the studies was undertaken using the Joana Briggs Qualitative Assessment and Review Instrument, the National Institutes of Health (NIH) checklist, and the Authority, Accuracy, Coverage, Objectivity, Date, Significance (AACODS) checklist. Resilience and well-being scales used in the studies for inclusion were also assessed using pre-defined criteria. Nineteen studies met the inclusion criteria. Poverty alleviation policies were important in strengthening resilience and well-being outcomes. Resilience and well-being were connected by old age, gender, race, adaptive farming and livelihoods diversification, security, and knowledgeability. Resilience and well-being outcomes were advanced by the synergistic effect of household, community and governance level capacities encapsulated in knowledgeability. This systematic review is critical to improving southern Africa context-specific resilience, and well-being policies and interventions.

Keywords: resilience; recurrent disaster; drought; rural; subsistence farming; southern Africa

---

1. Introduction

Disasters have increasingly become regular and omnipresent, with devastating effects on humans and ecosystems. In this study, we define a disaster as a catastrophe resulting in injury, loss of life, and social and economic disruption that exceeds the coping capacity of the affected people and the ecology [1,2]. There are two forms of disasters: natural and human-induced. Naturally occurring disasters can be classified into five groups, namely, geophysical: earthquakes, landslides, tsunamis, and volcanic activity; hydrological: avalanches and floods; climatological: extreme temperatures, droughts, and wildfires; meteorological: cyclones and storms/wave surges; and biological: disease epidemics such as Ebola and insect infestation such as locust invasions [3]. In contrast, human-induced disasters include armed conflicts and wars, famine, ethnic conflicts and displaced populations, industrial and transport accidents, environmental degradation such as pollution, as well as anthropogenic intentional hazards such as terrorism or weapons of mass destruction [3,4].

People cannot effectively stop natural disasters such as droughts but they can mitigate disaster risks and reduce their negative impacts through information sharing, behaviour change, effective governance and technological innovations [1]. While humans cannot stop natural disasters, frameworks such as that proposed by Birnbaum and colleagues [5], suggest that we can create a resilience to disasters by identifying and experiencing disaster risks, and we can learn from them to predict the future and selectively choose the most likely risks to address. The framework further posits that choosing the risks to address accompanied by the identification of existing resilience standards and their evaluation; identification of gaps and commensurate interventions; preparing work plans, execution and appraisal collectively strengthen disaster resilience capabilities [5]. Similarly, the Sendai framework for disaster risk reduction 2015–2030 proposed that nations can create and strengthen disaster resilience capabilities by gaining an understanding of disaster risk; enhancing disaster risk governance; investing in disaster risk reduction and; building back better after a disaster event [1]. The Sendai framework for disaster risk reduction succeeded in the Hyogo Framework for Action (HFA) 2005–2015 which sought to build the resilience of nations and communities to disasters. The HFA came after the Yokohama Strategy for a Safer World which provided the basis for the 1999 international strategy for disaster reduction [6].

There is no universal definition of resilience. Attempts to define resilience have confined it to the parameters for specific study areas that seek to investigate resilience to what, how, and by whom [7]. For this systematic review, resilience is defined as the capability to leverage the environment to expect, withstand, recover, and adjust to disaster-induced distress [8]. The capabilities exist in isolation or in tandem at the individual, household, and collective level. Therefore, we examine resilience at all levels so as to frame it within the collective nature of the study area's way of life. This approach enables relevant contextually and culturally appropriate study outcomes. It is anticipated that recurrent drought leaves some form of adaptive capabilities at the various levels which makes resilience to drought an important subject of interest. We define well-being as an agreeable state characterised by the absence of ill health.

This systematic review focuses on resilience to climate-induced disasters, especially drought in southern Africa for various reasons. Foremost, southern Africa experiences recurring droughts. Evidence suggests that southern Africa experienced droughts in the early 1900s [9–11]. However, in the 1980s, there was a remarkable spike in the frequency, intensity, and impact of droughts across the region [12,13]. Since then, naturally occurring disasters, especially droughts that are induced by the El Nino southern oscillation, have occurred almost every two years [10,14,15]. Recurrent droughts devastate livelihoods and induce humanitarian interventions that help communities cope, thus, promoting a false and unsustainable sense of defiance against droughts [16]. Humanitarian interventions are critical enablers of recovery but their prescriptive nature and externality often ignore inherent capacities such as the traditional knowledge of the communities they seek to help [17,18]. Evidence suggests that traditional knowledge and culture are vital and enabling elements of disaster resilience [19]. Governments and their partners across the region have a responsibility to leverage inherent capacities to build and strengthen resilience, especially in response to recurrent threats such as droughts which have become a 'new normal.' However, the stakeholders are yet to work out a comprehensive approach to building drought resilience. The synthesised information from this systematic review will provide the foundation that informs the approach.

Secondly, unlike the rest of sub-Saharan Africa, which also experiences droughts, southern Africa countries are classified as middle-income development status. This development status is expected to be leveraged in building and demonstrating resilience to disasters. Moreover, recurring droughts in the region are no longer unexpected but a reality. Countries in other sub-Saharan Africa regions are of a low-income development status and are expected to have less disaster coping capacities compared to southern Africa. Lastly, natural disasters in other sub-Saharan Africa regions attract quick donor attention and large funding compared to southern Africa [20–22]. The differences enumerated above are contextual to the region and affect the timely and effective disaster response. This uniqueness has compelled us to confine our systematic review to the southern Africa region, anticipating context-specific findings that will inform the region's disaster management strategies and policies.

Evidence suggests that southern African governments have not sufficiently prioritised drought resilience building; instead, they are caught in cyclical responses to recurring droughts [23,24]. This could be attributed to underlying vulnerabilities such as a weak governance and institutional capacity, accompanied by a high inequality, poverty, and environmental degradation [24–26]. Drought response strategies usually tend to be humanitarian in nature, which is critical in disaster recovery of the predominantly rural and subsisting communities. Recovery deals with the planning and allocation of resources to restore capabilities lost or degraded by a disaster event. During emergency operations, humanitarian assistance focuses on emergency needs and often neglect building and strengthening resilience capabilities. More so, because political interference with local processes and the long time required implementing resilience interventions make it difficult for humanitarian responses to focus on resilience. The underlying vulnerabilities such as weak governance, land degradation, and poverty remain unaddressed, yet they are critical to resilience building. For example, over 70% of the population in the region is subsisting and rural based, and almost half of these live on less than one US dollar a day [27]. Drought-combating strategies that do not address rural poverty and inequality affecting such a large proportion of the population would be ineffective. Such interventions create a trajectory of communities bouncing back to their pre-disaster state of poverty and vulnerability. Nonetheless, southern Africa has exhibited some form of drought resilience activities such as land reclamation and rangeland management in Lesotho, crop and livestock diversification in Namibia and South Africa. Another example is the regional vulnerability assessment and analysis program (RAAV) which monitors ongoing integrated food security classification and vulnerability as well as member states' disaster management capabilities [28–31].

There are gaps in the research on how resilience to droughts relates to the well-being of rural subsistence communities. The gaps are perpetuated by the lack of adequate contextual resilience measures to inform resilience policies and interventions. Generating evidence to bridge this gap has the potential to mitigate the negative impact of droughts on rural communities and help them recover in the most rapid and sustainable way. In addition, it will enable governments and humanitarian and development agencies to reduce expenditure on repetitive and costly drought interventions. The evidence will also inform the implementation of the United Nation's Sustainable Development Goals (SDGs) in the region, specifically those that address poverty (SDG1), hunger (SDG2), and health and well-being (SDG3) [32]. Therefore the purpose of this study is to assess the relationship between resilience to drought and well-being; and to identify gaps where further research is needed to inform a standard and contextual measure of resilience. However, resilience has been conceptualised differently and there is no single definition, hence, it was important to assess the suitability of the instruments used to measure resilience.

2. Methods

This systematic review was planned, implemented, and reported in accordance with the Preferred Reporting Items for Systematic Reviews and Meta-Analyses (PRISMA) guidelines (S 1). The PRISMA statement is a checklist with 27 essential items for ensuring reporting transparency [33]. Details of this systematic review's methods were registered by the PROSPERO international prospective registry for systematic reviews, reference CRD42017064396 [34]. Additionally, a protocol has been published in BMC Systematic Reviews [16].

2.1. Search Strategy

A librarian experienced in systematic reviews assisted in the development of the search strategy (see Acknowledgements). Thereafter, a comprehensive search was conducted from 1 January 1980 through to 10 August 2018. The following 13 electronic bibliographic databases were searched: Africa Journal Online (AJOL), CINAHL, MEDLINE, Academic Search Complete, Environment Complete, Humanities International Complete, Psychology and Behavioral Sciences Collection, PsycINFO, Embase, Web of Science, Applied Social Science Index and Abstracts, ProQuest Central, and Scopus. Additionally, multi-disciplinary databases and key organisational websites such as FAO, Google Scholar, Global Health Library, OECD, the World Bank, IFRC, USAID, and World Vision were searched. The following combination of search terms and keywords was used in the search:

Resilien* OR adapt* OR coping OR adjustmen* OR coheren*)
AND (drought* OR disaster*) AND (Well-being* OR wellbeing* OR disparit* OR status)
AND (Southern Africa* OR Botswana* OR Lesotho* OR Namibia* OR Swaziland* OR South Africa*)

Search terms varied slightly for each database. Studies were extracted into an EndNote library where they were subjected to further screening, as explained under 'Data extraction and quality assessment'.

2.2. Types of Participants

This systematic review is not limited by the participants' age, gender, social status, or ethnicity. Participants are drawn from the Southern Africa region where a large proportion of the region's population is rural, subsists on agriculture, and is faced with recurrent food shortages due to droughts [16].

2.3. Inclusion and Exclusion

Due to the nature and purpose of the study, we established wide inclusion criteria to broaden the literature coverage. This was mainly because disaster resilience is increasingly becoming a policy issue for governments across southern Africa. Therefore, studies were included if they (1) were published between January 1980 and 10 August 2018; (2) were peer-reviewed articles, dissertations, books and book chapters, working papers, technical reports, discussion papers, and conference papers; (3) were written in English and their full texts were available and accessible as we did not have the logistical and financial capacity to search for, retrieve and translate literature published in languages other than English; (4) measured resilience and its relationship to well-being; (5) were conducted in the southern Africa region. Reference lists of studies included were perused to identify relevant studies; those that met the criteria were included in the review. We define southern Africa as a geographical region comprised of Botswana, Lesotho, Namibia, South Africa, and Swaziland, as delineated by the United Nations geographical regions [35]. A search log was developed and used for accountability and transparency.

Studies were excluded if (1) they were carried outside the stated time frame; (2) conducted in countries other than the southern Africa region; (3) published in languages other than English; (4) were reviews, editorials, letters to editors, and opinion pieces; (5) and/or did not assess the relationship between drought resilience and well-being.

2.3.1. Data Extraction and Quality Assessment

Studies retrieved from databases were imported into an EndNote library and screened by title to eliminate duplicates. This was followed by a screening of the study abstracts to determine relevance. Thereafter, full texts of the remaining studies were read for eligibility and studies that met the inclusion criteria were retained. The extraction and appraisal of retrieved studies was conducted by one author (JKK) and independently reviewed by a second author (BJA). The two authors perused the reference lists of the retained studies to identify additional relevant studies. A third reviewer (AR) adjudicated the differences that emerged in the selection of the final studies for inclusion.

Piloted forms informed by the Cochrane Handbook for Systematic Reviews and the Joanna Briggs Institute (JBI) reviewers manual, 2014 edition, were used in the extraction of quantitative and qualitative data [36,37]. Extracted studies were identified by their author, year of publication, country, characteristics, design and data collection methods, setting, objectives, resilience outcome measures, instrument strength, and well-being (Table 1).

The quality assessment of the studies included involved two parts. Foremost was the analysis of the methodological quality of the studies. This enabled the evaluation of limitations and appropriateness of the studies' methods in addressing their research questions and objectives, and outcomes. Thereafter, we assessed the psychometric properties of the tools used in the studies.

2.3.2. Methodological Quality Assessment

We assessed the studies' designs, methods of data collection and analysis, selection bias, integrity, confounders, and reporting and summarised the findings as high medium or low using the appropriate tools. We appraised the dependability of the qualitative studies using the Joanna Briggs Institute Qualitative Assessment and Review Instrument (JBIQARI) [37]. The JBIQARI is an effective tool for assessing the risk of bias and a study's methodological quality. The results were assessed and scored as <4 points (low), 5–7 points (medium), or 8–10 points (high) (Table S2). Thereafter, we appraised the quality of grey literature using the Authority, Accuracy, Coverage, Objectivity, Date, Significance (AACODS) checklist [38]. The AACODS tool has been widely used in the quality assessment of grey literature by various studies and was found to produce rigorous results [39,40]. The use of AACODS enabled us to grade the studies as high (24–32 points), medium (15–23 points) or low ($\leq$14 points) (Table S3).

We did not encounter peer-reviewed studies that were experiments, quasi-experiments, or evaluations of interventions as anticipated in the protocol. Therefore, we used the National Institutes of Health (NIH) checklist to assess peer-reviewed observational studies that were quantitative. The NIH checklist measures 14 unique criteria to assess the internal validity of studies [41]. Studies were considered as good if they met the 10–14 criteria, fair if they met the 5–9 criteria and poor if they met the <4 criteria (Table S4). A high-quality rating implies a low risk of bias and vice versa [41]. Emerging evidence suggests that the NIH checklist is a robust tool for assessing risk bias in observational and cross-sectional studies [42–44].

We used a combined framework informed by Nukunu, Tolley, and colleagues for the thematic analysis of qualitative studies [45,46]. This enabled the identification of common threads of how resilience and well-being were conceptualised in the studies. The process involved first identifying patterns in the data. The second step was to search for relationships, interactions, and connections between patterns and themes. The third step was to ponder on the several meanings given to the same terms, and the fourth step involved giving meaning and significance to patterns observed in the data. The fifth step was to explore reasons to support the patterns and, lastly, the sixth step involved examining the relevance of emerging patterns to our research question.

2.3.3. Psychometric Properties Quality

With the exception of qualitative studies, the psychometric properties of the rest of the study scales were assessed for content validity, reliability, criterion validity, and construct validity using the Cyril and colleagues framework [47]. The components were chosen because of the breadth of reach in determining the strength of psychometric properties. For example, content validity analyses the extent to which a specific measure addresses all aspects of a given construct. We undertook the content validity to examine the extent to which the different facets of the scales used in the studies measured resilience. This involved assessing whether the study instruments were informed by a literature review, a panel of experts and empirical studies, and whether the target study audience had the opportunity to review the instruments. For each facet addressed, a point was awarded. We assessed the instrument reliability to establish if the scales used in studies consistently measured resilience. This was achieved by assessing whether the studies reported on the use of Cronbach Alpha and the test-retest measures. The Cronbach Alpha were scored as unacceptable <0.50 (0 points); poor ≥0.50 and <0.70 (1 point); acceptable ≥70 and <0.80 (2 points); and good ≥0.80 (2 points). The results of the test-retest were assessed as poor <0.40 (0 points); fair ≥0.40 and <0.60 (1 point); good ≥0.60 and <0.75 (2 points); and very good ≥75 (3 points).

We assessed the criterion validity of the scales to test the extent to which the latter related to well-being outcomes. This was done by establishing the correlation indices between resilience scores with well-being outcomes determined by grading the indices, whereby ≥0.70 meant a strong linear relationship (3 points), 0.50 meant moderate linear relationship (2 points), 0.30 meant a weak linear relationship (1 point), and 0 meant no linear relationship (0 points). We used the construct validity to assess if the instruments actually measured resilience, to what extent they did, and to identify the structure in the association between resilience subscales [16]. We examined whether the study instruments were subjected to exploratory and/or confirmatory factor analyses and whether the least factor analysis threshold was met in the subscales. This was done by determining if the extracted factors explained ≥50% of the variance; each extracted factor had at least three items; each variable loaded strongly on only one factor (≥0.35) and had two or more strong loadings (≥0.70); and was based on at least 10 cases per variable. For each criterion met, a point was awarded. The total psychometric properties scale oscillated from 0 to 17 (Table 2). Study instruments were graded as poor (<4 points), acceptable (5–9 points), good (10–13 points), or very good (>13 points) (Table S5).

2.4. Data Analysis

We did not carry out a meta-analysis because the retained studies were mainly observational by design and heterogeneous. Instead, we provide a narrative summary of the findings based on tables of ratings and frequencies. Several studies including systematic reviews have successfully used this approach to present their findings [47–49]. Nonetheless, an inductive thematic analysis of the qualitative studies' findings was carried out to identify resilience and well-being themes. The analysis was iterative and involved reading the retained studies to become familiar with their content, the coding of the retained studies' findings, grouping the codes into common areas to create potential themes, reviewing the themes to generate a thematic map, defining and naming the themes, and linking themes back to the review purpose to generate insight on resilience and well-being. A similar approach to qualitative data analysis in systematic reviews was proposed by Thomas and Harden [50].

Table 1. The study characteristics.

Author (Year) [Ref]	Study Design & Data Collection	Sample Characteristics	Study Setting	Study Objectives	Main Resilience Determinants	Assessment Outcome
Rankoana (2016) [51]	A qualitative study using open-ended questions.	n = 100 participants Male = 52; Female = 48	Drought prone Mogalakwena community in the Limpopo province of South Africa	Explore community perceptions of climate variability and the capabilities to adapt livelihoods	Household capacities, community capacities, and Indigenous/local knowledge	Medium (JBI QARI)
Van Riet (2012) [30]	A qualitative control case study of black communal and white commercial farmers using the Mmogo method.	n = 37 participants (FGD = 7), KIs (farmers = 4, State officials = 7), Farmers aged <60 years	Drought-prone North-West province, South Africa	Disaster risk management, legislative compliance, and accompanying political legacy	Political and governance capacities, and household capacities	High (JBI QARI)
Vogel et al. (2010) [17]	A retrospective longitudinal study using secondary data (policy reports) supplemented by primary data collection.	n = 27 subject matter expert interviews and focus group discussions (n = not given).	Subject matter experts working within the SADC regional bodies, commercial farmers, and members of the African Farmers Union	Assessment of drought governance for resilience enhancement	Political and governance capacities	High (JBI QARI)
Rankoana (2016) b [52]	A qualitative study through focus group discussions.	n = 50 participants Age = 35–78 years	Dikgale community in Limpopo, South Africa	Define how agricultural women-specific rituals enhance food security	Community capacities and Indigenous/local knowledge	High (JBI QARI)
Ngwenya et al. (2016) [53]	A participatory rural appraisal (PRA). Additional data was sourced through field observations, unstructured interviews and secondary data.	n = 18 FGDs. The FGD groups comprised of males only = 3 groups, females only = 3 groups, combined males and females = 12 groups	Farming communities in Okavango Delta, Botswana	Examine the influence of hydro-climatic change on health, food security, and livelihoods	Community capacities; Indigenous/local knowledge; household capacities	High (JBI QARI)

Table 1. *Cont.*

Author (Year) [Ref]	Study Design & Data Collection	Sample Characteristics	Study Setting	Study Objectives	Main Resilience Determinants	Assessment Outcome
Newsham et al. (2011) [28]	An ethnographic study of knowledge, farming, and climate change adaptation.	n = 8 FGDs. Each FGD comprised of 10–15 participants. Farmers and extension workers	Rural drought-prone Omusati region of north-west Namibia	Establish the need for adaptation policy to engage with the agro-ecological knowledge of farmers; capture how agro-ecological knowledge and science are combined to foster a climate change adaptive capacity	Household capacities; Indigenous/local knowledge; and political and governance capacities	Medium (JBI QARI)
Renzaho et al. (2016) [18]	Mixed methods with non-equivalent control groups' post-test only quasi-experimental design. Qualitative data collection through FGD. Quantitative data collection using a structured questionnaire and systematic sampling.	Qualitative data involved 16 FGDs, n = 197 (93 in Swaziland and 104 in Lesotho). For quantitative data, n = 3324 households (1789 in Swaziland and 1535 in Lesotho)	Drought-prone farming households in rural Lesotho and Swaziland	Examine resilience to droughts and develop an evidence-based framework to inform community resilience interventions	Household capacities, community capacities; and Indigenous/local knowledge	High (AACODS)
Bahta et al. (2016) [54]	Cross-sectional survey. Data collection using a semi-structured questionnaire, purposive sampling method procedures, and the creation of a perception index.	n = 87 participants Male = 62 Female = 25 Mean age = 51 years	Communal farmers in OR Tambo district, Eastern Cape province in South Africa	Examine farmers' awareness of drought, their vulnerabilities and relationships with gender, networks, stress, security and the role of government	Governance capacities and community capacities	Fair (NIH)
Bareki et al. (2017) [55]	Mixed methods. Qualitative data collection through in-depth face to face interviews. Quantitative data collection using a semi-structured questionnaire.	n = 85 participants	Nguni cattle development project members in North-West province in South Africa	Assess drought preparedness of intervention beneficiaries and identify factors of drought-preparedness among Nguni cattle farmers	Governance capacities, and household capacities	Fair (NIH)

Table 1. *Cont.*

Author (Year) [Ref]	Study Design & Data Collection	Sample Characteristics	Study Setting	Study Objectives	Main Resilience Determinants	Assessment Outcome
Bunting et al. (2013) [56]	Cross-sectional survey Data collection using semi-structured open-ended questionnaires, convenience sampling.	n = 330 households	Households in seven arid/semi-arid villages across the Okavango, Kwando and Zambezi catchments in Botswanan and Namibia	Explore perceptions of livelihood risk in the semi-arid Savanah and Zambezi catchments and how perceived risk mirrors the changing ecosystem in Botswana and Namibia	Governance capacities and household capacities	Fair (NIH)
Kolawole et al. (2016) [57]	Mixed methods. Qualitative data collection through key informant interviews, FGDs, and a stakeholder workshop. Quantitative data collection using a closed-end questionnaire. A multi-stage sampling procedure was used.	n = 592 households 27 FGDs Mean age = 51 years	Eight rural communities in the Okavango Delta in the Ngamiland district of Botswana	Investigate the impacts of climate variability on agriculture and identify adaptation strategies	Indigenous/local knowledge and household capacities	Fair (NIH)
Belle et al. (2015) [29]	A mixed methods cross-sectional survey.	Household survey (n = 102); KIs (n = 3)	Subsistence farmers in the drought-prone Koiti-Se-Phola community, Mafeteng district of Lesotho	Investigate the community's vulnerability to agricultural drought to inform resilience building	Household capacities and community capacities	Fair (NIH)
Thomas et al. (2007) [58]	A mixed methods observational study base on secondary rainfall data using Self-Organising Maps (SOMs) and primary data gathered through FGDs and KIs.	Secondary rainfall data Primary data: FGDs (n = 50); KIs (n = 30)	Natural resource dependent communities in three regions of Limpopo, KwaZulu Natal and north-west provinces	Analyse rainfall variability, the community's awareness of the variability and their adaptive capacities	Household capacities and community capacities, and indigenous/local knowledge	Fair (NIH)

Table 1. *Cont.*

Author (Year) [Ref]	Study Design & Data Collection	Sample Characteristics	Study Setting	Study Objectives	Main Resilience Determinants	Assessment Outcome
Mlenga et al. (2015) [59]	Mixed methods. Qualitative data collection through structured and unstructured interviews and FGDs. Quantitative data collection using a questionnaire. A random sampling technique was used.	n = 200 households	Drought-vulnerable farming households that benefited from NGO climate change and drought mitigation interventions in the Lowveld agro-ecological zone of Swaziland	To understand the determinants of conservation agriculture (CA) in the Lowveld agro-ecological zone of Swaziland	Household capacities	Fair (NIH)
Mlenga et al. (2016) [60]	A knowledge, attitudes, and practices (KAP) survey conducted in the low veld agro-ecological zone of Swaziland.	n = 450	Drought-prone beneficiaries of a water sanitation and hygiene (WASH) intervention	Evaluate the effectiveness of a WASH intervention in mitigating disaster risk and enhancing community resilience	Household capacities and community capacities and health	Fair (NIH)
Akpalu (2005) [61]	Mixed methods. Qualitative data collection through an open-ended questionnaire. Quantitative data collection using closed-ended questionnaire. A random sampling technique was used.	n = 34 participants Male = 10 Female = 24 Age = 26–85 years	Drought-affected Thorndale located in the Bushbuckridge region of the Limpopo province in South Africa	Assess the effects of the 2002/2003 drought, the responses, constraints encountered and the implications of the drought on HHs	Household capacities and community capacities	Medium (AACODS)
Hudson (2002) [62]	Mixed methods. Qualitative data collection through interviews. Quantitative data collection using questionnaires.	Commercial farmers (n = 25); Communal farmers (n = 35)	Commercial and communal livestock farmers in the North-West province in South Africa	Assess and compare commercial and communal livestock farmers' drought management strategies	Political and governance capacities, and household capacities	High (AACODS)

Table 1. *Cont.*

Author (Year) [Ref]	Study Design & Data Collection	Sample Characteristics	Study Setting	Study Objectives	Main Resilience Determinants	Assessment Outcome
Shongwe et al. (2014) [63]	A cross-sectional study Quantitative data collection through questionnaires.	$n = 350$	Rain-dependent farming households on Swazi communal land in Mpolojeni in the Lowveld of Swaziland.	Identify household adaptation strategies and determinants of the choice of strategies	Household capacities and community capacities	Fair (NIH)
Mason (2005) [64]	An analysis of secondary epidemiological data drawn from national and subnational surveys such as demographic health surveys (DHS) and multiple indicator cluster surveys (MICS) in southern Africa.	Secondary anthropometric and HIV prevalence data drawn from six countries with UNICEF support	Children of 0–5 years in Lesotho and Swaziland	Explore child malnutrition trends in relation to HIV/AIDS and the 2001–2003 drought	Household capacities and health factors	Good (NIH)

Table 2. The quality assessment of scales.

Author Year [Ref]	Content Validity				Reliability		Criterion Validity	Construct Validity (EFA and/or CFA)				Total Points
	Informed by Literature Review	Panel of Experts	Empirical Study	Reviewed by Target Population	Internal Consistency	Test-Retest		Factors Explained ≥50% of the Variance	Included at Least 3 Items	Variables Loading	Based on 10 Cases per Variable	
	Yes = 1 No = 0	Yes = 1 No = 0	Yes = 1 No = 0	Yes = 1 No = 0	0–3 Points	0–3 Points	0–3 Points	Yes = 1 No = 0	Yes = 1 No = 0	Yes = 1 No = 0	Yes = 1 No = 0	Maximum Points = 17
Renzaho et al., 2016 [18]	1	1	1	1	3	0	3	0	0	0	0	10
Bahta et al., 2016 [54]	0	0	0	0	0	0	3	0	0	0	0	3
Bareki et al., 2017 [55]	0	0	0	0	0	0	0	0	0	0	0	0
Bunting et al., 2013 [56]	0	0	0	0	0	0	3	0	0	0	0	3
Kolawole et al., 2016 [57]	1	0	1	1	0	1 *	1	0	0	0	0	5
Belle et al., 2015 [29]	1	1	0	0	2	0	2	0	0	0	0	6
Thomas et al., 2007 [58]	0	0	1	0	0	0	2	0	0	0	0	3
Mlenga et al., 2015 [59]	0	0	0	0	0	0	1	0	0	0	0	1
Mlenga et al., 2016 [60]	1	0	1	0	0	0	3	0	0	0	0	5
Akpalu et al., 2005 [61]	0	0	0	0	0	0	0	0	0	0	0	0
Hudson et al., 2002 [62]	1	0	0	0	0	0	1	0	0	0	0	2
Shongew et al., 2014 [63]	0	0	0	0	0	0	1	0	0	0	0	1
Mason 2005 [64]	0	0	1	0	0	0	3	0	0	0	0	4

* Denotes item mentioned in the report without stating details.

3. Results

We report our findings within the confines of the Preferred Reporting Items for Systematic Reviews and Meta-Analyses (PRISMA) guidelines [30]. Our search yielded 3950 studies. Our criteria excluded duplicates (n = 747) and magazines, and newspapers (n = 227). Screening of titles and abstracts excluded 2913 studies. The full texts of the remaining 63 studies were retrieved and read for eligibility and relevance, which led to a further exclusion of 48 studies. Fifteen remaining studies (n = 15) met our inclusion criteria. Reference lists of studies retained were screened and yielded four (n = 4) more studies, resulting in a total of 19 studies included in this systematic review (Figure 1).

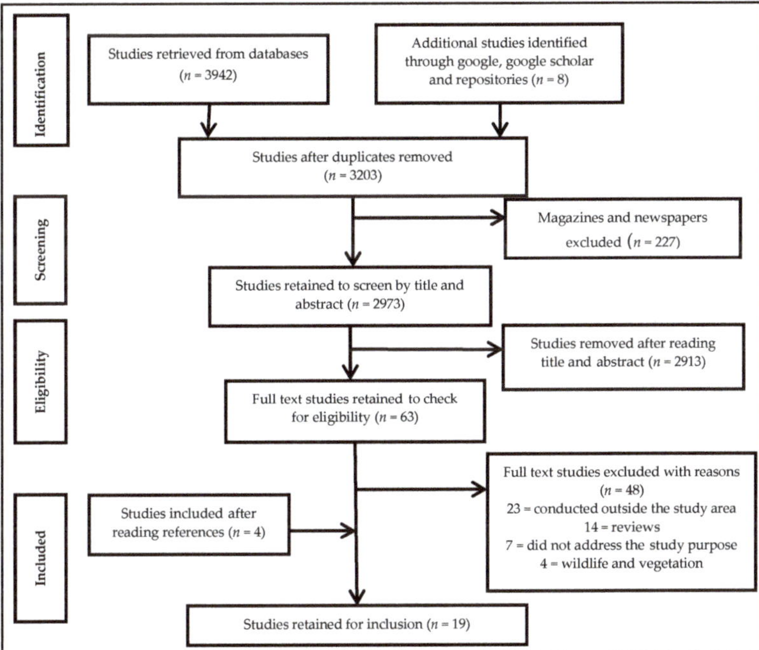

Figure 1. The Preferred Reporting Items for Systematic Reviews and Meta-Analyses (PRISMA) flow diagram.

3.1. Study Characteristics

The sample sizes of the retained studies varied from 10 to 3324. Six of the studies used qualitative methods, two applied quantitative methods and the remaining studies used mixed methods. The rural farming communities were the predominant study population except for two studies, one of which focused on drought subject matter experts and the other on anthropometry in children <5 years [17,64].

Included studies had a range of objectives, from rainfall and climate variability to food security, coping, and adaptation (Figure 2). Nonetheless, all studies aimed to demonstrate the relationship between drought resilience and well-being across southern Africa.

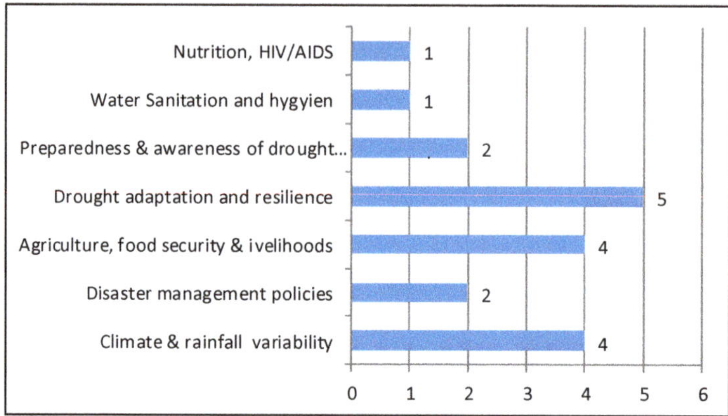

Figure 2. The variability of the studies' objectives.

3.2. *Summary of Findings*

Our findings suggest that the most prevalent determinants of drought resilience were political and governance, indigenous and local knowledge, community and household capacities.

3.2.1. Political and Governance Capacities

Eight of the nineteen studies [17,28,30,54–56,58,62] examined the political and governance determinants of drought management and response. These studies observed that local politics and governance determined the nature of drought response and resilience outcomes. For example, Van Riet found political and historical legacies such as the 1913 Land Act and tenure racialised farming into predominantly well-resourced white commercial farming and poorly resourced black subsistence farming [30]. The study observed that drought compounded environmental degradation, job and crop losses, as well as low-income levels. However, black subsistence farmers were negatively affected more than their commercial counterparts. Subsistence farmers relied on rudimentary coping mechanisms such as old age pensions, community-saving schemes and burial societies, and sought temporary grazing rights from neighbouring traditional leaders. Burial societies are informal community-saving schemes where members make periodical financial contributions that are drawn from to facilitate funerals. Subsistence farmers experienced deprivation, hunger, helplessness, and structural barriers such as inaccessibility to resources and agricultural land. Commercial farmers owned the best agricultural land and in large quantities, with multiple private water sources such as boreholes. They also enjoyed government subsidies prior to the 1990s in order to support their farming activities. Farmers unable to sustain farming without subsidies left farming for non-farming occupations.

A similar politicisation of farming along the racial divide was observed in a study of commercial and communal farmers in North-West province, South Africa [62]. It was observed that commercial farming was dominated by white farmers to whom farming was a profitable business. They proactively understocked and destocked early enough before the drought conditions worsened to optimise their returns. They also had access to vast pasture land that enabled rotational grazing and reared sheep to supplement income from cattle sales during droughts. During the drought, commercial farmers earned more livestock from their communal counterparts, who rented the former's pasture land and paid with livestock. The commercially viable farming business enabled the diversification of livelihoods into off-farm business ventures to reduce their drought exposure risk. Black communal farmers relied on unconventional approaches. For example, they shared limited food crops with livestock, allowed livestock to be undernourished in anticipation for recovery after the drought, and combined cattle rearing with goats, which required less water and pasture but was of less economic value. Communal farmers sought wage-based incomes on commercial farms and other businesses but encountered fewer employment opportunities, which affected their purchasing power as well as their food and nutrition needs. Interestingly, commercial farmers were motivated by profit while their communal counterparts practised livestock farming as a cultural value. Both farmer groups highlighted the absence of social support to cope with the negative effects of droughts [62].

However, this claim of lack of social support was contradicted by the rainfall variability study. This study cited social cohesion and support as tenets of the farmers' resilience to frequent droughts that had devastated farming livelihoods [58]. The study participants claimed that persistent drought led to crop and livestock losses, hunger, tiredness, sickness, indebtedness, and reliance on welfare. However, out of their misery emerged intra-community collective action that enabled government intervention with extension services. The services included the fusion of drought-tolerant indigenous livestock and crop breeds with new varieties for increased productivity. Other government schemes that were introduced included group poultry, piggery and horticultural interventions, which enabled livelihood diversification as well as the supplementation of staple foods [58]. Similar livelihood diversification schemes were observed by Van Riet, who noted that government-inspired hydroponics, piggery, poultry, community bakery, and food plots interventions were effective in mitigating drought effects [30]. However, the beneficiaries were too few compared to the need. Nonetheless, those who benefited had better incomes and access to food and other necessities throughout the drought seasons.

Vogel and colleagues noted that reactive state-led drought risk governance was entrenched in various policy frameworks [17]. The policies covered emergency relief and agricultural subsidies (1982/83), regional drought cooperation (1991/92), consolidated drought appeal for SADC (1994/95), joint crop assessments and early warning (1995), the establishment of country-level vulnerability assessment committees and the regional vulnerability assessment committee in 2000/01 [17]. The policies focused on food aid to reduce macro-level cereal deficits and prevent starvation at a community level. However, they were unable to proactively and holistically mitigate the effects of recurring drought. The policies were singled out as promoting dependence on humanitarian assistance and weakening resilience building because they remained delinked from development interventions [17]. The government inability to mainstream disaster management into development was corroborated by another study which noted that drought management was outsourced to consultants within the confines of assessment reports and plans for legislative compliance [30].

In a different study, Bahta and colleagues observed that inadequate government involvement negatively affected communal farmers' drought resilience [54]. The study noted poor service delivery, insufficient and late drought relief, lack of training and lack of timely early warning information as key government failures in resilience building. It was reported that the government failed to provide security to prevent farm attacks and high stock thefts that escalated in drought periods. Inadequate government intervention aggravated drought vulnerability that was linked to psychological stress. For example, some farmers committed suicide due to the inability to cope with the drought impacts [54]. Separate studies by Akapalu and Van Riet observed stock thefts and security incidences on farms [30,61]. Drought periods corresponded with increased insecurity on farms. This was associated with aggravated unemployment and hunger, and compromised livelihoods that inhibited household capacities to adequately deal with drought effects [30,61].

An observational study conducted in northern Botswana and the Caprivi Strip of Namibia observed that government intervention with social services was critical in the adaptation to climate variability [56]. The study associated hunger, employment, human and wildlife interactions, and ill health as the main risks to livelihoods during drought. The risks were mitigated through government interventions such as wage labour, piped water, loaning farming machinery, and education and skills. The resilience and well-being outcomes observed were increased prosperity, financial stability, diversified livelihoods, access to clean water, and social change with transformed drought adaptation and coping measures [56]. Nonetheless, the study noted that some households which were still subsisting experienced two to five months of hunger and food insecurity annually.

A drought-preparedness study among Nguni cattle farmers in North-West province in South Africa observed that inadequate government support and a lack of capital, credible, and timely early warning information were the main barriers to drought preparedness [55]. There was regular contact between farmers and government extension workers, but this was never leveraged to disseminate information and educate farmers on drought mitigation. More than half of the study participants did not have drought plans, which they blamed on the inadequacy of early warning, a responsibility of the government. However, a small proportion of the farmers had fodder banks and some leased extra grazing land to mitigate the drought effects. Nonetheless, the absence of early warnings compromised farming stocks and the farmers' socioeconomic status as they did not have alternative livelihoods. Conversely, an ethnographic study in drought-vulnerable northern Namibia credited adaptive capacity to the joint efforts of the government extension workers and the farmers [28]. The study highlighted the intrinsic success of skilled extension workers who creatively harnessed different information sources to disseminate useful and timely early warnings. The study also noted that the government was actively involved in disaster mitigation, albeit using ineffective top-down approaches that often did not recognise the different contexts and inherent capacities in the communities.

3.2.2. Indigenous and Local Knowledge

Eight studies [18,28,51–53,57,58,62] identified indigenous and local knowledge as a determinant of resilience. They emphasised that communities with rich indigenous and local ecological knowledge and practices had good resilience outcomes than those without them for example, a study in Mogalakwena community in Limpopo, South Africa, noted that indigenous knowledge of seasons and early warnings, as well as traditional practices such as mixed cropping, the use of livestock manure, and the use of early maturing seeds, enabled the community to adapt to droughts [51]. Similarly, another study pointed out that women used indigenous knowledge and culture to promote drought adaptation behaviour [52]. Coping and adaptation practices observed were seed dressing, traditional crop maintenance, and rain-making rituals that promoted food security and a constant seed supply. Other practices noted were supplicatory rain making and communal crop protection rituals performed to invoke supernatural interventions for rain and the protection of crops from animals and birds [52].

A study of resilience in Swaziland and Lesotho observed that the application of traditional knowledge complemented with contemporary knowledge and skills improved health-related behaviour and practices [18]. It was found that knowledgeable communities were those informed about their inherent capacities and services. Such communities knew when and where to seek assistance [18]. A study of agro-ecological knowledge among Ovambo farmers in north-central Namibia suggested that mixing traditional agro-ecological knowledge with scientific agricultural knowledge co-produced hybrid knowledge without the limitations of either knowledge base [28]. The resulting hybrid agro-ecological knowledge imbued farming with drought adaptation practices such as early maturing crops, the use of donkey traction to plough large expanses of land, destocking, hunting, and gathering, and sharing food among households [28]. Interestingly, the adoption of cattle post-grazing from the predominantly traditional transhumance was noted to exacerbate land degradation.

A study of disaster-prone communities in Ngamiland District in Botswana submitted that adverse weather effects such as droughts led to a reduction in farming output and food availability, ultimately decreasing human welfare [57]. The study pointed out that the indigenous knowledge of weather forecasting (ethnometeorology) was a critical factor in adaptation and resilience. Households relied on the old tradition of observing the natural phenomena within their environment to inform their agricultural decisions. Some of the natural phenomena highlighted were the behaviour of particular plants, the presence of particular insects, wild animal migrations, and the position and brightness of particular stars. Changes in the patterns of natural phenomena symbolised good rains, poor rains, or droughts, and forewarned communities to prepare for adversity and adjust their livelihoods accordingly [57]. Similar views were observed in a study of commercial and communal farmers [62]. Farmers pointed to wind and rainfall patterns, the presence of poisonous plants in early spring, termite behaviour, and the absence of mole-mounds as drought predictors. They claimed that the observation of the natural phenomena enabled them to adjust their farming practices in anticipation of adverse weather conditions [62].

A PRA study in the Okavango Delta in north-western Botswana identified traditional community structures such as Kgotla (a traditional meeting place) and chieftaincy as strong mechanisms for mobilising adaptation to climate variability and change [53]. Traditional institutions mediated access to resources and promoted adaptation based on local ecological knowledge. Kgotla orchestrated local learning processes that empowered people to adapt or adjust their livelihoods based on the nature of adversity. Households with diversified livelihoods were cushioned from the extreme impacts of floods, human and livestock disease outbreaks, and frequent droughts. Both Kgotla and chieftaincy incentivised collective action and community participation in decision-making to mitigate periodic droughts and floods that negatively affected livelihoods and well-being. The institutions guided the development committees and volunteer associations for socio-health activities such as malaria and tsetse fly prevention. They mobilised farmer groups into traditional *malapo* (flood recession) farming which was an important livelihood in the harsh environment. Farmers adapted to planting quick maturing crops in the flood recession plains or dry river beds where soils retained moisture from seasonal floods. Traditional institutions and knowledge were credited with maintaining community cohesion and promoting adaptation to climate variability and were the central government's heartbeat of consultation on public policy [53]. The application of traditional knowledge was also observed in a rainfall variability study in South Africa [58]. The study submitted that farmers who assimilated indigenous drought-resistant livestock breeds and crop species were able to prevent drought-induced losses [58]. However, indigenous species had lower yields but were better adapted to drought conditions than other varieties. Farmers claimed that regardless of the low yields, the crops required short growing time and reduced farming risks as well as food insecurity in drought periods. Farmers pooled their knowledge and resources to leverage scale and market opportunities which, in turn, increased their income and all-year food supply [58].

Conversely, traditional institutions and knowledge were slowly being eroded by western-modelled education and external assistance [18,28,30,53,62]. People who had acquired education undervalued traditional early warnings and some simply dismissed them in favour of scientific early warnings [53,57,62]. This was compounded by the humanitarian and development interventions by non-governmental organisations (NGOs) that inadvertently undermined intrinsic community capacities. The interventions discouraged community efforts in self-sustainment in anticipation of handouts. For example, Renzaho and colleague observed that disregard for intrinsic capacities and poor community engagement by humanitarian actors discouraged communities from anticipating and preparing for disasters [18].

3.2.3. Community Capacities

Nine studies profiled the importance of community capacities in drought resilience [18,29,51–53,55,58,60,61]. The main elements identified were knowledge sharing, social networks, participation, cohesion, and connectedness. For example, Renzaho and colleague underscored community cohesion and support, social networks, empowerment and participation, psychological well-being and community ownership of disaster preparedness as collective elements that enhanced resilience [18]. Community cohesiveness was again identified as a resilience factor in a rainfall variability study which noted that cohesion in the community facilitated collective adaptability, including diversion from rain-fed agriculture to other livelihoods [58]. Cohesiveness and unanimity enabled the establishment of joint small-scaled commercial initiatives such as poultry and drought-resistant horticultural projects, and the establishment of a cooperative group to improve collective bargaining power and economies of scale, and address market risks [58]. Cooperation, sharing of information, costs, and risks were reported to have facilitated a drought-resilient community to emerge [58]. Similarly, a study in Thorndale in South Africa earmarked social solidarity practices such as drought committees, kinship ties, and social interaction as enhancing cohesiveness during difficult periods [61]. For example, people joined efforts to work on their community gardens where they learnt new farming ideas that they adapted in their homes. Additionally, joint efforts enabled the communities to obtain amenities such as water reservoirs and community standpipes using economies of scale.

A survey of knowledge, attitudes, and practices (KAP) in the low veld of Swaziland stated that joint community efforts led to ownership of the water infrastructure and enhanced knowledgeability and capacity to manage and maintain the infrastructure [60]. The clean water initiative attracted community participation in its functionality and maintenance. The study credited the water intervention for promoting joint learning and improvement of health outcomes such as improved hygiene and sanitation. Specifically, there was a notable increase of households with and using latrines (34.9–71.3%), and good hand-washing practices (75.5%) which were linked to hygiene and sanitation intervention by an NGO. The study associated improvements in knowledge, attitudes, and community practices in sanitation and hygiene with enhanced resilience [60]. Collective efforts were again captured in a study carried out in the Limpopo province in South Africa [51]. The study suggested that a community's collective understanding of seasonal changes and cropping practices limited the impact of droughts on crop production and promoted adaptation. For example, short-season crops were adapted by entire communities instead of their well-liked but late maturing crops [51]. This had cascading effects on livelihoods, which also changed due to productivity and production changes in a subsistence dominated area.

A study in the Okavango Delta of Botswana found that the community management of rangelands was critical in rangeland preservation and the community's adaptation to climate change [53]. The study highlighted that rangelands were important community resources that supported livelihoods such as livestock grazing, crafting, and hunting and gathering wild foods. Community members set, agreed on, and monitored adherence to procedures for rangelands utilisation. Rangelands were fragile and exposed to recurrent droughts and floods, as well as degradation resulting from high livestock and wildlife populations. Focusing on the nexus between people and the environment was a viable approach to risk management and the sustainability of community livelihoods and well-being in a fragile environment [53]. The relationship between rangeland management and resilience was affirmed by a 2015 study in Lesotho [29], which suggested that the poor management of the rangelands by the communities led to massive degradation and exacerbated drought effects. Specifically, the degradation led to the deterioration of crops and livestock output, which further cascaded into food insecurity and socioeconomic challenges. The study pointed to deforestation, a high old-age ratio and low education levels as key vulnerabilities in the community; these were reflected in weak coping and adaptation strategies [29].

3.2.4. Household Capacities

Overwhelmingly, 16 studies submitted that household capacities were critical elements in resilience building [18,28–30,51,53,55–64]. The main household elements that instigated adaptation, resilience and well-being were diversified livelihoods, socioeconomic status, education levels, access to resources, and soft skills. Three studies profiled household socioeconomic status, household assets and livelihoods [29,53,56]. For example, Bunting and colleagues related household socioeconomic status to access resources [56]. The authors determined that financial assets, access to water, health and employment opportunities were the main risks to household livelihoods and well-being. Households with access to these resources coped better with adversity. The absence of or limited access to resources curtailed livelihoods, exacerbated food shortage, hunger, and poor health. For example, wage-based employability was a key factor in offsetting yearly household crop loss due to droughts and floods. Households with access to water standpipes had better water security and did not experience the burden of waterborne diseases compared to those without and those who competed with the wildlife for water sources in drought periods [56]. Likewise, Ngwenya and colleagues noted that household capital such as access to land and land use, knowledgeability, and multiple home ownership in rural and urban locations were important elements of adaptation [53]. During harsh periods, such as droughts or disease outbreaks, households escaped adversity in rural farming homes by moving to urban areas where they had homes. Moreover, the movement between areas required households to diversify livelihoods to support their well-being in either place. In rural areas, households switched land use depending on the conditions. For example, they alternated between *malapo* farming and dryland farming when the seasons changed. Correspondingly, households with more skills than farming opportunistically switched from crop production to different livelihoods such as fishing, harvesting aquatic foods, and wild plants in the delta depending on the environmental conditions. The study concluded that households' adaptation capacities were deeply intertwined with resilience and well-being outcomes [53].

Household demographics such as gender, age, education, and socioeconomic status were strong determinants of household resilience, healthiness, and well-being [18,29,63]. For example, Belle and colleagues acknowledged that households with low education levels and socioeconomic statuses had poor coping mechanisms that perpetuated inadequacy, helplessness, and poverty [29]. The authors found that during difficult drought periods, families sent their young children into manual labour to reduce the burden of household food requirements and earn income to subsidise family needs. Another study acknowledged that cattle farming was a male's domain and that old age was a factor in access to farming capital and grazing land [55]. The majority of the surveyed farmers were aged >60 years; youth participation was limited by the unaffordability of capital requirements and limited access to grazing land. The study further suggested that limited education among elderly farmers was a factor in the lack of drought preparedness and compromised incomes and livelihoods [55].

Similarly, Shongwe and colleagues observed in Swaziland that the ability to perceive and prepare for adversity was dependent on the age of the household [63]. The authors noted that adaptation required labour intensive agricultural activities which old people were unable to provide. Almost 62% of the household heads were aged >50 and more than 55% were illiterate, making it difficult to comprehend and apply new and improved farming systems. They continued to grow drought-intolerant crops such as maize (>90%), which further aggravated their food insecurity and health [63]. Age was also highlighted in a resilience survey that revealed elderly-headed households were less resilient to droughts than other households. Elderly-headed households also experienced weak socio-political empowerment that limited their participation and self-confidence to bring about the desired changes in their well-being [18]. Bahta and colleagues noted that gender was influential in decision making [54]. The authors observed that key decisions on drought adaptation were a male domain, with limited participation from women. Women who were responsible for food preparation did not have the bargaining power on drought-related agricultural activities. However, women were perceived to be more resilient; they knew how to search for food and ensured their children's nutrition and well-being through drought periods [54].

Soft skills such as self-organisation, information access, ability to perceive and prepare against adversity, communication and connectedness were influential elements for household preparedness and adaptation. For example, a study of Nguni farmers attributed the lack of drought preparedness in households to inadequate access to early warning information and knowledge [55]. The regular contact between farmers and extension workers was never leveraged to disseminate information and educate farmers on drought mitigation. The lack of preparedness resulted in significant farming losses and compromised livelihoods [55]. Another study that examined the state of disaster preparedness, mitigation, and response plans found 84% and 91% of households lacked disaster preparedness plans in Lesotho and Swaziland [18]. Barriers to disaster preparedness were poor collaboration, limited resources, inability to volunteer, inability to perceive the importance of preparedness, competing priorities, poor community governance and communication, lack of funding opportunities, and dependence on humanitarian assistance. The absence of drought preparedness plans deprived households of sufficient esteem to self-determine their response and recovery strategies. It made them reliant on humanitarian assistance for survival [18].

Household connectedness and cohesion were profiled as important resilience and well-being elements. For instance, Akapalu [61] and Newsham and colleagues [28] suggested that kinship ties enabled families without access to farming land and livestock to benefit from food and livestock products from their kinsmen during difficult periods. Sharing resources through kinship ties, spousal connections and other family connectedness helped to spread drought risk across households to minimise the negative effects. Additionally, kinship ties enabled the easy flow of goods and services such as fodder, herbal medicine, and labour, which were shared among families depending on their needs [28,61].

3.3. Methods Used in the Development of Included Study Scales

The scales of studies included were informed by empirical studies (n = 5) [18,57–59,64] and literature review (n = 5) [18,29,57,59,62]. Two studies used a combination of a literature review and empirical studies (n = 2) [57,59]. One study (n = 1) was informed by a literature review, an empirical study, and the target population [57]. Interestingly, only one study (n = 1) combined all the four steps [18]. The remaining studies were silent on how their scales were developed (Table 2).

Quality Rating of Scales

We examined scales for reliability, content validity, reliability, criterion validity and construct validity, and applied a 17-point-based measure. We assessed the scales' reliability by examining whether the test-retest and the internal consistency measured by the Cronbach Alpha were performed. Two studies (n = 2) [18,29] measured the internal consistency of tools. Of these, Renzaho and colleague [18] had a Cronbach Alpha $\geq$0.80 and was scored as good (3 points). The other study by Belle and colleague [29] had a Cronbach Alpha $\geq$0.764 and was scored as acceptable (2 points). The remaining studies were silent on their internal consistency.

None of the studies demonstrated having undertaken a test-retest reliability except one study (n = 1) [57], which suggested having undertaken it without stating details on how it was done or the outcome. We performed a criterion validity assessment to examine the relationship between the scales used and well-being outcomes. Five studies [18,54,56,59,64] showed a strong linear relationship and scored 3 points on our assessment framework informed by Cyril et al. [48] (Table 2). Two studies [60,61] showed moderate linear relationships (2 points) and three studies [57,59,62,63] were assessed to have a weak linear relationship (1 point). The rest of the studies showed no linear relationships (Table 2).

Overall, 17 psychometric properties were measured and only one study met the good criteria with a score of 10 points [18]. Three studies were assessed to be of acceptable quality (5–9 points) [29,57,60]. The remaining studies scales were assessed as poor (0–4 points) as reflected in Table 2.

3.4. Methodological Assessment of Studies Included

Different approaches commensurate with study types were used to assess the methodological quality of studies included. For example, we used the AACODS checklist to assess the quality of three non-peer reviewed studies included [18,61,62]. Two studies were assessed to be of high quality [18,62]. A third study was assessed to be of medium quality [61] (Table S3). The remaining 10 studies were observational and were assessed with 14-point criteria informed by the NIH checklist. One study met 11 of the 14 methodological criteria points and was assessed as good [64]. The remaining nine studies scored between 6–9 criteria points and were assessed as fair on the NIH checklist [29,54–60,63,64] (Table S4).

3.5. Quality Assessment of Qualitative Studies

Six of the studies included in the review used qualitative methods [17,28,30,51–53]. Their quality was assessed with a 10-point quality assessment framework informed by the Joana Briggs Qualitative Assessment and Review Instrument [37] (Table S2). Three of the studies scored between 8–10 points and were assessed as high quality [28,52,53]. The remaining three were medium quality (5–7 points) as reflected in Table S2 [17,30,51].

We conducted a thematic analysis to identify the common threads in how resilience was conceptualised in the included studies. The common resilience threads that emerged were broken into four main themes, as profiled in the summary of findings. The themes were: (i) community capacities, (ii) household capacities, (iii) indigenous/local knowledge, and (iv) political and governance capacities (Figure 3).

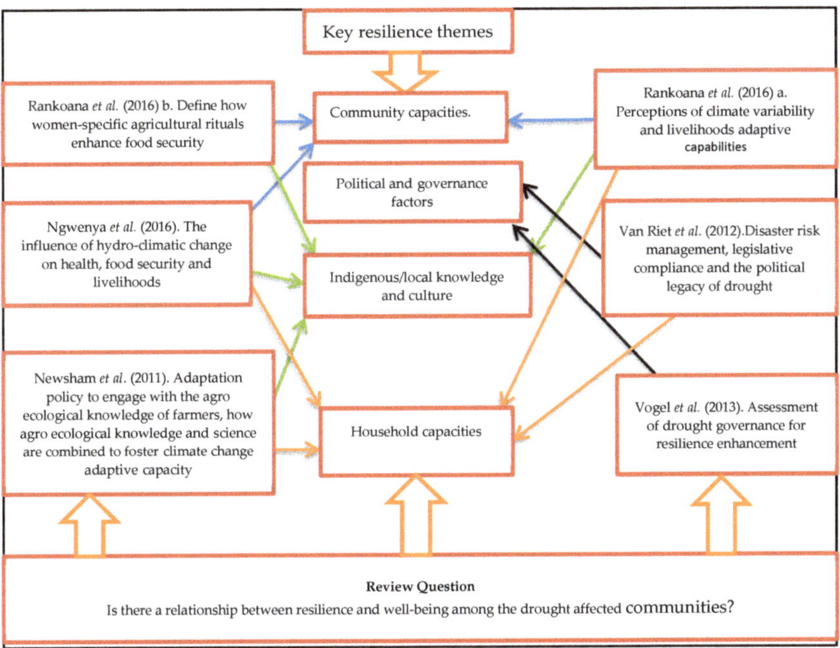

Figure 3. The synthesis of qualitative resilience themes adopted from Reference [46].

4. Discussion

Southern Africa experiences recurrent droughts that continuously erode livelihoods and affect the well-being of communities. Nonetheless, the affected communities have adopted resilience mechanisms to cope with and adapt to the periodic episodes of drought. We sought to understand the relationship between resilience to drought and well-being, examine the suitability of the resilience instruments and their psychometric properties, and identify gaps and unanswered questions in order to enhance the resilience theory in the region. We determined that 4 out of the 13 studies that applied quantitative and mixed methods [18,29,57,60] yielded acceptable to good relationships between the resilience scales and well-being (Table 2). This finding affirms that the scales used in the identified studies actually measured resilience. However, gaps in the robustness of the tools still remain, as reflected in those studies with weak or no relationships. Interestingly, all the assessed studies were silent on the construct validity of their scales, which made it difficult to determine if the scales were a result of exploratory and confirmatory analyses and whether the subscales met the minimum threshold for factor analyses. Furthermore, the internal consistency of the scales was assessed in only two studies (n = 2) [18,29] with good outcomes; the rest of the studies seemed not to have applied this critical measure to their scales. The lack of evidence of internal consistency in most studies suggests key gaps in the scale constructs and their subsequent outcomes. Testing the internal consistency of scales is a critical component of the accuracy and validity of data interpretation [65]. None of the qualitative studies stated their scales for us to determine their appropriateness in measuring resilience. We applied a thematic synthesis of the findings and their corresponding discussions to identify common themes as a proxy for understanding their scales. Four common themes of community capacities, household capacities, indigenous/local knowledge, and political and governance capacities emerged. Similar themes emerged from the quantitative and mixed methods studies, with an extra theme of HIV/AIDS. This finding is consistent with studies from other regions that acknowledged a combination of a few themes or individual themes with spatial variations as resilience factors [66,67]. Banding these themes together makes this study unique and provides evidence to construct a contextual composite index for benchmarking resilience interventions in southern Africa. A contextual resilience index would guide interventions to specifically apply approaches that reflect the realities of the region. In the long run, this would increase the effectiveness and efficiency of resilience interventions.

The resilience capacities at the different levels function synergistically; for example, traditional institutions of governance were critical in mobilising communities and households for adaptation to climate-induced hazards [53]. Traditional governance institutions functioned in tandem with modern governance across the region to collectively manage resources, biodiversity, and adaptation [68]. The dualism of the traditional and the modern can be further leveraged to promote hybrid knowledge, behaviour, crops, and livestock species that enhance the resilience and well-being of recurrent drought-affected people. Besides traditional knowledge pre-dating scientific knowledge, its merits in drought adaptation and resilience cannot be understated. Studies from other regions found that the rich knowledge of traditional early warnings and their application minimised disaster-induced fatalities, injuries, and livelihood losses [69–71]. Harnessing and blending traditional knowledge with scientific knowledge will increase understanding and acceptability among different segments of society. In addition, it will produce localised information that addresses threats to livelihoods and well-being in specific contexts. However, there is a risk of traditional knowledge disappearing or becoming redundant as more people acquire formal western education where they inadvertently get cultural miseducation. Traditional practices are indicative of people's attachment to land and mastery of the environment. Their disappearance would lead to loss of centuries-old, rich knowledge and practices, as well as the detachment from land and the environment. Scholars have observed that detachment from land and environment aggravates its unsustainable exploitation, the loss of a community's adaptation capacities, and poor well-being outcomes [72–74].

Humanitarian interventions to mitigate disasters focused on welfare, a costly approach that provided only temporary relief [18,75]. While such interventions assist households to cope, they do not necessarily enhance resilience [14]. Our findings suggest multi-sectoral poverty alleviation interventions reinforced household and community level capacities to create resilient communities. This challenges the findings from other regions that confined resilience and well-being to household and community level capacities [76–79]. We advance that household level capacities work in tandem with community and governance level capacities to grow resilience and advance well-being outcomes.

Interestingly, only one study included in the review associated HIV/AIDS with droughts, yet evidence suggests that southern Africa has one of the world's highest HIV/AIDS burdens [80]. This mismatch suggests that drought-resilience interventions may be missing the nexus between the burden of HIV/AIDS and drought resilience. Addressing the burden of HIV/AIDS in the context of drought resilience would go a long way in reducing vulnerabilities and enhancing the well-being of households. It would also create a synergistic and comprehensive resilience framework that optimises resources and well-being outcomes.

Limitations

Firstly, the variability of study designs made meta-analysis inapplicable to this review. Secondly, we used common quality assessment tools that focus on specific areas of quality that could have differed from the aims and objectives of included studies. Thirdly, the generalisability and transferability of the findings beyond the study area should be taken with caution because our study parameters were restricted to southern Africa. We could have inadvertently excluded eligible studies that were not accessible, so only studies available and accessible were included in this review.

5. Policy Implications

This synthesis of evidence to identify the relationship between resilience to drought and health and well-being is timely and will assist to stimulate appropriate planning and policy interventions. Moreover, because the evidence suggests that there is strong likelihood of continuous occurrence of drought-induced disasters across the region. This calls for a serious review and update of regional and national disaster management policies which mostly aim to resist and/or mitigate disaster effects. New and revised policies that focus on the transformation of communities' capabilities and equip them in such a way as to cope and adapt to recurring drought conditions are urgently needed. Such policies should perceive resilience as a culture and a way of life just like droughts are quickly becoming. To achieve this, further research is necessary to establish the regional context specific resilience measurement constructs that will benchmark resilience policies and interventions. Such measurement constructs can be yielded from nurturing and supporting local-led research initiatives to ensure the outcomes are evidence-driven and not just transplanted from other regions without validation. There is an urgent need for a regional resilience institute to continuously generate evidence to inform regional and national policies. Such a structure will significantly reduce the cost and burden of droughts on the regional economies, agriculture, and people.

Additionally, there is need for policymakers to have clarity on the difference between resilience and disaster risk reduction interventions. Disaster risk reduction deals with the identification of hazards, analysis of hazard impacts and causes, and the removal or reduction of vulnerabilities [81]. On the contrary, resilience deals with the transformation of people's capacities to cope, overcome, and recover from disaster effects. Differentiating between the two would generate a paradigm shift and re-orient disaster governance from the conventional disaster management in the region to a new culture of resilience building. Equally important is the need for the external assistance to be focussed on boosting inherent resilience capacities rather than the periodical emergency responses.

6. Conclusions

Droughts remain a serious threat to well-being, and cannot be effectively stopped. However, peoples' capacities to cope, adapt, and live with it can be improved. This systematic review highlights the critical factors that can improve and unlock people's capacities to live with droughts. Our evidence suggests that resilience capacities are vested in households, communities, and at a government level. Poverty alleviation policies were important in strengthening resilience and well-being outcomes. Equally important was the need to leverage blended traditional knowledge with modern scientific knowledge to enhance resilience and optimise well-being outcomes. However blending traditional and scientific knowledge and processes remains a research gap, which, when addressed, will create a wider pool of disaster resilience information and knowledge. Additionally, it will preserve centuries of old traditions and increase acceptability and uptake by the segments of society.

We suggest that age, gender, race, and diversified livelihoods were central in mediating access to resources that unlocked household and community resilience. However, persistent drought-induced stress, food insecurity, hunger, age, racialised farming, and insecurity on farms undermined people's well-being. The need for resilience policies and interventions to focus on these key aspects cannot be understated.

Supplementary Materials: The following are available online at http://www.mdpi.com/1660-4601/15/11/2375/s1, Table S1: The PRISMA checklist, Table S2: Quality assessment of qualitative studies based on JBIQARI, Table S3: Quality assessment for grey literature based on AACODS, Table S4: Quality of peer-reviewed studies included based on NIH quality assessment checklist, Table S5: Rating of scales based on framework by Cyril and colleagues.

Author Contributions: J.K.K. and A.R. conceptualised the study; J.K.K. performed the searches, data selection, data extraction, and quality assessment; and wrote the manuscript. B.A. cross-validated the search and data extraction, independently performed the quality assessment, and enhanced the manuscript's intellectual content. A.R. reviewed and adjudicated papers about which there was disagreement as to whether they should be included. A.R. also revised the manuscript and made important contributions. K.A. reviewed the manuscript for intellectual content. All authors reviewed drafts of the manuscript and approved the final version.

Acknowledgments: Kaysha Carroll, University of Western Sydney, assisted in crafting the search strategy.

Conflicts of Interest: The authors declare no conflict of interest.

References

1. United Nations Office for Disaster Risk Reduction. *Sendai Framework for Disaster Risk Reduction 2015–2030*; UNISDR: Geneva, Switzerland, 2015; p. 32.
2. Dombrowsky, W.R. Again and again: Is a disaster what we call a 'disaster'? *Int. J. Mass Emerg. Disasters* **1995**, *13*, 241–254.
3. International Federation of the Red Cross and Red Crescent Societies. Types of Disasters: Definition of Hazard. Available online: http://www.ifrc.org/en/what-we-do/disaster-management/about-disasters/definition-of-hazard/ (accessed on 15 May 2018).
4. Chen, R.; Zhang, Y.; Xu, D.; Liu, M. Climate change and coastal megacities: Disaster risk assessment and responses in shanghai city. In *Climate Change, Extreme Events and Disaster Risk Reduction*; Springer: Berlin, Germany, 2018; pp. 203–216, ISBN 978-203-319-56468-56465.
5. Birnbaum, M.L.; Daily, E.K.; O'Rourke, A.P.; Loretti, A. Research and evaluations of the health aspects of disasters, part ix: Risk-reduction framework. *Prehosp. Disaster Med.* **2016**, *31*, 309–325. [CrossRef] [PubMed]
6. United Nations International Strategy for Disaster Risk Reduction. *Hyogo Framework for Action 2005–2015: Building the Resilience of Nations and Communities to Disaters. Extract from the Final Report of the World Conference on Disaster Reduction (a/conf.206/6)*; UN/ISDR: Geneva, Switzerland, 2007; p. 28.
7. Walsh-Dilley, M.; Wolford, W. (Un) defining resilience: Subjective understandings of 'resilience' from the field. *Resilience* **2015**, *3*, 173–182. [CrossRef]
8. Acosta, J.D.; Chandra, A.; Madrigano, J. An agenda to advance integrative resilience research and practice: Key themes from a resilience roundtable. *RAND Health Q.* **2017**, *7*, 5. [PubMed]
9. Manatsa, D.; Chingombe, W.; Matsikwa, H.; Matarira, C. The superior influence of Darwin sea level pressure anomalies over enso as a simple drought predictor for Southern Africa. *Theor. Appl. Climatol.* **2008**, *92*, 1–14. [CrossRef]
10. Manatsa, D.; Mushore, T.; Lenouo, A. Improved predictability of droughts over southern Africa using the standardized precipitation evapotranspiration index and enso. *Theor. Appl. Climatol.* **2017**, *127*, 259–274. [CrossRef]
11. Msangi, J. Drought hazard and desertification management in the Drylands of southern Africa. *Environ. Monit. Assess.* **2004**, *99*, 75–87. [CrossRef] [PubMed]
12. Campbell, D.J. Strategies for coping with severe food deficits in Rural Africa: A review of the literature. *Food Foodways* **1990**, *4*, 143–162. [CrossRef]
13. Tyson, P.D. *Climatic Change and Variability in Southern Africa*, 1st ed.; Oxford University Press: Cape Town, South Africa, 1986; p. 220, ISBN 0195704304.
14. Masih, I.; Maskey, S.; Mussá, F.; Trambauer, P. A review of droughts on the African continent: A geospatial and long-term perspective. *Hydrol. Earth Syst. Sci.* **2014**, *18*, 3635–3649. [CrossRef]
15. Mason, J.B.; Chotard, S.; Bailes, A.; Mebrahtu, S.; Hailey, P. Impact of drought and HIV on child nutrition in eastern and Southern Africa. *Food Nutr. Bull.* **2010**, *31*, S209–S218. [CrossRef] [PubMed]
16. Kamara, J.K.; Wali, N.; Agho, K.; Renzaho, A.M. Resilience to climate-induced disasters and its overall impact on well-being in Southern Africa: A mixed-methods systematic review protocol. *Syst. Rev.* **2018**, *7*, 127. [CrossRef] [PubMed]
17. Vogel, C.; Koch, I.; Van Zyl, K. "A persistent truth"—Reflections on rrought risk management in Southern Africa. *WCAS* **2010**, *2*, 9–22. [CrossRef]
18. Renzaho, A.M.; Kamara, J.K. *Building Resilience in Southern Africa: A Case Study of World Vision in Swaziland and Lesotho*; World Vision International: Johannesburg, South Africa, 2016; p. 96.

19. Gómez-Baggethun, E.; Reyes-García, V.; Olsson, P.; Montes, C. Traditional ecological knowledge and community resilience to environmental extremes: A case study in Doñana, SW Spain. *Glob. Environ. Chang.* **2012**, *22*, 640–650. [CrossRef]
20. Australian Government. Humanitarian Support for Crises in Africa. Available online: http://dfat.gov.au/aid/topics/investment-priorities/building-resilience/humanitarian-preparedness-and-response/Pages/humanitarian-support-for-crises-in-africa.aspx (accessed on 16 May 2018).
21. Office for Coordination of Humanitarian Assistance. *Riasco Action Plan for Southern Africa: Response Plan for the el Niño Induced Drought in Southern Africa May 2016–April 2017*; OCHA: Johannesburg, South Africa, 2016.
22. United States Agency for International Development. Dollar to Results: Usaid Investments and Illustrative Results. Available online: https://results.usaid.gov/results (accessed on 16 May 2018).
23. Office for the Coordination of Humanitarian Assistance. *Riasco Action Plan for Southern Africa: Review of the Regional Response Plan for the el Nino Induced Drought in Southern Africa*; OCHA: Johannesburg, South Africa, 2017.
24. Holloway, A. Disaster risk reduction in Southern Africa: Hot rhetoric—Cold reality. *Afr. Secur. Rev.* **2003**, *12*, 29–38. [CrossRef]
25. Vyas-Doorgapersad, S.; Lukamba, T. Disaster risk reduction policy for sustainable development in the Southern African development community: A policy perspective. *J. Public Adm.* **2012**, *47*, 774–784.
26. Villholth, K.G.; Tøttrup, C.; Stendel, M.; Maherry, A. Integrated mapping of groundwater drought risk in the Southern African development community (SADC) region. *Hydrogeol. J.* **2013**, *21*, 863–885. [CrossRef]
27. United Nations. *The United Nations Millenium Development Goals Report*; United Nations: New York, NY, USA, 2012.
28. Newsham, A.J.; Thomas, D.S. Knowing, farming and CLIMATE change adaptation in North-Central Namibia. *Glob. Environ. Chang.* **2011**, *21*, 761–770. [CrossRef]
29. Belle, J.; Hlalele, M. Vulnerability assessment of agricultural drought hazard: A case of koti-se phola community council. *J. Geogr. Nat. Disast.* **2015**, *5*, 143–149. [CrossRef]
30. Van Riet, G. Recurrent drought in the dr ruth segomotsi mompati district municipality of the north west province in South Africa: An environmental justice perspective. *Jàmbá* **2012**, *4*, 1–9. [CrossRef]
31. Southern Africa Development Community (SADC). Regional Vulnerability Assessment and Analysis Programme (RVAA). Available online: https://www.sadc.int/sadc-secretariat/directorates/office-deputy-executive-secretary-regional-integration/food-agriculture-natural-resources/regional-vulnerability-assessment-analysis-programme-rvaa/ (accessed on 29 September 2018).
32. Lim, S.S.; Allen, K.; Bhutta, Z.A.; Dandona, L.; Forouzanfar, M.H.; Fullman, N.; Gething, P.W.; Goldberg, E.M.; Hay, S.I.; Holmberg, M. Measuring the health-related sustainable development goals in 188 countries: A baseline analysis from the global burden of disease study 2015. *Lancet* **2016**, *388*, 1813–1850. [CrossRef]
33. Moher, D.; Liberati, A.; Tetzlaff, J.; Altman, D.G. Preferred reporting items for systematic reviews and meta-analyses: The PRISMA statement. *Ann. Intern. Med.* **2009**, *151*, 264–269. [CrossRef] [PubMed]
34. Kamara, J.K.; Dhingra, N.; Renzaho, A. Resilience to Climate Induced Disasters and Its Overall Impact on Well-Being in Southern Africa: A Systematic Review. Available online: http://www.crd.york.ac.uk/prospero/DisplayPDF.php?ID=CRD42017064396 (accessed on 10 October 2018).
35. United Nations. Standard Country or Area Codes for Statistical Use (m49): Geographic Regions. Available online: https://unstats.un.org/unsd/methodology/m49/ (accessed on 10 August 2018).
36. Higgins, J.P.; Green, S. Cochrane Handbook for Systematic Reviews of Interventions. Available online: http://handbook.cochrane.org (accessed on 11 August 2018).
37. Institute, J.B. *Joanna Briggs Institute Reviewers Manual*; Joan Briggs Institute: Adelaide, Australia, 2011.
38. Tyndall, J.; Flinders University. Aacods Checklist. Available online: https://dspace.flinders.edu.au/xmlui//bitstream/handle/2328/3326/AACODS_Checklist.pdf;jsessionid=AC42DFAFF5785B12B2822D1320159067?sequence=4 (accessed on 18 May 2018).
39. Toppenberg-Pejcic, D.; Noyes, J.; Allen, T.; Alexander, N.; Vanderford, M.; Gamhewage, G. Emergency risk communication: Lessons learned from a rapid review of recent gray literature on ebola, zika, and yellow fever. *J. Health Commun.* **2018**, 1–19. [CrossRef] [PubMed]
40. Hurley, C.; Shiely, F.; Power, J.; Clarke, M.; Eustace, J.A.; Flanagan, E.; Kearney, P.M. Risk based monitoring (RBM) tools for clinical trials: A systematic review. *Contemp. Clin. Trials* **2016**, *51*, 15–27. [CrossRef] [PubMed]

41. National Heart Lung and Blood Institute (NIH). Quality Assessment Tool for Observational Cohort and Cross-Sectional Studies. Available online: https://www.nhlbi.nih.gov/health-topics/study-quality-assessment-tools (accessed on 22 May 2018).
42. Mangin, D.; Stephen, G.; Bismah, V.; Risdon, C. Making patient values visible in healthcare: A systematic review of tools to assess patient treatment priorities and preferences in the context of multimorbidity. *BMJ Open* **2016**, *6*. [CrossRef] [PubMed]
43. Ward, J.L.; Harrison, K.; Viner, R.M.; Costello, A.; Heys, M. Adolescent cohorts assessing growth, cardiovascular and cognitive outcomes in low and middle-income countries. *PLoS ONE* **2018**, *13*. [CrossRef] [PubMed]
44. Woolford, M.H.; Weller, C.; Ibrahim, J.E. Unexplained absences and risk of death and injury among nursing home residents: A systematic review. *J. Am. Med. Dir. Assoc.* **2017**, *18*, 366.e1–366.e5. [CrossRef] [PubMed]
45. Nukunu, A.N. *A Critical Analysis of Decentraliastion and Community-Based Irrigation Water Resource Governance in Ghana*; University of New England: Armidale, Australia, 2014.
46. Tolley, E.E.; Ulin, P.R.; Mack, N.; Succop, S.M.; Robinson, E.T. *Qualitative Methods in Public Health: A Field Guide for Applied Research*, 2nd ed.; John Wiley & Sons: San Francisco, CA, USA, 2016; p. 344, ISBN 7981118834657.
47. Cyril, S.; Oldroyd, J.C.; Renzaho, A. Urbanisation, urbanicity, and health: A systematic review of the reliability and validity of urbanicity scales. *BMC Public Health* **2013**, *13*, 513. [CrossRef] [PubMed]
48. Jamnadass, R.; Dawson, I.; Franzel, S.; Leakey, R.; Mithöfer, D.; Akinnifesi, F.; Tchoundjeu, Z. Improving livelihoods and nutrition in sub-saharan africa through the promotion of indigenous and exotic fruit production in smallholders' agroforestry systems: A review. *Int. For. Rev.* **2011**, *13*, 338–354. [CrossRef]
49. Gulliver, A.; Griffiths, K.M.; Christensen, H. Perceived barriers and facilitators to mental health help-seeking in young people: A systematic review. *BMC Psychiatry* **2010**, *10*, 113. [CrossRef] [PubMed]
50. Thomas, J.; Harden, A. Methods for the thematic synthesis of qualitative research in systematic reviews. *BMC Med. Res. Methodol.* **2008**, *8*, 45. [CrossRef] [PubMed]
51. Rankoana, S.A. Perceptions of climate change and the potential for adaptation in a rural community in Limpopo province, South Africa. *Sustainability* **2016**, *8*, 672. [CrossRef]
52. Rankoana, S.A. Rainfall scarcity and its impacts on subsistence farming: The role of gender and religious rituals in adaptation to change. *Agenda* **2016**, *30*, 124–131. [CrossRef]
53. Ngwenya, B.; Thakadu, O.; Magole, L.; Chimbari, M. Memories of environmental change and local adaptations among Molapo farming communities in the Okavango delta, Botswana—A gender perspective. *Acta Trop.* **2017**, *175*, 31–41. [CrossRef] [PubMed]
54. Bahta, Y.T.; Jordaan, A.; Muyambo, F. Communal farmers' perception of drought in South Africa: Policy implication for drought risk reduction. *J. Disaster Risk Reduct.* **2016**, *20*, 39–50. [CrossRef]
55. Bareki, N.P.; Anitwi, M.A. Drought preparedness status of farmers in the Nguni cattle development project and the sire subsidy scheme in North West province, South Africa. *Appl. Ecol. Environ. Res.* **2017**, *15*, 589–603. [CrossRef]
56. Bunting, E.; Steele, J.; Keys, E.; Muyengwa, S.; Child, B.; Southworth, J. Local perception of risk to livelihoods in the semi-arid landscape of Southern Africa. *Land* **2013**, *2*, 225–251. [CrossRef]
57. Kolawole, O.D.; Moseki, R.M.; Ngwenya, B.N.; Thakadu, O.; Mmopelwa, G.; Donald Letsholo, K. Climate variability and rural livelihoods: How households perceive and adapt to climatic shocks in the Okavango Delta, Botswana. *WCAS* **2016**, *8*, 131–145. [CrossRef]
58. Thomas, D.S.G.; Twyman, C.; Osbahr, H.; Hewitson, B. Adaptation to climate change and variability: Farmer responses to intra-seasonal precipitation trends in South Africa. *Clim. Chang.* **2007**, *83*, 301–322. [CrossRef]
59. Mlenga, D.H.; Maseko, S. Factors influencing adoption of conservation agriculture: A case for increasing resilience to climate change and variability in Swaziland. *J. Environ. Earth Sci.* **2015**, *5*, 2224–3216.
60. Mlenga, D.H. Towards community resilience, focus on a rural water supply, sanitation and hygiene project in Swaziland. *AJRD* **2016**, *4*, 85–92. [CrossRef]
61. Akapalu, D.A. *Response Scenarios of Households to Drought-Driven Food Shortage in a Semi-Arid Area in South Africa*; University of Witwatersrand: Johannesburg, South Africa, 2005.
62. Hudson, J.W. *Responses to Climate Variability of the Livestock Sector in the North- West Province, South Africa*; Colorado State University: Fort Collins, CO, USA, 2002.

63. Shongwe, P.; Masuku, M.B.; Manyatsi, A.M. Factors influencing the choice of climate change adaptation strategies by households: A case of Mpolonjeni area development Programme (ADP) in Swaziland. *JAS* **2014**, *2*, 86–98. [CrossRef]
64. Mason, J.B.; Bailes, A.; Mason, K.E.; Yambi, O.; Jonsson, U.; Hudspeth, C.; Hailey, P.; Kendle, A.; Brunet, D.; Martel, P. Aids, drought, and child malnutrition in Southern Africa. *Public Health Nutr.* **2005**, *8*, 551–563. [CrossRef] [PubMed]
65. Tavakol, M.; Dennick, R. Making sense of cronbach's alpha. *Int. J. Med. Educ.* **2011**, *2*, 53–55. [CrossRef] [PubMed]
66. Lebel, L.; Anderies, J.; Campbell, B.; Folke, C.; Hatfield-Dodds, S.; Hughes, T.; Wilson, J. Governance and the capacity to manage resilience in regional social-ecological systems. *Ecol. Soc.* **2006**, *11*, 19. [CrossRef]
67. Cutter, S.L.; Burton, C.G.; Emrich, C.T. Disaster resilience indicators for benchmarking baseline conditions. *JHSEM* **2010**, *7*. [CrossRef]
68. Holzinger, K.; Kern, F.G.; Kromrey, D. The dualism of contemporary traditional governance and the state: Institutional setups and political consequences. *PRQ* **2016**, *69*, 469–481. [CrossRef]
69. Hiwasaki, L.; Luna, E.; Shaw, R. Process for integrating local and indigenous knowledge with science for hydro-meteorological disaster risk reduction and climate change adaptation in coastal and small island communities. *Int. J. Disaster Risk Reduct.* **2014**, *10*, 15–27. [CrossRef]
70. Audefroy, J.F.; Sánchez, B.N.C. Integrating local knowledge for climate change adaptation in Yucatán, Mexico. *IJSBE* **2017**, *6*, 228–237. [CrossRef]
71. Walshe, R.A.; Nunn, P.D. Integration of indigenous knowledge and disaster risk reduction: A case study from Baie Martelli, Pentecost Island, Vanuatu. *IJDRS* **2012**, *3*, 185–194. [CrossRef]
72. Beckford, C.L.; Jacobs, C.; Williams, N.; Nahdee, R. Aboriginal environmental wisdom, stewardship, and sustainability: Lessons from the Walpole island first nations, Ontario, Canada. *J. Environ. Educ.* **2010**, *41*, 239–248. [CrossRef]
73. Kingsley, J.; Townsend, M.; Henderson-Wilson, C.; Bolam, B. Developing an exploratory framework linking Australian aboriginal peoples' connection to country and concepts of wellbeing. *IJERPH* **2013**, *10*, 678–698. [CrossRef] [PubMed]
74. Booth, A.L.; Skelton, N.W. "You spoil everything!" indigenous peoples and the consequences of industrial development in British Columbia. *Environ. Dev. Sustain.* **2011**, *13*, 685–702. [CrossRef]
75. Waters, T. *Bureaucratizing the Good Samaritan: The Limitations of Humanitarian Relief Operations*; Routledge: New York, NY, USA, 2018; ISBN 9780429970498.
76. Elrick-Barr, C.E.; Preston, B.L.; Thomsen, D.C.; Smith, T.F. Toward a new conceptualization of household adaptive capacity to climate change: Applying a risk governance lens. *Ecol. Soc.* **2014**, *19*, 12. [CrossRef]
77. Van Der Vegt, G.S.; Essens, P.; Wahlström, M.; George, G. Managing risk and resilience. *Acad. Manag. J.* **2015**, *58*, 971–980. [CrossRef]
78. Tanner, T.; Lewis, D.; Wrathall, D.; Bronen, R.; Cradock-Henry, N.; Huq, S.; Lawless, C.; Nawrotzki, R.; Prasad, V.; Rahman, M.A. Livelihood resilience in the face of climate change. *Nat. Clim. Chang.* **2015**, *5*, 23. [CrossRef]
79. Fielke, S.J.; Srinivasan, M. Co-innovation to increase community resilience: Influencing irrigation efficiency in the waimakariri irrigation scheme. *Sustain. Sci.* **2018**, *13*, 255–267. [CrossRef]
80. Murray, C.J.; Ortblad, K.F.; Guinovart, C.; Lim, S.S.; Wolock, T.M.; Roberts, D.A.; Dansereau, E.A.; Graetz, N.; Barber, R.M.; Brown, J.C. Global, regional, and national incidence and mortality for hiv, tuberculosis, and malaria during 1990–2013: A systematic analysis for the global burden of disease study 2013. *Lancet* **2014**, *384*, 1005–1070. [CrossRef]
81. United Nations International Strategy for Disaster Reduction. *United Nations International Strategy for Disaster Reduction*; United Nations: Geneva, Switzerland, 2009.

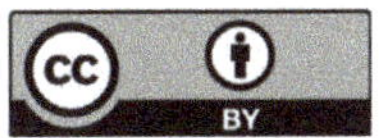

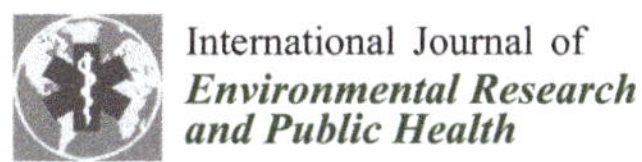

International Journal of
Environmental Research and Public Health

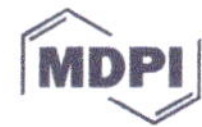

Article

Health Consequences of an Armed Conflict in Zamboanga, Philippines Using a Syndromic Surveillance Database

Miguel Antonio Salazar [1,2,*], Ronald Law [3,4] and Volker Winkler [1,*]

1 Institute of Global Health, University of Heidelberg, Im Neuenheimer Feld 324, 69120 Heidelberg, Germany
2 Graduate School, Angeles University Foundation, Angeles City, Pampanga 2009, Philippines
3 Department of Health, Health Emergency Management Bureau, Sta. Cruz, Manila 1003, Philippines; rplaw@doh.gov.ph
4 College of Public Health, University of the Philippines, Manila 1000, Philippines
* Correspondence: mike.salazar@uni-heidelberg.de (M.A.S.); v.winkler@uni-heidelberg.de (V.W.); Tel.: +63928-6582700 (M.A.S.); +49-6221-56-5031 (V.W.)

Received: 3 November 2018; Accepted: 26 November 2018; Published: 29 November 2018

Abstract: The Zamboanga armed conflict was a 19-day long encounter in the Philippines in 2013 that displaced 119,000 people from their homes. This study describes the health consequences of this complex emergency in different age groups, time periods, and health facilities using data from Surveillance in Post Extreme Emergencies and Disasters (SPEED). This is a descriptive study of the SPEED database spanning 196 days of observation post-disaster and 1065 SPEED reports from 49 health facilities. Evacuation centers and village health centers, both primary care facilities, had the highest number of consults. Common infections and noncommunicable diseases were the most common reasons for consultations, namely, acute respiratory infections, fever, watery diarrhea, skin disease, and hypertension. Infections can be associated with environmental conditions in displaced populations, while hypertension has a high prevalence in the country and implies long-term care. Conflict-related injuries and deaths were not frequently observed due to the volatile situation that influenced health-seeking behavior as well as possible reporting gaps. In conclusion, in complex emergencies, as in natural disasters, wherein early alert and warning for potential outbreaks is crucial, SPEED can assist decision makers on response and recovery interventions. Linkages between SPEED and other surveillance and reporting systems need to be explored.

Keywords: disasters; armed conflict; complex emergencies; syndromic surveillance

---

1. Introduction

On September 9, 2013, in the city of Zamboanga, Philippines, a gun battle ensued between the Philippine Armed Forces and the Moro National Liberation Front (MNLF). The MNLF engaged government forces in five villages, or barangays, the country's smallest governance division. The hostilities ended 19 days after the start of the encounter. During the course and in the aftermath of the military skirmish, 118,819 individuals were affected and evacuated from their homes [1]. Six months after the encounter, only half of the affected population were able to return to their homes. The conflict compromised the nutrition and hygiene of the 20,000 internally displaced people in the two largest evacuation sites [2]. The Zamboanga armed conflict may be considered a complex emergency, as it fits the definition of a humanitarian event due to armed conflict, political destabilization, food supply shortages, displacement of populations, and health systems disruption [3].

Conflict and the resulting displacement of affected residents leads to health consequences. Traditionally, communicable diseases have been the focus of disaster management and refugee health [4,5]. Displaced populations are particularly susceptible to communicable diseases because of risk factors such as cramped housing, environmental damage, economic difficulty, lack of hygiene and clean water supply, inadequate nutrition, and lack of basic health services. Diarrhea and acute respiratory infections are the two most common causes of morbidity and mortality in displaced populations [5]. Measles, on the other hand, is a highly deadly disease in situations where shelter is poorly planned, people live in close proximity to each other, and immunization rates are low [4–7].

Furthermore, noncommunicable diseases (NCDs) have been seen to have a significant burden on health services post-disaster regardless of whether the event is due to natural hazards or conflict [5,8,9]. NCDs, due to prolonged treatment and the need for coordinated long-term care, pose a challenge during disaster response and recovery because of the resulting disrupted and unresponsive health system [8]. NCD treatment may either be neglected or inadequate in a disaster setting if response is poorly planned and NCDs are not considered a priority [9].

Complex emergencies are situations where livelihood and life are threatened by war, civil disturbance, and migration of people in the midst of political instability and security threats, all of which make emergency response difficult [10]. The types of injuries observed from complex emergencies may be different from disasters due to natural hazards such as typhoons and earthquakes. Violent trauma comprises one of the major direct health impacts in armed conflicts. Its effects may vary from the type and location of the conflict. In complex emergencies in Eastern Europe, violent trauma contributed to the majority of direct morbidity and mortality; however, its significance in complex emergencies in Asia and Africa was typically less due to the predominance of infectious diseases [3]. Natural hazards due to typhoons and earthquakes cause more deaths from injuries, which may be due to drowning and crush injuries, respectively [11–13]. For morbidity, minor injuries such as bruises, cuts, and burns played a more significant role compared to fractures in natural hazards in the Philippines in 2013 [14,15].

Surveillance for Post Extreme Emergencies and Disasters (SPEED) is a syndromic surveillance system deployed specifically after disasters and emergencies and is a joint project of the Philippine Department of Health (DOH) and the World Health Organization established in 2011 [16,17]. Disease surveillance and early warning systems have the ability to inform decision makers on possible disaster risks [18]. Multi-hazard early warning systems are integral parts of understanding disaster risk—one of the priorities under the Sendai Framework for Disaster Risk Reduction 2015–2030 [19]. Health Emergency and Disaster Risk Management (H-EDRM) is a concept that covers the intersection between disaster risk reduction management and health. It is suggested that research in this field should include needs assessments, monitoring, and evaluation and reporting systems that can measure health indicators in all phases of disasters: mitigation, preparedness, response, and recovery [20]. SPEED is an example of a reporting system in H-EDRM focused on disaster response and recovery.

Previous studies in the Philippines have looked into the health effects of natural hazards using SPEED. In the aftermath of the natural hazards in the Philippines in 2013, namely a flood, typhoon, and an earthquake, SPEED data showed that infectious diseases still dominated in morbidity; however, NCDs had a substantial burden to the health systems of the affected populations [14,15,21]. Although SPEED was also deployed in the Zamboanga armed conflict, the health effects of this complex emergency have yet to be studied using SPEED data. This study aims to describe the health consequences of the Zamboanga armed conflict on consultations for communicable diseases, injuries, and NCDs in different age groups, time periods, and health facility types using data from SPEED and their health system implications.

2. Materials and Methods

This study analyzed the SPEED database specifically for the Zamboanga armed conflict in 2013. SPEED was activated in Zamboanga City from 11 September 2013 to 24 March 2014, thereby beginning two days after the onset of the Zamboanga siege and spanning 196 days in total. The SPEED reports are comprised of all disease consultations for a particular day fitting the case definitions regardless of attribution to the disaster for a specific health facility, which includes village health centers, evacuation centers, hospitals, and community health centers. SPEED reports can be submitted to the system on a daily basis either manually, via Short-Messaging System (SMS), or through the internet by the designated public health nurse or data encoder [17].

Similar to previous studies done for SPEED, the 21 disease entities were divided into three groups: communicable diseases, NCDs, and injuries [14,15]. Communicable diseases included in SPEED are acute bloody diarrhea, acute flaccid paralysis, acute hemorrhagic fever, acute jaundice syndrome, acute respiratory infection (ARI), acute watery diarrhea, animal bites, conjunctivitis, fever, fever with other symptoms (FOS), suspected leptospirosis, skin disease, suspected measles, suspected meningitis, and tetanus. Fractures and wounds (including bruises and burns) make up the injury group, while noncommunicable diseases are comprised of acute asthmatic attack, acute malnutrition, high blood pressure, and known diabetes mellitus. Descriptions for each of the 21 syndromes have been mentioned by Salazar et al. in 2016 and in the SPEED Operations Manual [14,17].

The database is composed of reports with disease or syndrome counts for a particular health facility per day. There were two observed age groups: individuals under the age of five and those aged five and older. Rates were established with the denominator as either the population of the village or municipality, depending on the health facility type. Village health centers and evacuation centers used the village population, while hospitals and community health centers used the city population. The 2010 Philippine census data for villages was used for the denominator for village health center and evacuation center rates, while municipality census data was used for hospital and community health center rates. Rates were presented as per 10,000 population, similar to other studies conducted on SPEED [14,15,22].

Similar to the analysis of SPEED for typhoon Haiyan, the Bohol earthquake, and the Luzon flood in the Philippines, two time periods, less than or equal to two months and greater than two months post-disaster, were compared in this study. These time periods corresponded to disaster response and recovery, respectively [14]. To compare rates for the two disaster time periods, Poisson regression was used [23]. Consultation rates for health facility types and the mean difference between age groups (under five and five and older) were presented as mean rates with 95% confidence intervals. To illustrate total daily consultation rates among the four health facility types across the observed time period, models for each of the health facility types were derived using the multivariable fractional polynomial method [24]. Day zero for this study was pegged at the onset of the conflict.

This is a descriptive study of the SPEED database managed by the Health Emergency Management Bureau (HEMB) of the DOH. SPEED uses aggregated and anonymized data from health facilities and evacuation centers affected by emergencies and disasters. The SPEED data for the Zamboanga armed conflict was requested from the director of HEMB and the authors had exclusive access to the data.

3. Results

3.1. Health Facilities

There were 1065 SPEED reports during the Zamboanga armed conflict within a 196-day period of observation post-disaster. The first SPEED report was transmitted on the second day of the armed conflict. There was a decrease in the number of SPEED reports after the first day of reporting; however, the most notable drop happened around the 60th to 80th day, where the number of reports thereafter plateaued (see Figure 1).

Among the 49 reporting health facilities, 21 were evacuation centers, 15 were village health centers, nine were hospitals, and four were community health centers. Evacuation centers (448) had the most reports, followed by village health centers (297), hospitals (266), and community health centers (54). Comparing the total rates of consultations seen per day for the four facilities, evacuation centers (32.3 per 10,000 population) were on top, with village health centers (24.8 per 10,000 population), hospitals (0.3 per 10,000 population), and community health centers (0.2 per 10,000 population) following suit. For all health facility types, there were more daily consultations in the response period than during the recovery period (see Table 1).

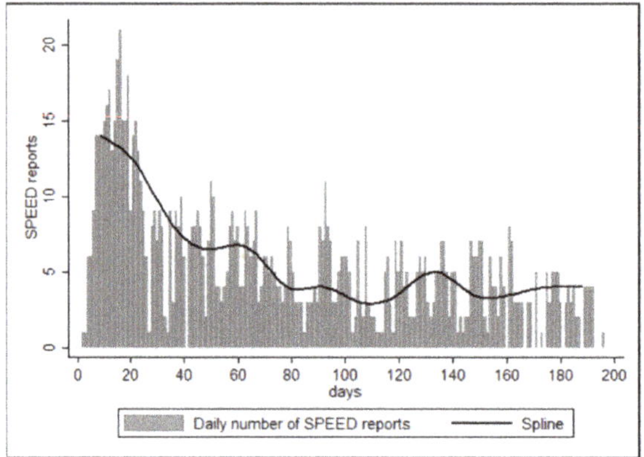

Figure 1. Bar graph of daily number of Surveillance in Post Extreme Emergencies and Disasters (SPEED) reports with spline.

Table 1. Total consultation rates per 10,000 individuals for health facility types comparing time post-disaster.

Health Facility Type	Mean Number of Consultations per Day (95% Confidence Intervals) (*n*)	≤2 Months (Response) (*n*)	>2 Months (Recovery) (*n*)	Difference between ≤2 Months and >2 Months (*p*-value)
Evacuation center	32.3 (27.9–36.7) (*n* = 448)	34.3 (*n* = 373)	22.4 (*n* = 75)	11.9 (<0.01)
Village health center	28.5 (24.5–32.5) (*n* = 297)	65.5 (*n* = 70)	17.1 (*n* = 227)	48.4 (<0.01)
Hospital	0.3 (0.2–0.3) (*n* = 266)	0.5 (*n* = 68)	0.2 (*n* = 198)	0.3 (<0.01)
Community health center	0.2 (0.1–0.2) (*n* = 54)	0.4 (*n* = 13)	0.1 (*n* = 41)	0.3 (0.03)
Regardless of facility type	21.6 (19.3–23.9) (*n* = 1065)	33.2 (*n* = 524)	10.3 (*n* = 541)	22.9 (<0.01)

Modeled rates for hospitals and community health centers showed little variability. Evacuation centers and village health centers differed considerably in their modeled rates. For village health centers, there was an exponential decrease in the total daily consultation rates, while evacuation centers had a delayed peak with a less profound decline (see Figure 2).

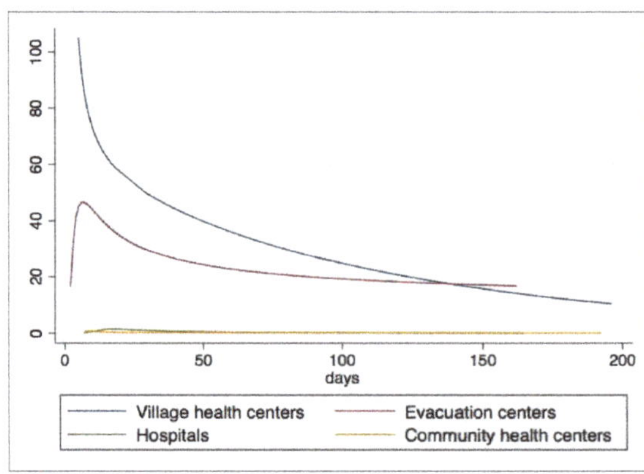

Figure 2. Poisson regressions for daily total consultations per 10,000 individuals across time for different health facility types.

There was a notable difference between the time periods, within two months (response) and after two months (recovery), regardless of health facility type. There were similar numbers of SPEED reports for both the response (524) and recovery (541) periods. When disaggregated by health facility type, evacuation centers had more reports in the response period. The other three health facility types had more SPEED reports during the recovery period. Similar to the visualized models, village health centers had the highest difference between the rates of the two time periods. The disaster response period had significantly higher rates for all four health facilities when comparing total consultation rates (see Table 1).

3.2. Syndrome Rates

Communicable diseases such as acute respiratory infections (11.3 per 10,000 population), fever (3.5), acute watery diarrhea (2.3), and skin disease (1.7) had the highest syndrome rates among all 21 syndromes. Hypertension was the only disease entity that had a syndrome rate ≥1 per 10,000 population and was not communicable in nature (see Table 2). Injuries such as fractures and wounds had daily rates below 1 per 10,000 individuals, but there were more cases of wounds (1982) than of fractures (154) in terms of absolute number of cases.

Table 2. Top syndrome rates per 10,000 individuals separated by time post-disaster and by age.

Syndrome	Total n = 1065	≤2 Months (Response) n = 524	>2 Months (Recovery) n = 541	Difference between ≤2 Months and >2 Months (p-value)	<5 Years of Age	≥5 Years of Age	Difference between <5 Years and ≥5 Years (95% Confidence Interval)
				Communicable diseases			
Acute respiratory infection (ARI)	11.3	18.0	4.8	13.2 (<0.01)	41.8	7.2	34.7 (30.7–38.6)
Fever	3.5	4.9	2.2	2.7 (<0.01)	14.0	2.1	11.8 (10.1–13.6)
Acute watery diarrhea	2.3	3.8	0.9	2.9 (<0.01)	8.5	1.5	7.0 (5.9–8.1)
Skin disease	1.7	2.4	1	1.4 (<0.01)	5.7	1.2	4.5 (3.7–5.3)
Fever with other symptoms (FOS)	0.3	<0.1	0.1	0.5 (<0.01)	*0.3*	*0.3*	<0.1 (−0.1–0.2)
Communicable disease total	19.4	29.9	9.3	20.6 (<0.01)	71.1	12.5	58.6 (52.0–65.2)
				Injuries			
Open wounds and bruises/burns	0.7	0.9	0.4	0.4 (<0.01)	0.9	0.6	0.3 (0.1–0.5)
Injury total	0.7	0.9	0.4	0.4 (<0.01)	0.9	0.6	0.3 (0.1–0.5)
				Non-communicable diseases (NCDs)			
High blood pressure	1.0	1.8	0.3	1.4 (<0.01)	<0.1	1.2	1.2 (1.0–1.4)
Acute asthmatic attack	0.4	0.6	0.2	0.4 (<0.01)	1.1	0.3	0.8 (0.6–1.0)
NCD total	1.5	2.4	0.6	1.8 (<0.01)	1.4	1.5	0.1 (−0.3–0.5)

The majority of the disease entities had higher rates in the disaster response period compared to the recovery period. Comparing the two disaster phases, among the 21 diseases, 13 had p-values less than 0.05. For communicable diseases, these were ARI, fever, acute watery diarrhea, skin disease, FOS, conjunctivitis, suspected measles, acute bloody diarrhea, and animal bites. ARI, fever, acute watery diarrhea, skin disease, acute bloody diarrhea, and animal bites had higher rates for the disaster response period compared to the recovery period. FOS, suspected measles, and acute bloody diarrhea, on the other hand, had higher rates for the disaster recovery period. The other four were wounds, bruises, and burns for injuries and high blood pressure, acute asthmatic attack, and diabetes for NCDs (See Table 2). Acute flaccid paralysis had no consults for the whole period of observation.

All the disease entities for communicable diseases had higher rates for the under-five age group, except for FOS, tetanus, and suspected meningitis. High blood pressure, diabetes mellitus, and fractures were the other diseases with higher rates for those five years and older. Of these six syndromes, the communicable diseases, FOS, tetanus, and suspected meningitis had 95% confidence intervals crossing zero.

3.3. Syndromes of Outbreak Potential

The DOH has a list of diseases of epidemic potential that are classified as either an immediately notifiable or a weekly notifiable disease or syndrome [25]. Among the diseases and syndromes in SPEED, acute flaccid paralysis, tetanus, animal bites (proxy for rabies), and suspected measles warrant immediate notification based on the directives of the DOH. Notifiable diseases for weekly reporting included in SPEED are the following: acute bloody diarrhea, suspected meningitis, acute watery diarrhea (which could be cholera), suspected leptospirosis, and FOS (which could be either typhoid or malaria) [25,26]. For the whole observation period, looking at the actual number of cases, there was no consult for acute flaccid paralysis, 12 for tetanus, 235 for animal bites, 60 for suspected measles, 60 for acute bloody diarrhea, 4 for suspected meningitis, 4781 for acute watery diarrhea, 31 for suspected leptospirosis, and 794 for FOS.

When visualized across time, the top immediately notifiable and weekly notifiable diseases were seen to have differing characteristics. Again, looking at the actual number of cases per day, there were more reported cases of acute watery diarrhea and FOS, which are weekly notifiable diseases, compared to animal bites and suspected measles, which are immediately notifiable diseases. Suspected measles had spikes in both the response and recovery periods, while animal bite cases had a peak in the end of the disaster response period (around the 2-month mark) and decreased thereafter. Acute watery diarrhea consistently had a higher number of cases during the disaster response period, while there were variable peaks for FOS across the observed time period (see Figure 3).

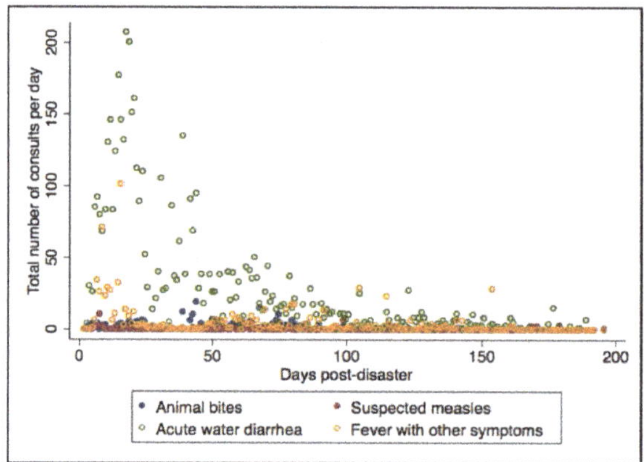

Figure 3. Total daily consultations of the most common immediately notifiable syndromes (animal bites and suspected measles) and the most common weekly notifiable syndromes (acute watery diarrhea and fever with other symptoms) across time among all reporting health facilities.

4. Discussion

4.1. Common Syndromes

In complex emergencies, communicable diseases are the usual primary care conditions [5,27]. The Zamboanga armed conflict was no exception. The top five syndromes observed can be managed in primary care settings. Similarly, in disasters in the same year (Bohol earthquake, typhoon Haiyan, and the Luzon flood), acute respiratory infections were also the most common followed by fever, acute water diarrhea, and skin disease. NCDs were also part of the top six syndromes in the form of hypertension [14,15]. However, compared to the disasters ensuing from natural hazards, wounds did not figure prominently in the disease burden in this armed conflict [14].

The top communicable disease in the Zamboanga armed conflict, ARI, reflected the yearly morbidity profile of the Zamboanga peninsula [28]. This was not the case for fever, acute watery diarrhea, and skin disease, which garnered the succeeding top numbers of consultations during the response and recovery periods post-disaster. However, the three syndromes can be associated to the environmental conditions experienced by the displaced individuals in the aftermath of the conflict, namely loss of shelter, decreased food security, and compromised access to water, sanitation, and hygiene [5,10]. The conflict displaced 80,757 individuals who were placed in 60 evacuation centers while 38,062 displaced people went to the homes of their families or relatives [1]. Those living in evacuation centers were faced with difficulties in accessing food, clean water, sanitation, and proper shelter [29]. All top four disease syndromes are communicable in nature and may be attributed to conditions in evacuation areas or temporary homes where basic services are sub-optimally provided [5,30].

NCDs represented by hypertension, the fifth most common syndrome seen in this study, are included in the top morbidities in the Zamboanga region and the Philippines in general [28]. Hypertension had been previously studied in disasters in the Philippines. In Typhoon Haiyan, hypertension was also the most common NCD and the third most common among the 21 syndromes of SPEED [15,21]. In another study done after Haiyan, hypertension was included in the top three diagnoses for adults seeking consult from mobile medical teams in 40 villages in the provinces of Samar and Leyte [31]. In 2013, hypertension was the third most common cause of morbidity in the general Philippine population, while in the Zamboanga Peninsula, the region of Zamboanga City, it was the second highest [28]. As the population is moving towards increased food availability and having sedentary work environments during normal times, people already have an increased risk of having NCDs [32]. When displaced populations who are exposed to protracted emergencies or a prolonged rehabilitation process such as in Zamboanga [29] are given packaged food with low nutritional value, have limited space for free movement, and have decreased physical activity, vulnerability to NCDs is further magnified.

Compared to other studies looking at natural hazards also using the SPEED database, the Zamboanga armed conflict had lower rates for injuries, namely wounds and fractures. In typhoon Haiyan and the Bohol earthquake, injuries resulted in rates of 1.4 and 1.2 consultations per 10,000 population, respectively. The Zamboanga armed conflict witnessed 0.7 consultations per 10,000 for injuries. The injuries seen in the typhoon and the earthquake were mostly minor in nature [14]. These injuries could be attributed to the magnitude and force of the disaster, where the affected population sustained direct injuries because of fallen structures and debris as a result of the earthquake or flying and floating debris brought about by typhoons and floods. Susceptibility to injuries is inversely related to the capacity for physical protection [33,34]. In contrast, the injuries in conflict can be attributed to gunshots or other forms of violence; however, it is hypothesized that not all people displaced by the conflict actually dealt with hazards such as gunshots, bombings, or grenades, or if they did, SPEED was not able to capture it. The consultations seen in SPEED reflected this disparity, where minor injuries were not as common in the conflict compared to natural hazards. However, these rates may also be underestimated because not all people who are injured will seek medical care or will be brought to health facilities because of several factors unique in the context of complex emergencies [35].

4.2. Mortality

Deaths related to violence are usually the perceived hallmark of conflicts. In Eastern Europe, trauma-related deaths predominated in the conflict in Bosnia-Herzegovina. In Asia and Africa, on the other hand, deaths due to infectious diseases and those related to malnutrition predominated [3]. In total, there were 13 deaths reported in SPEED across the observed time period ranging from day 2 to day 196. There were five deaths within the response period and eight deaths in the recovery period. There were 11 deaths reported from hospitals, while there was one death each for village health centers and community health centers. Fever was the cause of the most number of deaths among disease syndromes, with six deaths, followed by four for leptospirosis, two for hypertension, and one for wounds. The deaths reflected in SPEED, mostly communicable in nature, do not give a comprehensive picture of deaths that occurred as a consequence of the conflict.

There were differences in the deaths reported through SPEED to that of the DOH's official mortality tally. According to the DOH, there were 268 deaths due to gunshot wounds in the Zamboanga armed conflict; however, these were not reflected in SPEED [36]. As these deaths were direct effects of the 19-day long conflict and may not have been treated in a health facility, these records could not be captured by SPEED, a health facility-dependent reporting system. In addition, as health facilities did not report daily, there were deaths that could have been missed on days in which the health facility did not send a SPEED report. Nevertheless, the reporting of deaths in the SPEED database should be further scrutinized. A time series analysis on the different systems of certifying and registering deaths after disasters, whether natural or human-induced, is suggested. Also, a delineation between direct and indirect causes of deaths will be essential. These would give a more complete picture of the impact of complex emergencies and natural disasters on mortality, such as the causes of deaths and the temporality or the relation to time post-disaster.

4.3. Health Facility Type

Evacuation centers had the highest number of consults per health facility per day regardless of time period post-disaster. However, during the response period to the Zamboanga armed conflict, there were more consults during the first two months post-disaster in village health centers. This may be the time when the situation had stabilized. It also shows the importance of evacuation centers as points for delivery of basic health services to the displaced population. It is hypothesized that the affected population was familiar with the village health centers, the frontline primary health care facilities, and their services, thus they sought health care in these facilities. However, as the population moved to temporary shelters, health services were delivered in the evacuation centers, explaining the large number of consultations reported from evacuation centers.

There were more SPEED reports and a higher number of consultations coming from village health centers and evacuation centers in the Zamboanga armed conflict compared to typhoon Haiyan, where SPEED was also used. In typhoon Haiyan, village health centers had the most consultations on average; however, village health centers comprised only a minority of the SPEED reports and had the highest variability. Furthermore, the distribution of consultations for health facilities across time were not discussed in publications on Haiyan using SPEED [15]. This study, on the other hand, gives a visualization of the consultations for evacuations centers and village health centers across time, showing the difference between disaster response and recovery. Reports from village health centers and evacuation centers also made up the majority of SPEED reports for this particular disaster. This study demonstrates the importance of evacuation centers and village health centers as health facilities being utilized by the displaced population to gain access to basic health services during response and recovery.

The magnitude of the disaster could have played a role in the predominance of reports from village health centers in the Zamboanga armed conflict, which was isolated to one city, compared to typhoon Haiyan, where nine regions of the Philippines were affected. The importance of community health centers in typhoon Haiyan could have reflected the need to optimize aid, since these were the main health facilities and seats of health governance of the municipalities affected [15]. Since the health system disruption of the conflict was less than typhoon Haiyan and localized within one city, relief efforts could have been distributed more to village health centers and evacuation centers.

4.4. Policy and Health System Implications

As part of its mandate of informing the decisions of health policy makers and providing them with early warning systems to detect possible outbreaks of conditions expected in disasters and emergencies [17], SPEED's performance during the Zamboanga armed conflict showed that it was able to detect possible measles and cholera outbreaks. Episodes of animal bites were also recorded, which could have prompted public health measures to control stray dogs and other animals in the city. However, syndromic surveillance was shown to have limited capacity in investigating conditions that are not part of the case definitions. As disease entities are not specific and are not confirmed in the laboratory, these reported cases must be investigated further.

Event-based surveillance can feed from the real-time, location-specific reports from SPEED and lead surveillance teams to areas with unusual increases in syndrome consultations. As event-based surveillance entails rapid detection and assessment of public health events and emergencies, the team can further examine and respond to possible outbreaks identified from SPEED [37].

For SPEED to be fully utilized by public health decision makers and H-EDRM researchers, the system has to be integrated with other surveillance systems already used by the DOH. The suggestions by Foldy in 2004 to improve outcomes of surveillance systems adapted to SPEED are the following: (1) the SPEED database should be available to be mined, (2) the results from SPEED should have user-friendly visual displays or a SPEED dashboard, (3) there should be capacity for diverse technical inputs to understand complex data, (4) surveillance should be linked to response, and (5) there should be institutional capacity to confirm the diagnosis, both clinical and laboratory [38]. This entails coordination among different bureaus within the DOH. SPEED is under the Health Emergency Management Bureau, while the other surveillance systems are under the Epidemiology Bureau of the DOH. Moreover, it was observed that health facilities were not consistent in sending daily SPEED reports. The gaps in the reporting in SPEED, whether in terms of morbidity and mortality, shows the need for further validation through different data sources within and outside government to get the best picture of the complex emergency or disaster. It is also prudent to assess the reporting system for deaths post-disasters in health facilities and investigate the process of certification and reporting. These can provide information on the mechanisms of death, classification, and possible public health interventions.

Since disasters from natural hazards and complex emergencies amplify health systems' weaknesses and needs [10,14], other health services should be monitored aside from infectious diseases, non-communicable diseases, and injuries. Mental health services during and after conflicts are essential during disaster response and recovery. In a humanitarian setting, mental health conditions could be preexisting, trauma-induced, or triggered by failures in basic services during response and recovery [39,40]. On the other hand, women still needed to access maternal health services during the on-going conflict in Zamboanga. Consultations for antenatal, delivery, and postnatal care were seen in evacuation centers and in health facilities [41]. Aside from emergency obstetric care, the minimum initial service package in humanitarian emergencies also includes other interventions under reproductive health, such as those for sexual violence, contraception, and HIV [42]. When it was first developed in 2011, SPEED did not include syndromes or diseases pertaining to mental health or maternal health. The inclusion of mental health and reproductive health in SPEED can be further studied by the DOH to be able to capture important concerns that can guide provision of more specific health services.

4.5. Limitations

The SPEED database is dependent on the use of the health workforce who may be preoccupied and overworked during times of emergencies and disasters. The use of the system and its activation is dependent on the decisions of either the local chief executive, health officer, or the DOH. This in turn affects the allocated human resources and logistics deployed to support SPEED's operational requirement [17]. The required continued monitoring and governance by health officials coupled with other external stressors in disaster response and recovery could have led to the inconsistencies in the reporting of health facilities in the aftermath of the complex emergency.

The data quality of SPEED needs to be further evaluated even though SPEED results are initially validated by HEMB [14]. As a secondary data source without confirmed diagnoses, results from SPEED can only be used for descriptive studies and not for confirming the need for declaring outbreaks [17]. Furthermore, as SPEED is housed in HEMB and isolated from other disease surveillance systems, coordination among DOH bureaus needs to be improved in order to have an integrated disease surveillance and response system both in disasters and in normal times.

5. Conclusions

The SPEED data for the Zamboanga armed conflict showed that primary care conditions such as common infections and NCDs were the most prevalent reasons for consultations. Evacuation centers had the highest rates and the highest number of SPEED reports, thus highlighting the importance of the health facilities nearest to the population affected. Common infectious diseases, such as ARI, fever, watery diarrhea, and skin disease, may be associated with environmental conditions of displaced populations in contexts wherein essential health services are lacking or inadequate. Hypertension, on the other hand, is a common condition needing chronic and long-term care. These forms of considerations validate the emphasis that must be placed on primary health care in the immediate aftermath of disasters, whether natural or human-induced. Lastly, SPEED was able to assist decision makers on identifying possible outbreaks, which were averted; however, it did not pick up a high number of injuries and deaths due to violence expected from complex emergencies. SPEED is also in isolation from other reporting systems. It is suggested that linkages between SPEED and other surveillance systems, such as event-based surveillance and indicator-based surveillance and other reporting systems used especially for trauma and deaths, be strengthened to better illustrate the public health impacts of complex emergencies. Coordination within the DOH needs to be improved in order to have a truly integrated disease surveillance system.

Author Contributions: The authors of this manuscript were involved in the conception and design of the study or have contributed to the acquisition, analysis, or interpretation of the data of the study. They took part in its critical revision. They have agreed to be accountable for all aspects of the work. M.A.S. wrote the manuscript, conceptualized the study, interpreted the results, and collated the responses and comments from other authors. R.L. was vital in the acquisition of data and was part of the analysis of the results and the revision of the manuscript. V.W. contributed to the writing of the manuscript, conceptualization of the study, and the analysis of the results.

Funding: We acknowledge financial support by Deutsche Forschungsgemeinschaft within the funding programme Open Access Publishing, by the Baden-Württemberg Ministry of Science, Research and the Arts and by Ruprecht-Karls-Universität Heidelberg.

Acknowledgments: The authors would like to thank the leadership and staff of the Health Emergency Management Bureau of the Department of Health for their technical support and guidance in the completion of this study. The views stated in this article are those of the authors and do not necessarily reflect the official policy or position of the Health Emergency Management Bureau or the Philippine Department of Health.

Conflicts of Interest: The authors declare no conflict of interest.

References

1. National Disaster Risk Reduction and Management Council. *Final Report Re Armed Conflict in Zamboanga City and Basilan Province*; National Disaster Risk Reduction and Management Council: Quezon City, Philippines, 2013.
2. United Nations Office for the Coordination of Humanitarian Affairs. *Philippines: Zamboanga Action Plan 2014 (Revision)*; United Nations Office for the Coordination of Humanitarian Affairs: Makati, Philippines, 2014; Volume 30.
3. Brennan, R.J.; Nandy, R. Complex Humanitarian Emergencies: A Major Global Health Challenge. *Emerg. Med.* **2001**, *13*, 147–156. [CrossRef]
4. Médecins, S.F. *Refugee Health: An Approach to Emergency Situations*; Médecins Sans Frontières: Geneva, Switzerland, 1997.
5. Connolly, M.A.; Gayer, M.; Ryan, M.J.; Salama, P.; Spiegel, P.; Heymann, D.L. Communicable Diseases in Complex Emergencies: Impact and Challenges. *Lancet* **2004**, *364*, 1974–1983. [CrossRef]
6. Lam, E.; McCarthy, A.; Brennan, M. Vaccine-Preventable Diseases in Humanitarian Emergencies among Refugee and Internally-Displaced Populations. *Hum. Vaccin. Immunother.* **2015**, *11*, 2627–2636. [CrossRef] [PubMed]
7. Kouadio, I.K.; Kamigaki, T.; Oshitani, H. Measles Outbreaks in Displaced Populations: A Review of Transmission, Morbidity and Mortality Associated Factors. *BMC Int. Health Hum. Rights* **2010**, *10*, 5. [CrossRef] [PubMed]
8. Slama, S.; Kim, H.J.; Roglic, G.; Boulle, P.; Hering, H.; Varghese, C.; Rasheed, S.; Tonelli, M. Care of Non-Communicable Diseases in Emergencies. *Lancet* **2016**, *389*, 326–330. [CrossRef]

9. Demaio, A.; Jamieson, J.; Horn, R. Non-Communicable Diseases in Emergencies: A Call to Action. *PLoS Curr.* **2013**, *5*. [CrossRef] [PubMed]
10. Wisner, B.; Adams, J. *Environmental Health in Emergencies and Disasters*; World Health Organization: Geneva, Switzerland, 2002.
11. Centers for Disease Control and Prevention (U.S.). Deaths Associated with Hurricane Sandy—October–November 2012. *Morb. Mortal. Wkly. Rep.* **2013**, *62*, 393–397.
12. Ochi, S.; Murray, V.; Hodgson, S. The Great East Japan Earthquake Disaster: A Compilation of Published Literature on Health Needs and Relief Activities, March 2011–September 2012. *PLoS Curr.* **2013**, *5*. [CrossRef] [PubMed]
13. Ching, P.K.; de los Reyes, V.C.; Sucaldito, M.N.; Tayag, E. An Assessment of Disaster-Related Mortality Post-Haiyan in Tacloban City. *West Pacific Surveill. Response J.* **2015**, *6* (Suppl. 1), 34–38. [CrossRef]
14. Salazar, M.A.; Pesigan, A.M.; Law, R.; Winkler, V. Post-Disaster Health Impact of Natural Hazards in the Philippines in 2013. *Glob. Health Action* **2016**, *9*, 31320. [CrossRef] [PubMed]
15. Salazar, M.A.; Law, R.; Pesigan, A.; Winkler, V. Health Consequences of Typhoon Haiyan in the Eastern Visayas Region Using a Syndromic Surveillance Database. *PLoS Curr.* **2017**, *9*. [CrossRef]
16. Banwell, N.; Montoya, J.; Opeña, M.; IJsselmuiden, C.; Law, R.; Rutherford, S.; Chu, C.; Murray, V.; Balboa, G.J. Developing the Philippines as a Global Hub for Disaster Risk Reduction—A Health Research Initiative as Presented at the 10th Philippine National Health Research System Week Celebration. *PLoS Curr.* **2016**, *8*. [CrossRef] [PubMed]
17. Health Emergency Management Bureau. *Surveillance in Post Extreme Emergencies and Disasters Operations Manual for Managers*; Department of Health Philippines: Manila, Philippines, 2011.
18. Aitsi-Selmi, A.; Murray, V.; Wannous, C.; Dickinson, C.; Johnston, D.; Kawasaki, A.; Stevance, A.S.; Yeung, T. Reflections on a Science and Technology Agenda for 21st Century Disaster Risk Reduction: Based on the Scientific Content of the 2016 UNISDR Science and Technology Conference on the Implementation of the Sendai Framework for Disaster Risk Reduction 2015–2020. *Int. J. Disaster Risk Sci.* **2016**, *7*, 1–29.
19. UNISDR (United Nations International Strategy for Disaster Reduction). *Sendai Framework for Disaster Risk Reduction 2015–2030*; UNISDR: Geneva, Switzerland, 2015.
20. Lo, S.T.T.; Chan, E.Y.Y.; Chan, G.K.W.; Murray, V.; Abrahams, J.; Ardalan, A.; Kayano, R.; Yau, J.C.W. Health Emergency and Disaster Risk Management (Health-EDRM): Developing the Research Field within the Sendai Framework Paradigm. *Int. J. Disaster Risk Sci.* **2017**, *8*, 145–149. [CrossRef]
21. Martinez, R.E.; Quintana, R.; Go, J.J.; Marquez, M.A.; Kim, J.K.; Villones, M.S.; Salazar, M.A. Surveillance for and Issues Relating to Noncommunicable Diseases Post-Haiyan in Region 8. *West Pacific Surveill. Response J.* **2015**, *6* (Suppl. 1), 21–24. [CrossRef] [PubMed]
22. National Statistics Office. The 2010 Census of Population and Housing Reveals the Philippine Population at 92.34 Million. Available online: https://psa.gov.ph/content/2010-census-population-and-housing-reveals-philippine-population-9234-million (accessed on 30 November 2015).
23. Hutchinson, M.K.; Holtman, M.C. Analysis of Count Data Using Poisson Regression. *Res. Nurs. Health* **2005**, *28*, 408–418. [CrossRef] [PubMed]
24. Zhang, Z. Multivariable Fractional Polynomial Method for Regression Model. *Ann. Transl. Med.* **2016**, *4*, 174. [CrossRef] [PubMed]
25. Department of Health Philippines. *Adopting the 2008 Revised List of Notifiable Diseases, Syndromes, Health-Related Events and Conditions, AO 2008–0009*; Department of Health Philippines: Manila, Philippines, 2008.
26. Health Emergency Management Bureau. *Manual of Treatment Protocols of Common Communicable Diseases and Other Ailments During Emergencies and Disasters*, 2nd ed.; Banatin, C., Dominguez, N., Eds.; Department of Health Philippines: Manila, Philippines, 2013.
27. Gayer, M.; Legros, D.; Formenty, P.; Connolly, M.A. Conflict and Emerging Infectious Diseases. *Emerg. Infect. Dis.* **2007**, *13*, 1625–1631. [CrossRef] [PubMed]
28. Epidemiology Bureau. *The 2013 Philippine Health Statistics*; Asuncion, I., Benegas-Segarra, A., Timbang, T., Sinson, F., Rebanal, L., Eds.; Department of Health Philippines: Manila, Philippines, 2013.
29. Asian Institute of Journalism and Communication. *Zamboanga Learning Review on Post-Conflict Community Engagement*; Asian Institute of Journalism and Communication: Manila, Philippines, 2015.
30. Elfaituri, S.S. Skin Diseases among Internally Displaced Tawerghans Living in Camps in Benghazi, Libya. *Int. J. Dermatol.* **2016**, *55*, 1000–1004. [CrossRef] [PubMed]

31. Mobula, L.M.; Fisher, M.L.; Wood, T.; Plyler, W. Prevalence of Hypertension among Patients Attending Mobile Medical Clinics in the Philippines after Typhoon Haiyan. *PLoS Curr.* **2016**, *8*. [CrossRef] [PubMed]
32. WHO Regional Office for Europe. *Gaining Health: The European Strategy for the Prevention and Control of Noncommunicable Diseases*; WHO Regional Office for Europe: Copenhagen, Denmark, 2006.
33. Doocy, S.; Daniels, A.; Packer, C.; Dick, A.; Kirsch, T.D. The Human Impact of Earthquakes: A Historical Review of Events 1980–2009 and Systematic Literature Review. *PLoS Curr.* **2016**, *28*, 237–244. [CrossRef] [PubMed]
34. Doocy, S.; Dick, A.; Daniels, A.; Kirsch, T.D.; Hopkins, J. The Human Impact of Tropical Cyclones: A Historical Review of Events 1980-2009 and Systematic Literature Review Citation Abstract Authors. *PLoS Curr.* **2013**, *1*, 1–25.
35. Murray, C.J.L.; King, G.; Lopez, A.D.; Tomijima, N.; Krug, E.G. Armed Conflict as a Public Health Problem. *BMJ* **2002**, *324*, 346–349. [CrossRef] [PubMed]
36. Health Emergency Management Bureau. *Final Report: Armed Conflict in Zamboanga City*; Health Emergency Management Bureau: Manila, Philippines, 2014.
37. WHO Regional Office for the Western Pacific. *A Guide to Establishing Event-Based Surveillance*; WHO Western Pacific Regional Office: Manila, Philippines, 2008.
38. Foldy, S.L. Linking Better Surveillance to Better Outcomes. *Morb. Mortal. Wkly. Rep.* **2004**, *53*, 12–17.
39. World Health Organization; United Nations High Commissioner for Refugees. *MhGAP Humanitarian Intervention Guide (MhGAP-HIG): Clinical Management of Mental, Neurological and Substance Use Conditions in Humanitarian Emergencies*; WHO: Geneva, Switzerland, 2015.
40. Health Emergency Management Bureau. *Pocket Emergency Tool*, 4th ed.; Department of Health Philippines: Manila, Philippines, 2012.
41. United Nations Office for the Coordination of Humanitarian Affairs. *Philippines: Zamoanga and Basilan Emgerency Situtaion Report No. 8*; UN OCHA: Manila, Philippines, 2013.
42. Women's Refugee Commission. *Minimum Initial Service Package (MISP) for Reproductive Health in Crisis Situations: A Distance Learning Module*, 3rd ed.; Women's Refugee Commission: New York, NY, USA, 2011.

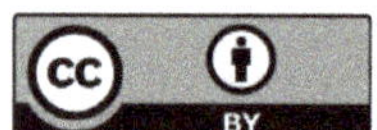

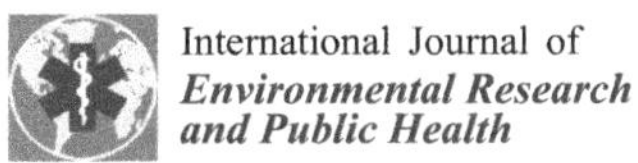

International Journal of
Environmental Research and Public Health

MDPI

Article

Health Emergency Disaster Risk Management of Public Transport Systems: A Population-Based Study after the 2017 Subway Fire in Hong Kong, China

Emily Ying Yang Chan [1,2,3,4,*], Zhe Huang [1], Kevin Kei Ching Hung [1,4], Gloria Kwong Wai Chan [1], Holly Ching Yu Lam [1], Eugene Siu Kai Lo [1] and May Pui Shan Yeung [1]

1 Collaborating Centre for Oxford University and CUHK for Disaster and Medical Humanitarian Response (CCOUC), JC (Jockey Club) School of Public Health and Primary Care, The Chinese University of Hong Kong, Hong Kong, China; huangzhe@cuhk.edu.hk (Z.H.); kevin.hung@cuhk.edu.hk (K.K.C.H.); gloria.chan@cuhk.edu.hk (G.K.W.C.); hollylam@cuhk.edu.hk (H.C.Y.L.); Euglsk@cuhk.edu.hk (E.S.K.L.); may.yeung@cuhk.edu.hk (M.P.S.Y.)

2 Nuffield Department of Medicine, University of Oxford, Oxford OX3 7BN, UK

3 François-Xavier Bagnoud Center for Health & Human Rights, Harvard University, Boston, MA 02138, USA

4 Accident and Emergency Medicine Academic Unit, The Chinese University of Hong Kong, Hong Kong, China

* Correspondence: emily.chan@cuhk.edu.hk; Tel.: +852-2252-8850

Received: 8 November 2018; Accepted: 11 January 2019; Published: 15 January 2019

Abstract: *Background:* Literature on health emergency disaster risk management (Health-EDRM) for urban public transport safety is limited. This study explored: (i) the confidence in public transport safety, (ii) the relationship between socio-demographic characteristics and risk perception of transport safety and (iii) the association between previous first-aid training and response knowledge. *Method:* This is a population-based cross-sectional telephone survey conducted in March 2017, one month after a major subway incident in Hong Kong. Respondents were randomly selected with the Random Digit Dialing method among Cantonese-speaking population ≥15 years. Sociodemographic information, type of transport used and the corresponding worries, response knowledge and previous first-aid training experience (as a proxy for individual skills in Health-EDRM training proxy) were collected. *Results:* Among the 1000 respondents, 87% used public transport daily. The self-reported confidence in subway safety was 85.6% even after a subway fire accident. Female, those with lower income and people unmarried were more likely to express worry about transport safety. About 46.1–63.2% respondents had the correct fire related health response knowledge. Previous first-aid training (32%) was found to be associated with fire response knowledge in a mixed pattern. *Conclusions:* Despite inadequacy in fire response knowledge, previous first-aid training appeared to be a beneficial factor for emergency response knowledge. Emergency responses education should be provided to the public to reduce health losses during emergencies.

Keywords: public transport; subway; safety; fire; risk perception; emergency response; Health-EDRM

---

1. Introduction

Global urbanization has led to the rapid development of public transportations in cities. Subways or metro systems are identified as a recommended mode of urban public transportation as those networks will increase population mobility, geographic connections, and reduce environmental impact from air pollution caused by automobiles [1]. Thus, urban metro systems have an important role in the socio-economic development of many active developing metropolises. About 22% of the world's

632 largest cities have developed metro systems, and 53 cities in the Asian region has the fasting growing infrastructure with predominant number metro systems when compared with 40 European, 30 North American, 14 South American and one African cities [2].

The heavy reliance of urban residents on metro systems potentially has major implications for health risks and public safety. Globally, numerous critical incidents in urban metro system, such as fire, have been reported to cause massive human impact in high-density cities [1,3,4]. For example, the 1987 King's Cross Fire in London, the 1990 subway fire in New York City, the 1995 Baku Metro Fire in Azerbaijan, and the 2003 Daegu Subway Fire in South Korea have all resulted in more than 100 casualties [5–7]. During emergencies, appropriate personal response may lower vulnerability health risks and even save lives [8]. According to the Sendai Framework, understanding disaster risk and enhancing preparedness are the priorities in risk reduction strategies [9]. Vulnerability is one of the key components in risk assessment [10] while sociodemographic characteristics have been recognized as underlying disaster health risk drivers [10]. Meanwhile, training, which is associated with awareness raising and knowledge enhancement, is defined as non-structural measures in disaster preparedness and resilience [10]. Studies have indicated urban population tends to misjudge their own actual health risk for disaster and emergency [11–15]. Ensuring public safety, education, and emergency preparedness will thus be immensely important to reduce potential harm during and immediately after an emergency incident. For example, an effective railway passenger evacuation during an onboard fire in Shanghai had resulted in no casualties in 2018 [16]. Better understanding of community's capacity to manage health risks will help to support evidence-based health emergency disaster risk management (Health-EDRM) [17,18] policies and bottom-up resilience capacity building.

Hong Kong, a metropolis in southern China, has a 7.4 million urban based population and has developed a metro system, the Mass Transit Railway (MTR), since 1979. With over five million daily trips made on underground subways and overhead railways, public safety is a priority in such a high density environment [19]. On 10 February 2017, a subway firebomb during the evening rush hour in Hong Kong caused 18 injuries and one death [20]. The accident was regarded as the most serious attack incident in 38 years since the commissioning of the MTR [19].

A telephone survey study was conducted after the Hong Kong MTR fire accident in February 2017 to understand the health emergency and disaster risk awareness and preparedness towards transport-related incidents. This study aimed to examine individual's emergency response and its possible associating factors such as risk perception, previous trainings and other personal characteristics. Factors that could improve personal emergency response and hypothesized that different modes of transport (which is related to risk perception), socio-demographic characteristics, and first-aid training may affect the awareness or knowledge of emergency response were identified. In particular, fire response knowledge in health risks was studied since fire was a common hazard reported in previous transport accidents [1,3,4]. This research paper will report study findings of three main study objectives which include: (i) public transport utilization pattern and confidence associated with public transport safety after a major emergency public incident, (ii) the relationship between socio-demographic characteristics with risk perception and expressed worry with public transport system and (iii) if previous first-aid training, as a proxy for individual skills in Health-EDRM, may be associated with fire injury-related response knowledge to assess potential management capacity to response health risks in a public transportation system. The findings will provide evidence for global metropolis when examining health risk perception for public transportation system and will further support public education and disaster risk reduction policy development to address Health-EDRM in these communities.

2. Materials and Methods

2.1. Collection

This is a population, cross-sectional telephone-based survey study, which was conducted in 2–12 March 2017, within 1 month after a major subway fire incident in Hong Kong. The study population is stratified according to age, gender and area of residence of the 2016 Hong Kong Census and a representative sample was randomly selected with the Random Digit Dialing method (RDD) through computer generation among the Hong Kong Cantonese-speaking population aged above 15. Each interview lasted between 15 and 25 min. The telephone interviews were conducted by trained interviewers from 6 pm to 10 pm on weekdays and from 10 am to 10 pm on weekends to prevent over representation of the unemployed population. Up to five calls were made to each number before it was considered unanswered. Respondents were chosen based on the "last birthday method" which referred to the household member with the birthday closest to the interview date [11–13,21].

Self-reported information was collected for socio-demographic background (gender, age, area of residence, marital status and education attainment, Comprehensive Social Security Assistance (CSSA) status), and a total of 12 questions (see Supplementary Materials) were asked to identify respondents' current pattern of daily transportation), risk perception, worry level of transport safety after a major incidence (expressed worry), knowledge and accuracy of fire emergency response to physical injury, first-aid training, and expressed willingness to learn about community disaster preparedness. Specifically, first-aid training was used as a proxy for Health-EDRM training in the community and CSSA status was used as a proxy to examine socio-economic deprivation and its relationship to the study patterns. Three questions were also asked to explore knowledge and accuracies in health risk and response to fire incidents. Question T1 assessed fire-related first-aid knowledge that is commonly included in first-aid hand book [22] (Should room temperature water or ice water and ice be used to treat the burn? (a) ice water/ice cube; (b) room temperature water). Question T2 assessed the knowledge of the use if a fire blanket which have been promoted by the Hong Kong Fire Services Department (If you are in a fire incident setting and you found someone was on fire, how would you use a fire blanket) (a) put out the fire directly with the fire blanket; (b) cover the victim with the fire blanket and ask them to roll until the fire stops). Question T3 assessed the knowledge of the use of a fire distinguisher in a scenario which was rarely found in official fire response materials nor in first-aid hand books. (If there is no fire blanket at the scene, should fire hoses or extinguishers be used on people) (a) Yes; (b) No).

This study was approved by the Survey and Behavioral Research Ethics Committee of The Chinese University of Hong Kong. Verbal consent was sought from each respondent before the interviews.

2.2. Analysis

Descriptive statistical analysis and Pearson's χ^2 test were conducted on the sociodemographic characteristics of the respondents and the demographic characteristics were further compared with the Hong Kong Population Census data in 2016 [23]. Multiple logistic regression models were constructed to examine associations between variables and the research enquiries. Analyses were conducted using R version 3.1.3 (R Foundation for Statistical Computing, Vienna, Austria). All statistical significance was set at $\alpha = 0.05$.

3. Results

3.1. Subjects' Characteristics

A total valid final study sample of 1000 were collected with a study response rate of 64.8%. Figure 1 detailed the data collection algorithm. The total sample was representative in terms of the distribution of gender, area of residence, and marital status as stated in the 2016 Hong Kong population census data (Table 1).

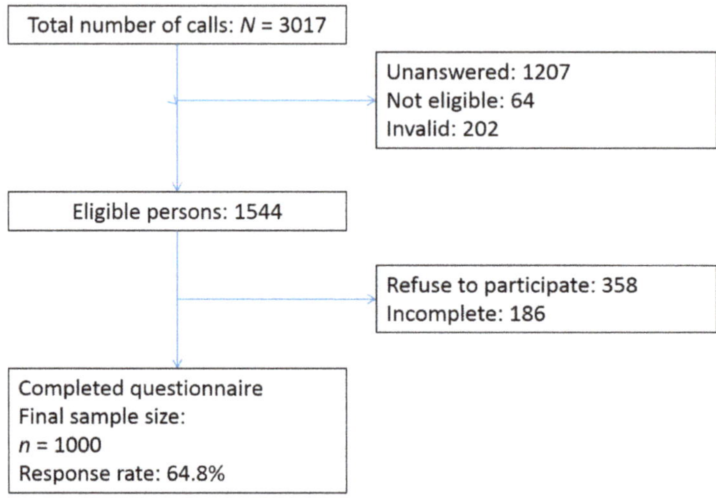

Figure 1. Study flow of the telephone survey.

Table 1. Sociodemographic characteristics of the survey respondents in March 2017 and the general population in Hong Kong in 2016.

Demographics		Sampled Respondents (*N* = 1000)		HK 2016 Population By-Census Data (*N* = 6,506,130)		Sample vs. Census *p*-Value [a]
		n	%	*n*	%	
Gender	Male	456	45.6%	2,947,073	45.3%	0.87 [b]
	Female	544	54.4%	3,559,057	54.7%	
Age	15–24	129	12.9%	785,981	12.1%	<0.01
	25–44	283	28.3%	2,228,566	34.3%	
	45–64	377	37.7%	2,328,430	35.8%	
	≥65	210	21.0%	1,163,153	17.9%	
Area of residence *	Hong Kong Island	182	18.2%	1,120,143	17.2%	0.70
	Kowloon	300	30.0%	1,987,380	30.6%	
	New Territories	517	51.8%	3,397,499	52.2%	
Education attainment	Primary and below	116	11.6%	1,673,431	25.7%	<0.01
	Secondary	474	47.5%	2,841,510	43.7%	
	Post-secondary	408	40.9%	1,991,189	30.6%	
Marital status	Single	439	44.2%	2,708,709	41.6%	0.11 [b]
	Married	554	55.8%	3,797,421	58.4%	

[a] χ^2 test was used to measure the overall difference between this survey and the 2016 Hong Kong Population Census data. *p*-Value < 0.05 indicates significant difference. [b] χ^2 test with continuity correction was used. * Marine population was excluded.

3.2. Daily Transport Utilization and Confidence in Transport Safety

Subway (43.9%) and buses (43.2%), were reported to be the two predominant modes of daily public transport in Hong Kong (Table 2). Analysis by age group showed that 15–24 years group regarded subway (62%) as their most preferred daily mode of transport. For non-motor vehicle based transport (walk/cycle), the elderly (10%) were found to be more likely than the younger groups to walk and cycle. Furthermore, people living in Hong Kong Island and those older than 65 would use other transport modes such as tram and taxi more often than other groups.

Table 2. Pattern of daily transport and level of perceived safety.

	n	%	1 Strongly Disagree	2 Disagree	3 Slightly Disagree	4 Slightly Agree	5 Agree	6 Strongly Agree	Mean	SD
Total	996	100%	1.4%	2.0%	14.1%	22.6%	38.9%	21.1%	4.59	1.11
Walk/cycle	57	5.7%	1.8%	1.8%	14.0%	17.5%	38.6%	26.3%	4.68	1.17
Subway	437	43.9%	1.4%	0.7%	12.4%	20.8%	41.0%	23.8%	4.71	1.07
Bus	430	43.2%	1.4%	3.3%	16.3%	25.6%	36.7%	16.7%	4.43	1.13
Private car	46	4.6%	2.2%	2.2%	8.7%	19.6%	32.6%	34.8%	4.83	1.20
Other modes	26	2.6%	0.0%	3.8%	15.4%	19.2%	50.0%	11.5%	4.50	1.03

Note: The question is "My daily transport is safe".

A Likert scale ranging from 1–6, 1 for the least safe and 6 for the safest, was used to measure respondents' rating on the safety level of the transport mode they used daily (defined as "perceived safety" below). Private cars were reported as the safest transport mode (mean = 4.83; standard deviation (SD) = 1.20) despite being ranked as the least utilized mode of transport (4.6%). Meanwhile, buses were regarded as the least safe mode (mean = 4.43; SD = 1.13). Subgroup analysis found no statistically significant differences for gender in perceived safety in the modes of daily transport (Figure 2).

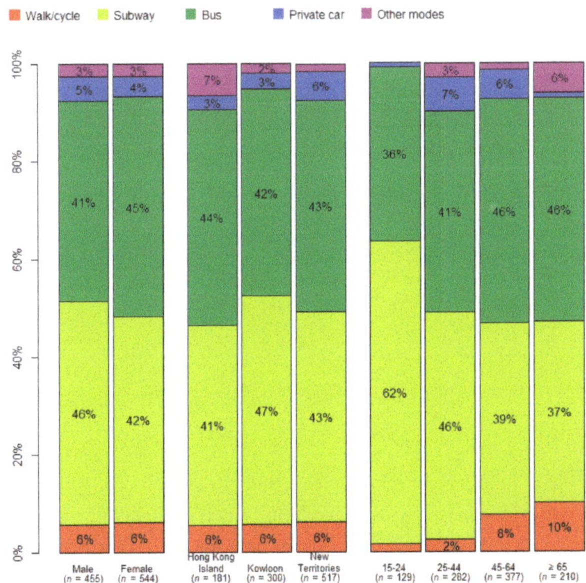

Figure 2. Subgroup analysis on daily transport mode.

Despite the survey study was conducted within a month after a major subway incident, 85.6% current subway users were satisfied with their transport routine and regarded their choice as safe (as expressed in "perceived safety", mean = 4.59; SD = 1.11). When respondents were asked whether they were worry about any disasters/ incidents would happen in the transport mode they used daily (defined as "expressed worry" below), about 35.0% (n = 348/981) of respondent expressed concern/worry about transport safety.

3.3. *Association Among Expressed Worry of Disaster/Incident Risk, Type of Transport Used and Socio-Demographic Factors*

Multiple logistic regression was used to examine the association between being worried about transport safety and socio-demographic variables including gender, age, education level, area of residence, CSSA status, marital status, as well as the form of daily transport. Being worried about daily transport use was initially regressed with all mentioned variables. Variables that showed an association with being worried (indicated by p-value < 0.1) in stage 1 of the model were included in the second stage (final model). The adjusted odds ratios (OR) and the corresponding 95% confidence interval (CI) are shown in Table 3. No statistically significant association was found between concern/worry about public transport and the mode of transport used. Final model, however, indicated the female gender and people who received CSSA were more likely to express worry about disaster/incident occurrence on their daily transport. Meanwhile, married individuals were less likely to expressed worry when compared with their unmarried counterparts.

Table 3. Factors associated with the expressed worry of disaster/incident occurring on my daily transport.

Characteristics		I am Worried that Disaster/Incident will Occur on the Daily Transport I Take (n = 990)			
		Stage 1 Model		Stage 2 Model	
		OR (95% CI)	p-Value	OR (95% CI)	p-Value
Gender	Male	1		1	
	Female	1.88 (1.44–2.46)	<0.01	1.92 (1.47–2.52)	<0.01
Age	15–24	1			
	25–44	1.33 (0.86–2.06)	0.20		
	45–64	0.90 (0.58–1.37)	0.61		
	≥65	1.24 (0.78–1.97)	0.36		
Area of residence	Hong Kong Island	1			
	Kowloon	0.92 (0.63–2.10)	0.66		
	New Territories	0.82 (0.58–1.16)	0.26		
Education	Primary or below	1			
	Secondary	0.91 (0.59–1.39)	0.66		
	Post-secondary or above	0.98 (0.64–1.50)	0.92		
Marital status	Single	1		1	
	Married	0.72 (0.55–0.93)	0.01	0.75 (0.57–0.98)	0.04
Form of daily transport	Walk/cycle	1			
	Subway	0.79 (0.45–1.39)	0.41		
	Bus	0.76 (0.43–1.34)	0.34		
	Private car	0.63 (0.28–1.43)	0.27		
	Others	1.23 (0.48–3.14)	0.67		
Accept Comprehensive Social Security Assistance	No	1		1	
	Yes	2.32 (1.23–4.38)	0.01	2.51 (1.30–4.83)	0.01

3.4. Association between Previous First-Aid Training and Fire Injury-Related Response Knowledge, and Willingness to Learn

Around 32.0% of respondents have at some point received first-aid training, the proxy variable which is used to describe individual skills in Health-EDRM. Multivariable logistic regression showed that those with a higher educational level were more likely to have received first-aid training (Table 4). About two-third of respondents (n = 671/993), were willing to learn about community disaster preparedness. Specifically, people who had expressed worry about transport safety were also more willing to learn (Table 4).

For the fire response questions, 47.0%, 53.8%, and 61.3% answered T1, T3, and T2 correctly respectively (Table 5). For T1, the first-aid related fire response question ("which ice water should not be used to treat the burn"), people with a higher educational level (OR = 2.55; 95% CI: 1.46–4.46) and had previously received first-aid training (OR = 1.97; 95% CI: 1.48–2.62) were more likely to answer correctly. However, people aged 65 or above (OR = 0.51; 95% CI: 0.30–0.89) were less likely to report a correct answer. Meanwhile, for the use of fire blanket (T2), a technical question that has been promoted by the local Fire Service Department, the female gender (OR = 1.61; 95% CI: 1.23–2.10) and people with a higher education level (OR = 2.16; 95% CI: 1.29–3.6) were more likely to answer correctly. For T3, the use of fire extinguisher, a question that is not related to first-aid nor promoted by the Fire Service Department, people aged 65 years or above (OR = 1.65; 95% CI: 1.01–2.69) and married people (OR = 1.40; 95% CI: 1.03–1.91) had higher rates of correct answers. Of note, the female gender (OR = 0.65; 95% CI: correctly.

Table 4. Factors associated with receiving first-aid training and willingness of learning more about community disaster preparedness.

Characteristics		Did You ever Receive First-Aid Training? n = 997				Willingness of Learning More about Community Disaster Preparedness n = 994			
		Stage 1 Model		Stage 2 Model		Stage 1 Model		Stage 2 Model	
		OR (95% CI)	p-Value	OR (95% CI)	p-Value	OR (95% CI)	p-Value	OR (95% CI)	p-Value
Gender	Male	1				1		1	
	Female	0.86 (0.66–1.12)	0.27			1.48 (1.13–1.93)	<0.01	1.51 (0.80–2.81)	0.20
Age	15–24	1		1		1		1	
	25–44	1.41 (0.90–2.18)	0.13	1.35 (0.87–2.11)	0.18	1.53 (0.98–2.40)	0.06	3.92 (0.95–16.09)	0.06
	45–64	1.03 (0.67–1.58)	0.9	1.29 (0.83–2.00)	0.26	1.14 (0.75–1.74)	0.55	1.08 (0.41–2.86)	0.88
	≥65	0.57 (0.35–0.94)	0.03	1.05 (0.61–1.79)	0.87	0.78 (0.49–1.23)	0.28	0.66 (0.23–1.91)	0.45
Area of residence	Hong Kong Island	1				1			
	Kowloon	1.04 (0.70–1.55)	0.86			0.96 (0.65–1.41)	0.83		
	New Territories	1.14 (0.79–1.64)	0.48			1.15 (0.80–1.64)	0.46		
Education	Primary or below	1		1		1		1	
	Secondary	3.96 (2.06–7.60)	<0.01	3.59 (1.83–7.07)	<0.01	1.40 (0.92–2.14)	0.12	1.45 (0.64–3.30)	0.38
	Post-secondary or above	6.82 (3.55–13.08)	<0.01	5.97 (2.96–12.03)	<0.01	1.60 (1.04–2.46)	0.03	2.37 (0.84–6.63)	0.10
Marital status	Single	1				1			
	Married	0.94 (0.72–1.23)	0.64			0.85 (0.65–1.12)	0.24		
Accept Comprehensive Social Security Assistance	No	1		1		1			
	Yes	0.42 (0.19–0.97)	0.04	0.65 (0.27–1.52)	0.32	1.08 (0.54–2.16)	0.83		
Worried about disaster/incident on the daily transport	No	1				1		1	
	Yes	1.08 (0.54–2.16)	0.3			2.93 (2.14–4.00)	<0.01	4.36 (1.69–11.25)	<0.01

In addition, 68.0% of the respondents said they did not know what to do when a fire incident occurs on public transportation. Of the 31.8% of the respondents who believed they had the ability to deal with fires on public transportation, there was no statistically significant association between their self-reported ability to deal with fires and accuracy of their fire response knowledge.

Table 5. Knowledge test of fire emergency response.

Fire Response Questions	Overall (n = 981)		Do not Know how to Deal with Fire in Transport (n = 627)		Know how to Deal with Fire in Transport (n = 354)		OR (95%CI) of Getting a Correct Answer (Know how to Deal with Fire vs. Do not Know)
	Incorrect	Correct	Incorrect	Correct	Incorrect	Correct	
T1: Room temperature water	53.0%	47.0%	52.7%	47.3%	53.3%	46.7%	OR = 0.98, 95% CI: 0.75–1.27, p = 0.86
T2: Fire blanket	38.7%	61.3%	37.4%	62.6%	40.3%	59.7%	OR = 0.91, 95% CI: 0.69–1.21, p = 0.52
T3: Fire Hose/ Extinguisher	46.2%	53.8%	48.1%	51.9%	44.0%	56.0%	OR = 1.18, 95% CI: 0.91–1.54, p = 0.22

Note: Specific question in knowledge test of fire emergency response: T1. Should room temperature water or ice water and ice be used to treat the burn? (a) ice water/ ice cube; (b) room temperature water; T2. If you are in a fire incident setting and you found someone was on fire, how would you use a fire blanket (a) put out the fire directly with the fire blanket; (b) cover the victim with the fire blanket and ask them to roll until the fire stops); T3. If there is no fire blanket at the scene, should fire hoses or extinguishers be used on people) (a) Yes; (b) No.

4. Discussion

The metro system is reported to be the most widely used daily transportation in Hong Kong. Meanwhile, private cars and buses are respectively perceived as the safest and the least safe transportation. Around one-third of respondents were worried that a disaster/incident will occur on their daily transport, in particular for the female gender, people receiving CSSA, and unmarried people. Consistent to the findings in another study in the same community [15], the respondents' knowledge accuracy was relatively low in the community. People with a higher educational level were more likely to report fire response knowledge that were either included in first-aid training or promoted by the local Fire Service Department. Older people and married individuals were more likely to correctly answer the fire response question which is not commonly included in first-aid handbooks or the promotion materials for fire responses. Only one-third of the respondents have received first-aid training and those with a higher educational level were more likely to have been trained. Approximately two-third of respondents were willing to learn about community disaster preparedness and respondents who expressed worries were more willing to learn.

Despite the 2017 MTR fire accident, the public's confidence in the MTR remained higher than buses, which is the other major mode of public transportation Hong Kong. Around 85% still considered the MTR as a safe mode of public transportation while only 79% agreed buses were safe. According to the Traffic Report 2016, public buses had the highest accident rate with 394 accidents per 1000 licensed vehicles. In the same year, nine percent of the bus accidents involved other vehicles (n = 2261) and majorities of the impact resulted in minor injuries (n = 1981) rather than serious ones (n = 276) or fatalities (n = 13) [24], which is consistent with the perceived safety from the study respondents. Another possible reason for the higher perceived risk of bus accidents may be due to previous major bus crashes and their media coverage, including the 2003 Tuen Mun Road Ting Kau bus accident resulting in 21 deaths and 20 injured [25] and 2008 Sai Kung Nam Wai Road bus crash which caused 18 deaths and 44 injured [26].

In this study, private cars were rated as the safest mode of transport. Yet, in Hong Kong, private cars caused more number of road accidents than trains and buses [24]. Savage's 2013 study about the United States also reported higher fatality risks for private cars relative to mainline trains, buses, and commercial aviation with the relative risks respectively at 17, 67 and 112 times [27]. A gap between people's risk perception and actual risk of private car safety has been observed in this study. However, the choice of transport is complex and was found not directly associated with the perceived safety level, which is consistent with previous studies [28–30]. Of note, the percentage of people choosing walking/ cycling was the highest among non-public transport modes. This may be associated with the increasing awareness in environmental protection in recently years. Other factors such as worry about unpleasant incidents [29], perceived control and trust in authorities [30] as well as other economic, convenience, and comfort factors come into deciding which transportation to take.

Among the 35% of respondents who expressed worry about disaster/incidents occurring during their daily transport experiences, the female gender, those receiving CSSA and unmarried people were found to be significant predictors. Women reported more worry than men, which is consistent with research which looked at gender differences in risk perception [31,32]. The result which showed people who received CSSA were more worried about disasters was also consistent with the finding that poverty is likely to be associated with frequent accidents and mental disorders [33]. On the other hand, it was uncertain why unmarried people expressed more concern about disaster/incidents on transportation, though Dugas and Robichaud suggested that individuals who are unmarried or divorced, receiving disability payments, and have very low annual incomes are associated with Generalized Anxiety Disorder [34].

Given perceived safety level appeared to have mild impact on the choice of transport mode, learning how to response to emergencies seems to be a good way to reduce health risks and dispel worries. First-aid training is a vital building block to the enhancement of personal disaster preparedness to Health-EDRM, and first-aid training was found to be positively associated with greater perceived knowledge on how to handle a medical emergency and demonstrate first-aid skills [8]. In this study, the relationship of first-aid training and knowledge accuracy in health risk management showed a mixed pattern. Those who had previously received first-aid training were more likely to correctly answer the first-aid related fire response question (T1), whilst no association or negative association were found for the accuracy of the other questions. Despite the mixed pattern, first-aid training was shown to be having beneficial effects in building fire emergency response knowledge among the general public. However, only 32.0% of the study respondents had previously received first-aid training and thus may potentially explain the small proportion of respondents who believed they are capable of responding to fire incidents on public transport and disasters in general. Promoting knowledge of emergency response (such as first-aid, general fire response as well as electrical fire response) and increasing awareness of personal vulnerability can be crucial for disaster preparedness in urban cities [35]. Other studies conducted that targeted specific sub-groups established similar conclusions [36].

The percentage of respondents who received first-aid training in a 2017 survey (32.0%) was slightly higher than that in 2012 (26.1%) [11]. The two most important reasons of receiving first-aid training were the relevance to job duty (39.1%) and personal interest (34.9%). First-aid training was also found to be associated with a higher educational level, which is consistent with previous studies [8,37]. However, the percentage of participants who received first-aid training in Hong Kong was much lower than Norway (90%) [38], Germany (80%) and Austria (80%) [39]. In Norway, first-aid training is part of the national school curriculum for grades 7 and 10, and is required by law for some occupations, such as drivers and employees in schools and kindergartens [38]. In addition, the gap between the low percentage of respondents who received first-aid training (32%) and willingness to learn more about disaster response (67.6%) indicates that urban residents, despite of the information access and resource availability, are inadequately prepared for individual self-help skills in Health-EDRM during emergencies and disasters. This finding suggests that there might be a gap and need in emergency response training.

Study limitations include the inability of cross-sectional studies to draw causative conclusion in their design. In addition, households which were not subscribed to land-based telephone service may be missed. However, the penetration rate of residential fixed line service in Hong Kong is more than 90% [40], which implied that most households have at least one home-based telephone a number of previous studies managed to provide valuable scientific evidence to the research community with telephone survey studies [41]. The valid sample size of 1000 and the comparability of the sample population with census data (stratified by key sociodemographic characteristics) will support the potential generalizability of the research findings. Furthermore, data collected in this study was based on self-reporting, which makes it difficult to validate the accuracy of the answers. The limited amount of time in each telephone survey had also restricted our ability to examine more detailed answers and the close-ended questions may limit answers from the respondents. Nevertheless, as the field data collection was completed within a short period after the subway fire incident, there should be minimal recall bias. According to the Travel Characteristics Survey 2011 [42], metro systems accounted for 30% for all trip purposes, while bus accounted for 49%. Although these results were different from our findings, it is possibly because of the expansion of the Hong Kong subway network after 2011. For instance, from 2014 to 2016, ten additional new transfer stations became operational. Therefore, despite the design limitations, the study findings provide evidence and an overview of how the urban residents may perceive their own health-related emergency risks as well the current attitude and knowledge gaps which might affect health and safety promotion in an urban community in Asia.

5. Conclusions

This study provides updated scientific evidence on general urban risk perception and Health-EDRM in a public transportation system [15]. In general, subway was the most popular public transport and respondents thought it was safe despite the event of a severe MTR fire accident. Perceived confidence in handling fire on transportation and fire response knowledge were relatively low. Previous first-aid training, the proxy indicator assess individual skills in Health-EDRM, was found to be an associating factor of better first-aid related fire response knowledge. However, the proportion of respondents who had previously received first-aid training was low. More than half of the respondents showed a willingness to learn more about community disaster preparedness, especially for those who expressed worry about transport safety. The promotion from local authorities about relevant knowledge and training on first-aid and other emergency response and preparedness activities may raise awareness, increase capacity for self-help, and reduce adverse health risks in times of emergencies and crisis, especially for people with low education level.

Supplementary Materials: The following are available online at http://www.mdpi.com/1660-4601/16/2/228/s1, Survey Questionnaire.

Author Contributions: Conceptualization, E.Y.Y.C., K.K.C.H., G.K.W.C. and H.C.Y.L.; Data curation, Z.H., H.C.Y.L. and E.S.K.L.; Formal analysis, E.Y.Y.C., Z.H., H.C.Y.L. and E.S.K.L.; Funding acquisition, E.Y.Y.C.; Investigation, H.C.Y.L. and M.P.S.Y.; Methodology, E.Y.Y.C. and H.C.Y.L.; Project administration, G.K.W.C. and H.C.Y.L.; Supervision, E.Y.Y.C., K.K.C.H., G.K.W.C. and M.P.S.Y.; Validation, K.K.C.H., G.K.W.C. and M.P.S.Y.; Visualization, Z.H. and E.S.K.L.; Writing—original draft, E.Y.Y.C. and Z.H.; Writing—review & editing, K.K.C.H., G.K.W.C., H.C.Y.L., E.S.K.L. and M.P.S.Y.

Funding: This research project was co-funded by the Chinese University of Hong Kong (CUHK) Focused Innovations Scheme—Scheme A: Biomedical Sciences (Phase 2) and the CUHK Climate Change and Health research project fund. The funders did not involve in the study.

Acknowledgments: The authors thank all the participants in this study. Special acknowledge to Chunlan Guo and Sida Liu for their support and comments during the study design and data collection process.

Conflicts of Interest: The authors declare no conflict of interest.

References

1. Fridolf, K.; Nilsson, D.; Frantzich, H. Fire evacuation in underground transportation systems: A review of accidents and empirical research. *Fire Technol.* **2013**, *49*, 451–475. [CrossRef]
2. Gonzalez-Navarro, M.; Turner, M.A. Subways and urban growth: Evidence from earth. *J. Urban Econ.* **2018**, *108*, 85–106. [CrossRef]
3. Garlock, M.; Paya-Zaforteza, I.; Kodur, V.; Gu, L. Fire hazard in bridges: Review, assessment and repair strategies. *Eng. Struct.* **2012**, *35*, 89–98. [CrossRef]
4. Brown, A.L.; Wagner, G.J.; Metzinger, K.E. Impact, fire, and fluid spread code coupling for complex transportation accident environment simulation. *J. Thermal Sci. Eng. Appl.* **2012**, *4*, 021004. [CrossRef] [PubMed]
5. Carvel, R.; Marlair, G. *A History of Fire Incidents in Tunnels*; Thomas Telford Publishing: London, UK, 2005.

6. Jeon, G.; Hong, W. Characteristic features of the behavior and perception of evacuees from the Daegu subway fire and safety measures in an underground fire. *J. Asian Archit. Build. Eng.* **2009**, *8*, 415–422. [CrossRef]
7. Tsukahara, M.; Koshiba, Y.; Ohtani, H. Effectiveness of downward evacuation in a large-scale subway fire using Fire Dynamics Simulator. *Tunn. Undergr. Space Technol.* **2011**, *26*, 573–581. [CrossRef]
8. Kano, M.; Siegel, J.M.; Bourque, L.B. First-Aid Training and Capabilities of the Lay Public: A Potential Alternative Source of Emergency Medical Assistance Following a Natural Disaster. *Disasters* **2005**, *29*, 58–74. [CrossRef]
9. United Nations Office for Disaster Risk Reduction. Sendai Framework for Disaster Risk Reduction. Available online: https://www.unisdr.org/we/coordinate/sendai-framework (accessed on 18 December 2017).
10. United Nations Office for Disaster Risk Reduction. Terminology. Available online: https://www.unisdr.org/we/inform/terminology (accessed on 18 December 2017).
11. Chan, E.Y.Y.; Yue, J.; Lee, P.; Wang, S.S. Socio-demographic predictors for urban community disaster health risk perception and household based preparedness in a Chinese urban city. *PLoS Curr.* **2016**. [CrossRef]
12. Chan, E.Y.Y.; Huang, Z.; Mark, C.K.; Guo, C. Weather Information Acquisition and Health Significance during Extreme Cold Weather in a Subtropical City: A Cross-sectional Survey in Hong Kong. *Int. J. Disaster Risk Sci.* **2017**, *8*, 134–144. [CrossRef]
13. Tam, G.; Huang, Z.; Chan, E.Y.Y. Household Preparedness and Preferred Communication Channels in Public Health Emergencies: A Cross-Sectional Survey of Residents in An Asian Developed Urban City. *Int. J. Environ. Res. Public Health* **2018**, *15*, 1598. [CrossRef]
14. Lam, R.P.K.; Leung, L.P.; Balsari, S.; Hsiao, K.-H.; Newnham, E.; Patrick, K.; Pham, P.; Leaning, J. Urban disaster preparedness of Hong Kong residents: A territory-wide survey. *Int. J. Disaster Risk Reduct.* **2017**, *23*, 62–69. [CrossRef]
15. Environment Bureau. Hong Kong Special Administrative Region. Climate Change Report 2015. Available online: http://www.enb.gov.hk/sites/default/files/pdf/ClimateChangeEng.pdf (accessed on 18 September 2017).
16. Zhang, L.; Lee, S.Y. Chinese High-Speed Train Fire Triggers Evacuation. Available online: https://www.reuters.com/article/us-china-accidents-train/chinese-high-speed-train-fire-triggers-evacuation-idUSKBN1FE13H (accessed on 18 September 2018).
17. Chan, E.Y.Y.; Murray, V. What are the health research needs for the Sendai Framework? *Lancet* **2017**, *390*, e35–e36. [CrossRef]
18. Lo, S.T.T.; Chan, E.Y.Y.; Chan, G.K.W.; Murray, V.; Ardalan, A.; Abrahams, J. Health Emergency and Disaster Management (H-EDRM): Developing the research field within the Sendai framework paradigm. *Int. J. Disaster Risk Sci.* **2017**. [CrossRef]
19. Hong Kong Special Administrative Region. LCQ19: Fire Incident at MTR Train and Public Transport Safety. 2017. Available online: http://www.info.gov.hk/gia/general/201703/01/P2017030100246.htm (accessed on 18 September 2017).
20. Kao, E. Hong Kong MTR Firebomb Suspect Dies in Hospital from 'Organ Failure'. Available online: http://www.scmp.com/news/hong-kong/law-crime/article/2094256/hong-kong-mtr-firebomb-suspect-dies-hospital-organ-failure (accessed on 18 September 2017).
21. Chan, E.Y.Y.; Wang, S.S.; Ho, J.Y.; Huang, Z.; Liu, S.; Guo, C. Socio-demographic predictors of health and environmental co-benefit behaviours for climate change mitigation in urban China. *PLoS ONE* **2017**, *12*, e0188661. [CrossRef] [PubMed]
22. Hong Kong St. John Ambulance. *First Aid Manual*; Hong Kong St. John Ambulance: Hong Kong, China, 2001.
23. Census and Statistics Department. Hong Kong Special Administrative Region. Available online: http://www.bycensus2016.gov.hk/en (accessed on 18 September 2017).
24. Hong Kong Police Force. Hong Kong Special Administrative Region. Available online: https://www.police.gov.hk/info/doc/statistics/traffic_report_2016_en.pdf (accessed on 18 December 2017).
25. China Daily. Bus Smash Kills 21 in Hong Kong. Available online: http://www.chinadaily.com.cn/en/doc/2003-07/11/content_244497.htm (accessed on 18 December 2017).
26. Ho, L.; Chan, P. Bus Crash Kills 18, Injures 44 in Sai Kung. Available online: http://www.chinadaily.com.cn/hkedition/2008-05/02/content_6656599.htm (accessed on 18 December 2017).
27. Ian, S. Comparing the fatality risks in United States transportation across modes and over time. *Res. Transp. Econ.* **2013**, *43*, 9–22.

28. Roche-Cerasi, I.; Rundmo, T.; Sigurdson, J.F.; Moe, D. Transport mode preferences, risk perception and worry in a Norwegian urban population. *Accid. Anal. Prev.* **2013**, *50*, 698–704. [CrossRef]
29. Backer-Grøndahl, A.; Fyhri, A.; Ulleberg, P.; Amundsen, A.H. Accidents and unpleasant incidents: Worry in transport and prediction of travel behavior. *Risk Anal. Int. J.* **2009**, *29*, 1217–1226. [CrossRef]
30. Rundmo, T.; Nordfjærn, T.; Iversen, H.H.; Oltedal, S.; Jørgensen, S.H. The role of risk perception and other risk-related judgements in transportation mode use. *Saf. Sci.* **2011**, *49*, 226–235. [CrossRef]
31. Sjöberg, L. Worry and risk perception. *Risk Anal.* **1998**, *18*, 85–93. [CrossRef]
32. Maccoby, E.E.; Jacklin, C.N. *The Psychology of Sex Differences*; Stanford University Press: Palo Alto, CA, USA, 1978.
33. Patel, V.; Kleinman, A. Poverty and common mental disorders in developing countries. *Bull. World Health Organ.* **2003**, *81*, 609–615.
34. Dugas, M.J.; Robichaud, M. *Cognitive-Behavioral Treatment for Generalized Anxiety Disorder: From Science to Practice*; Routledge: New York, NY, USA, 2012.
35. Paton, D. Responding to hazard effects: Promoting resilience and adjustment adoption. *Aust. J. Emerg. Manag.* **2001**, *16*, 47.
36. Loke, A.Y.; Lai, C.K.; Fung, O.W. At-home disaster preparedness of elderly people in Hong Kong. *Geriatr. Gerontol. Int.* **2012**, *12*, 524–531. [CrossRef] [PubMed]
37. Larsson, E.; Martensson, M.; Alexanderson, K. First-aid training could improve risk behavior and enhance bystander actions. *Prehospital Disaster Med.* **2002**, *17*, 134–141. [CrossRef] [PubMed]
38. Bakke, H.K.; Steinvik, T.; Angell, J.; Wisborg, T. A nationwide survey of first aid training and encounters in Norway. *BMC Emerg. Med.* **2016**, *17*, 6. [CrossRef]
39. Kureckova, V.; Gabrhel, V.; Zamecnik, P.; Rezac, P.; Zaoral, A.; Hobl, J. First aid as an important traffic safety factor–evaluation of the experience–based training. *Eur. Transp. Res. Rev.* **2017**, *9*, 5. [CrossRef]
40. Office of the Communications Authority. Hong Kong Special Administrative Region. Key Communication Statistics. Available online: http://www.ofca.gov.hk/en/media_focus/data_statistics/key_stat (accessed on 18 December 2017).
41. Lau, J.T.; Yang, X.; Pang, E.; Tsui, H.Y.; Wong, E.; Wing, Y.K. SARS-related perception in Hong Kong. *Emerg. Infect. Dis.* **2005**, *11*, 417. [PubMed]
42. Hong Kong Transport Department. Hong Kong Special Administrative Region. Travel Characteristics Survey 2011 Final Report. Available online: http://www.td.gov.hk/filemanager/en/content_4652/tcs2011_eng.pdf (accessed on 18 December 2017).

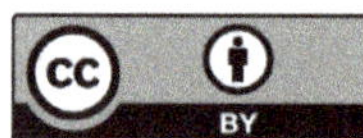

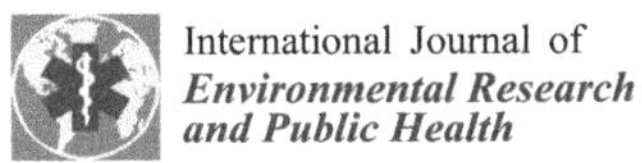
International Journal of
Environmental Research and Public Health

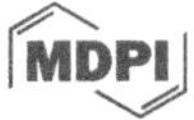

Article

Health Vulnerability Index for Disaster Risk Reduction: Application in Belt and Road Initiative (BRI) Region

Emily Yang Ying Chan [1,2,3,*], Zhe Huang [1], Holly Ching Yu Lam [1], Carol Ka Po Wong [1] and Qiang Zou [4]

1 Collaborating Centre for Oxford University and CUHK for Disaster and Medical Humanitarian Response (CCOUC), JC (Jockey Club) school of Public Health and Primary Care, Faculty of Medicine, Chinese University of Hong Kong, Hong Kong, China; huangzhe@cuhk.edu.hk (Z.H.); hollylam@cuhk.edu.hk (H.C.Y.L.); wongcarol@cuhk.edu.hk (C.K.P.W.)
2 Nuffield Department of Medicine, University of Oxford, Oxford OX3 7BN, UK
3 François-Xavier Bagnoud Center for Health & Human Rights, Harvard University, Boston, MA 02138, USA
4 Institute of Mountain Hazards and Environment, Chinese Academy of Science, Chengdu 610041, China; zouqiang@imde.ac.cn
* Correspondence: emily.chan@cuhk.edu.hk

Received: 27 December 2018; Accepted: 25 January 2019; Published: 29 January 2019

Abstract: Despite the importance of health vulnerability in disaster risk assessment, most of the existing disaster vulnerability indicators only emphasize economic and social vulnerability. Important underlying health risks such as non-communicable disease are not included in vulnerability measures. A three-phase methodology approach was used to construct a disaster risk model that includes a number of key health indicators which might be missing in global disaster risk analysis. This study describes the development of an integrated health vulnerability index and explains how the proposed vulnerability index may be incorporated into an all-hazard based disaster risk index in the Belt and Road Initiative (BRI), also known as the "Silk Road Economic Belt", region. Relevant indicators were identified and reviewed in the published literature in PubMed/Medline. A two-stage dimension reduction statistical method was used to determine the weightings of relevant dimensions to the construction of the overall vulnerability index. The proposed final health vulnerability index included nine indicators, including the proportion of the population below 15 and above 65 years, under-five mortality ratio, maternal mortality ratio, tuberculosis prevalence, age-standardized raised blood pressure, physician ratio, hospital bed ratio, and coverage of the measles-containing-vaccine first-dose (MCV1) and diphtheria tetanus toxoid and pertussis (DTP3) vaccines. This proposed index, which has a better reflection of the health vulnerability in communities, may serve as a policy and implementation tool to facilitate the capacity-building of Health-Emergency Disaster Risk management (Health-EDRM).

Keywords: Health vulnerability; Health-EDRM; disaster risk; Silk Road Economic Belt; map; Belt and Road Initiative

---

1. Introduction

Disasters have brought huge losses in human health and the economy globally. According to Economic Losses, Poverty & Disasters, 1998–2017 issued by the Centre for Research on the Epidemiology of Disasters and United Nations Office for Disaster Risk Reduction in 2018, climate-related and geophysical disasters alone have taken lives from 1.3 million people, and have affected 4.4 billion people in the world between 1998–2017. The report also highlighted a global direct economic loss of USD 2908 billion due to disasters within the same period [1]. Asia, similar to previous years, suffered from the highest disaster occurrence (more than 40% of the total) [2], while China, India, Indonesia, and the Philippines were four of the top five countries that were most frequently hit by natural disasters over the last decade [3]. Due to climate change, both the frequency and intensity of disasters have been predicated to increase in the 21st century [4]. Relevant risk assessment tools and disaster risk reduction plans are important for saving lives and reducing losses in the future.

Understanding disaster risk in all its dimensions is the first priority for Disaster Risk Reduction action in the Sendai Framework, which was the first major agreement endorsed by the United Nations (UN) General Assembly on Disaster Risk Reduction for policies and practices for disaster risk management [5]. Disaster risk can be conceptualized as a function of hazard, exposure, and vulnerability [6]. According to UNISDR [7], risk is defined as the harmful consequences resulting from interactions between hazards, exposure, and vulnerable conditions. Hazard refers to dangerous phenomena that may cause negative health impacts; exposure refers to the people who are present in hazard zones and subject to potential health losses; vulnerability refers to the characteristics and circumstances of a community that make it susceptible to the damaging effects of a hazard. Disaster risk assessment can be understood as quantifying these three components among the population.

There are major technical gaps in how to describe vulnerability, particularly to health risks, when constructing disaster risk indexes [8]. Existing vulnerability indicators/indexes mostly focus on economic and social vulnerability [9–11]. Most health vulnerability indexes were developed after 2010, and were related to human health vulnerability toward climate-related disasters such as heat wave [12–14], flooding [15], dengue fever [16], and climate change [17]. In addition, as the data used for index construction were largely based on the country's own capacity in data collection, multi-country comparisons are often difficult, as countries may have different data collection methods and capacities. The Index For Risk Management (INFORM), a collaborative work with the United Nations, and the World Risk Index, a joint work with the Integrated Research on Disaster Risk (IRDR), are sophisticated global disaster risk indexes that have accounted for health vulnerability [18,19]. However, the current indexes do not include important health-affecting factors such as chronic diseases. Chronic disease is an important aspect to be considered in disaster risk management, as discontinuous treatment and medicine, which is possible during a disaster event, can lead to adverse health consequences among chronic disease patients. For instance, the provision of insulin may sustain the well-being and survival of diabetes patients [20].

Under the influence of globalization, the spread of health risks is borderless, and the prevention and control of health emergencies (e.g., disasters) need to be managed collaboratively. China's Belt and Road Initiative (BRI), also known as the "Silk Road Economic Belt", was initiated in 2013 and aimed to connect the Asian, European, and African continents and their adjacent seas, and establish and strengthen partnerships among the countries along the Belt and Road [21]. Among these BRI countries, various types of disasters occur frequently, and the widespread damage and destruction caused by disasters seriously disrupts the functioning of a society, and poses a major socio-economic development challenge for the Belt and Road Initiative region. The BRI also provides a health cooperation platform to handle regional health emergencies, offers medical assistance, and disseminates experience in the field of health care [22]. Understanding disaster risk and vulnerability for the countries along the Belt and Road is crucial for resource allocation. Yet, current available health vulnerability indexes may not apply to the countries within Belt and Road Initiative.

Health-Emergency Disaster Risk Management (Health-EDRM) is an academic paradigm representing the intersection of health and disaster risk reduction that covers the systematic analysis and management of health risks surrounding emergencies and disasters [23]. This study falls into the primary Health-EDRM intervention category (prevention/preparedness) in the system (country) level.

The objective of this paper is to describe the development of a health vulnerability index that aims to be incorporated into the vulnerability index, and might be applied to the use of the all-hazard based disaster risk index in the BRI region. The developed index described in this study used open access data and proposed indicators that are available in most countries and make disaster risk comparison between countries possible. The proposed method can also be adopted by regions or populations that were not included in this study. The findings from this study provide evidence to support disaster risk reduction in the BRI regions, and serve as a basis for the development of a population-based disaster risk assessment tool.

2. Materials and Methods

A three-phase methodology approach was used to develop the final disaster risk model. Phase 1 of the approach focuses on the development of the health vulnerability index, which includes an extensive literature review to identify the relevant published indicators to construct health vulnerability. Phase 2 involves a two-stage dimension reduction statistical method to identify the weighting for the indicators that were included for the health vulnerability index development. Phase 3 aims to create the final disaster risk index by combining the three main component indexes (health vulnerability index, exposure, and hazard index), which can be described in the following equation: Risk = Exposure $\times$ Hazard $\times$ Vulnerability [6]. The health vulnerability index is combined with existing exposure and hazard indexes to form a disaster risk index at the national level. The exposure and hazard indexes were based and accessed through the Institute of Mountain Hazards and Environment at the Chinese Academy of Science (http://english.imde.cas.cn). As the mechanisms and the development of the two indexes were out of the scope of this study, they were not included in this paper's discussion.

2.1. Phase I

Data Scoping and Variable Selection

Variable selection criteria include: (1) any indicator that is conceptually relevant to health vulnerability or may capture the Health-EDRM risks of the community; (2) indicators that have been identified/suggested in relevant literatures or organizations (e.g., the World Health Organization (WHO), UN, INFORM model [18] and World Risk Index [19]), and (3) indicators that are available for open access from reliable sources (e.g., WHO and the World Bank) for all of the study regions. Since subsequent factor analysis cannot be performed with missing values, countries with missing values were excluded in the subsequent analysis. The countries/areas along the BRI region and countries/areas included in the analysis were listed in the supplementary material A1.

2.2. Phase II

Statistical Model for the Health Vulnerability Index

As this study made no assumption on the weighting for indicators, in order to determine the weightings and explore the importance of the underlying dimensions to the overall vulnerability, a two-stage dimension reduction statistical method was used. This method also increases robustness [10] and allows monitoring changes in the weighting of indicators over time. In stage one, factor analysis (FA) was used as the primary statistical procedure for dimension reduction. The observed and correlated indicators were assumed to be adequately explained by a lower number of unobserved and uncorrelated factors. Stage two modeling was based on the result of FA; the selected health indicators were used to produce a more compact representation of the indicators (factors).

Stage 1: Selected indicators are normalized and included in the FA analysis. The matrix of factor loadings was estimated via the maximum likelihood method, and the number of factors that is extracted should contribute cumulatively to the explanation of the overall variance by more than 60% [24]. The Chi-square test was used to examine whether the number of factors, k, are sufficient to account for the observed covariance [25]. A non-significant Chi-square test result ($p \geq 0.05$) indicates that k is sufficient to explain the observed covariance. The explanation power increases when k increases. To obtain the most efficient model, the smallest k that yielded a non-significant Chi-square test was chosen. The initial k tried was one, and then, k was increased by one at a time. Then, the process is repeated until the p-value of the Chi-square test ≥ 0.05 [25]. Factors identified from FA are sometimes expressed as a compound with a relative large number of non-zero weighting indicators, which may make factor interpretation hard. To make interpretations of factors easier, Varimax rotation [26] was conducted to obtain as few large loadings and as many near-zero loadings as possible.

Stage 2: The development of the Health Vulnerability Index (HVI) is based on the latent factors derived from the FA. Each latent factor has factor loading on every health indicator, measuring the correlation between the health factor and the health indicator. The construction of the weights of the selected health indicators is from the rotated matrix of factor loadings [24,27]: (1) the proportion on each latent factor of the total unit variance was extracted; (2) the intermediate weights of all of the health indicators were calculated from the factor loadings corresponding to the latent factor; (3) the proportion on each latent factor is multiplied by the intermediate weights of all the health indicators on each latent factor to generate the weights for all the selected health indicators. Finally, the weights were multiplied by the corresponding standardized health indicator, and were added together for every country's HVI. A higher value indicates a more vulnerable country. The HVI value of each country involved was categorized into five HVI clusters using the equal interval method for data presentation in the form of a vulnerability map. A five-level scale was selected, as it provides a good balance between risk-level differentiation and clarity, and has been widely adopted in risk-level presentations [28,29]. R version 3.4.1 and ArcMap version 10.4.1 were used.

2.3. Phase III

Disaster Risk Index Model

Exposure and Hazard

The exposure and hazard index were provided by the working dataset of The Institute of Mountain Hazards and Environment at The Chinese Academy of Science. The exposure index was estimated by using the population density data from the Socioeconomic Data and Applications Center [30] as a proxy. For hazard, the frequency of natural disaster was applied. Both indexes were in a pixel-based format, and can be illustrated using a map.

Disaster Risk Index

Raster values from the Exposure index, the Hazard index, and the Vulnerability index were multiplied to generate the final Risk index. Since both the exposure and the hazard indexes are pixel-based data, the vulnerability index was transformed from the country-based format to the pixel-based using ArcMap before combining with the other two indexes to form the final risk index.

$$\text{Calculation of Risk (Risk} = \text{Exposure} \times \text{Hazard} \times \text{Vulnerability)} \quad (1)$$

Logarithm transformations were applied for skewed data, including the exposure index and the hazard index. The log-transformed indexes and the vulnerability index were then transformed to a 0–1 scale using min–max normalization. The final disaster risk index was calculated by multiplying the three transformed components with equal weight (Formula (1)) [18,19]. The results were presented in the form of map in a scale with five risk levels.

3. Results

3.1. Key Indicators of Vulnerability

Based on the three evaluation criteria, nine health indicators were identified and included in the final index development. Table 1 describes the key health indicators included.

Table 1. Key indicators of health vulnerability and their relevance.

Dimension of Health Vulnerability	Indicator	Conceptual Relevance to Health Vulnerability
Vulnerable age [a]	1. Population ages 0–14 and population ages 65 and above (% of total)	Extreme age groups (children and elderly) are known to be more vulnerable to health risks and less likely to be resilient when a disaster strikes. This is an important component in the "dependency ratio". They are more likely to accumulate post-disaster health and service needs.
Premature mortality [b]	2. Under-five mortality rate (probability of dying by age five per 1000 live births)	Leading indicator of health in the United Nation (UN)'s Sustainable Development Goals (SDGs). It is closely linked to maternal health.
Preventable mortality [b]	3. Maternal mortality ratio (per 100,000 live births)	Leading indicator of health in the UN's Sustainable Development Goals (SDGs). In addition to preventable deaths, this indicator reflects the capacity of health systems to effectively prevent and address the complications occurring during pregnancy and childbirth.
Vaccination gap for measles [b]	4. Measles-containing-vaccine first-dose (MCV1) immunization coverage gap among one-year-olds (%)	Standard Expanded Program on Immunization (EPI) for common preventable Childhood Communicable Diseases for children <one year old. Coverage may be used to monitor immunization services as well as guide disease eradication and elimination efforts, and are a good indicator of health system performance. MCV1: Measles is one of the most contagious and mortality-causing diseases in displaced camps. DTP3: Tetanus is common preventable infection associated with injury/wound.
Vaccination gap for diphtheria, tetanus, and pertussis [b]	5. Diphtheria tetanus toxoid and pertussis (DTP3) immunization coverage gap among 1-year-olds (%)	
Chronic diseases status [b]	6. Raised blood pressure (SBP $\geq$140 OR DBP $\geq$90), age-standardized (%)	A proxy indicator for chronic non-communicable disease. Hypertension and heart disease are some of the leading causes of mortality and morbidity globally. Disease status and potential activity limitations among adults can impair one's ability to prepare, respond, or recover from a disaster.
Infectious disease [b]	7. Incidence of tuberculosis (per 100,000 population per year)	Tuberculosis (TB) is the second leading infectious cause of death, and one of the most burden-inflicting diseases in the world. SDGs include ending the TB epidemic by 2030. The incidence of tuberculosis gives an indication of the burden of TB in a population.
Coping capacity [b]	8. Hospital beds (per 10,000 population)	Health systems resources indicate the level of access to care and the provision of quality medical care, which are highly correlated with live-saving and health status.
	9. Physicians' density (per 1000 population)	

Source: [a] Data collected from the World Bank; [b] Data collected from the World Health Organization. DBP: diastolic blood pressure; SBP: systolic blood pressure.

The Health Vulnerability Index was constructed for the 147 countries along the Belt and Road region. Indicators one, six, and seven are related to population structure and health status; indicators four and five are used to monitor immunization services, which are good indictors of health system performance; indicators two and three are leading indicators of the level of child and maternal health, as well as the overall development in countries; and indictors eight and nine measure the availability of healthcare, and are important indicators of disaster coping capacity. The correlations between the nine health indicators were shown in Figure 1. All of the correlations presented are statistically significant (all p-values < 0.01).

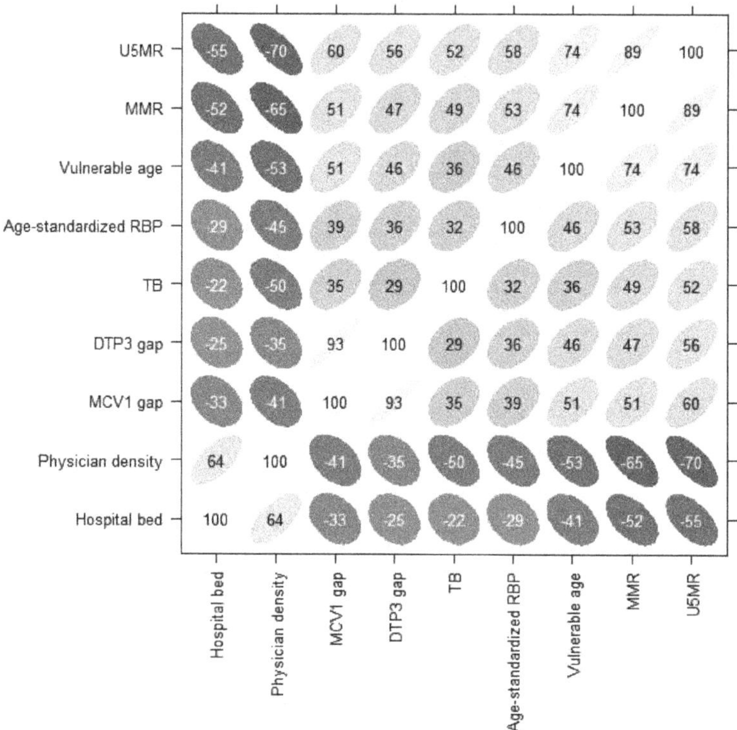

Figure 1. Correlation matrix of the proposed nine health indicators. Note: The figure depicts each correlation by an ellipse whose shape tends toward a line with a slope of one (or −1) for correlation coefficients near one (or −1), and toward a circle for a correlation coefficient near zero. In addition, 100 times the correlation coefficient is printed inside the ellipse (significance level at $\alpha = 0.05$).

3.2. Underlying Dimensions of Health Vulnerability

The results of the Chi-square test for the sufficiency of the number of factors suggested that a three-factor solution was adequate to account for the observed covariances in the data among the 147 countries. Both of the eigenvalues of the three-factor solution were larger than one, and the three factors counted for about 71% of the total variance. Factor loadings after rotation are shown in Figure 2.

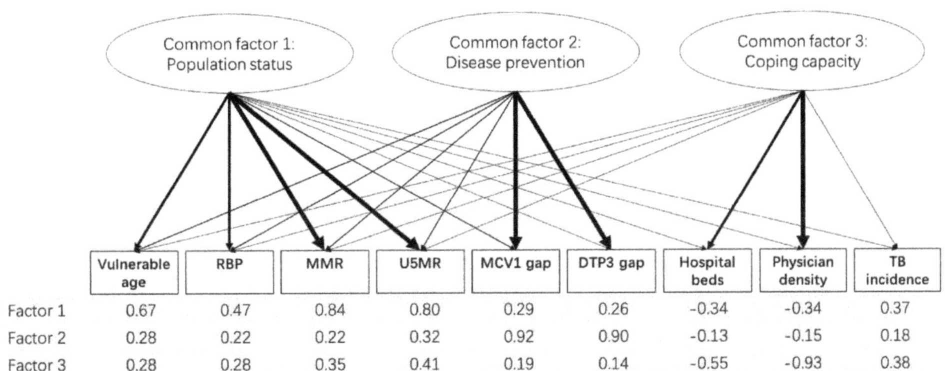

Figure 2. Factor loadings of the three latent factors. Note: Factor loadings are printed under the corresponding indicator. They are also indicated by the thickness of the arrow linking the factor and the indicator: the thicker the arrow, the higher the factor loading. Arrows are not shown if the absolute value of the factor loading is less than 0.2. Vulnerable age: people aged 0–14 or/and 65+ (%); RBP: Age-standardized raised blood pressure prevalence (%); MMR: Maternal mortality ratio (per 100,000 live births); U5MR: Under-five mortality rate (per 1000 live births); MCV1 gap: MCV1 Coverage Gap (%); DTP3 gap: DTP3 Coverage Gap (%); Hospital beds: Hospital beds density (per 10,000 population); Physician density: Physicians density (per 1000 population); TB incidence: Incidence of tuberculosis (per 100,000 population).

Since factor one is dominated by the maternal mortality ratio (per 100,000 live births) (MMR, 0.84) and the under-five mortality rate (per 1000 live births) (U5MR, 0.80), and moderately affected by vulnerable age (0.67) and age-standardized raised blood pressure prevalence (RBP) (0.47), this factor was labeled the "population status" factor. The second factor has its highest loadings on the measles-containing-vaccine first-dose (MCV1) gap (0.92) and diphtheria tetanus toxoid and pertussis (DTP3) gap (0.90), which was labeled the "disease prevention" factor. The third factor was highly correlated with physician density (0.92) and moderately with hospital beds (0.90), so it was labeled the "coping capacity" factor.

3.3. Factor Scores of Countries

The estimated scores of factors one to three for each country were calculated and categorized into five levels, as shown in Figure 3. Considering factor one, which reflects population status, Sierra Leone, Chad, and the Central African Republic are the most vulnerable countries, whilst Ukraine was shown to be the least vulnerable among all of the studied countries. For the second factor, Equatorial Guinea and Ukraine are prominent, because they had low MCV1 and DTP3 immunization coverage. For factor three, Thailand, the Solomon Islands, and Indonesia were at the highest end of the scale.

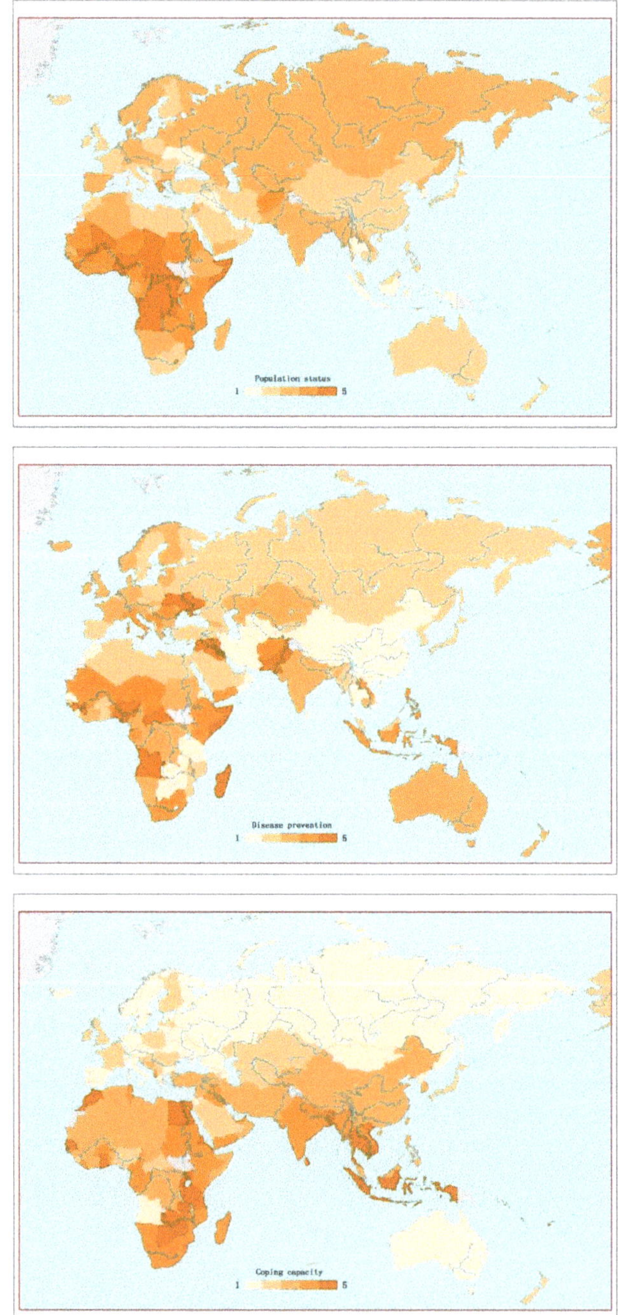

Figure 3. Factor scores of countries along the Belt and Road Initiative (BRI) region. Note: deeper color indicates a higher factor score and greater vulnerability.

3.4. Health Vulnerability Index of Countries

The development of the HVI was based on the FA model above, which captured the relative weights of the six health indicators. Weights for vulnerable age, RBP, MMR, U5MR, MCV1 gap, DTP3 gap, hospital beds, physician density, and incidence of tuberculosis (TB, per 100,000 population) were 0.10, 0.05, 0.14, 0.14, 0.15, 0.14, 0.07, 0.16, and 0.05, respectively. Greece, the Republic of Korea, and Belarus were the three least vulnerable countries, whereas countries labeled in the darkest color (the most vulnerable) were clustered in Africa, such as Somalia, the Central African Republic, and Chad (Figure 4).

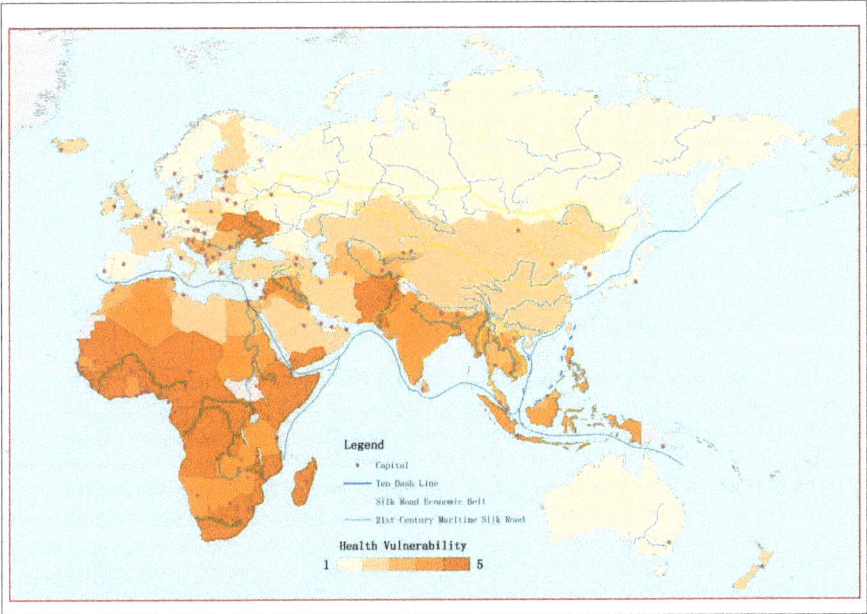

Figure 4. Health Vulnerability Index of countries along the Belt and Road Initiative (BRI) region. Note: deeper color indicates greater vulnerability.

3.5. Disaster Risk Mapping in Silk Road

The final disaster risk index along the Belt and Road region were calculated by combining the proposed vulnerability index, the hazard index, and the exposure index. The final index was in pixel-based format, and therefore was presented in a world map for illustration (Figure 5). The top five areas with the highest disaster risk that was identified in this study were in locations near the Philippines, Afghanistan, Bangladesh, Somalia, and Indonesia. Meanwhile, northwest China, North Africa, eastern Europe, and Australia were found to have relatively lower risks.

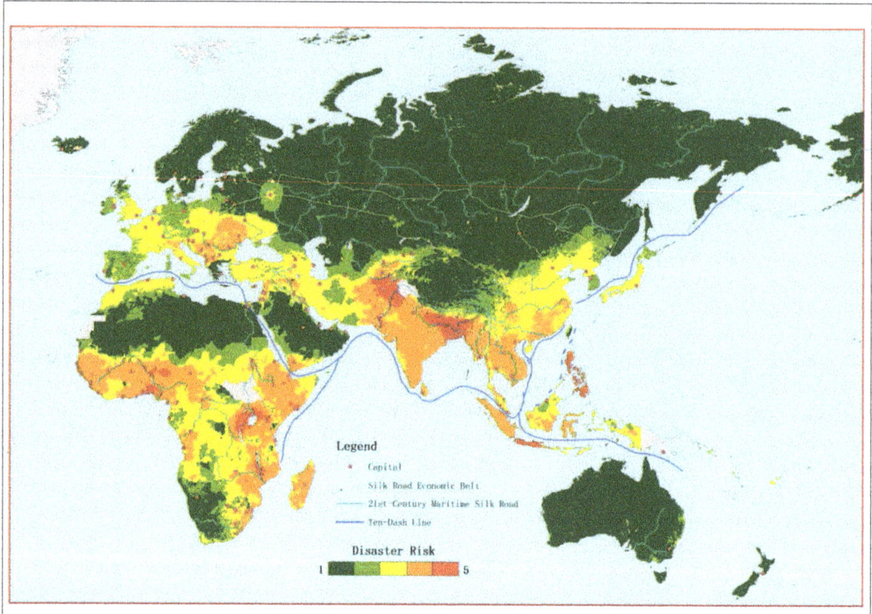

Figure 5. Health disaster risk of countries along the Belt and Road Initiative (BRI) region.

4. Discussion

This paper presents a three-phase methodology approach for disaster risk assessment that incorporated health vulnerability dimensions into an existing hazard-based disaster risk map development. The proposed health vulnerability assessment index covers seven health dimensions, including infectious disease, chronic disease, maternity, under five years old, healthcare services, immunization, and the dependency ratio. Under these seven dimensions, nine indicators were used for formulating the vulnerability index, namely: (1) proportion of population below 15 years and above 65 years, (2) under-five mortality ratio, (3) maternal mortality ratio, (4) prevalence of tuberculosis, (5) the age-standardized raised blood pressure, (6) physician ratio, (7) hospital bed ratio, and (8) coverage of the MCV1 and (9) DTP3 vaccines. Then, the vulnerability index that was formed was combined with an existing disaster risks index from the Institute of Mountain Hazards and Environment at The Chinese Academy of Science.

Based on the formula established in this study and the public data mentioned in the Methods session, Greece, the Republic of Korea, and Belarus were found to be the three least vulnerable countries, while Somalia, the Central African Republic, and Chad were the three most vulnerable countries. After combining the vulnerability index with the exposure and hazard indexes, areas close to the Philippines, Afghanistan, Bangladesh, Somalia, and Indonesia were shown to have the highest disaster risk among the 147 study countries along the BRI region.

The Index For Risk Management (INFORM) and the World Risk Index are global disaster risk indexes that have incorporated health related components for vulnerability. INFORM is a global risk assessment index that is a collaboration of the Inter-Agency Standing Committee Task Team for Preparedness and Resilience and the European Commission and is adopted in the Global Risk Map (https://globalriskmap.terria.io/About.html) (including 190 countries). These included tuberculosis prevalence, HIV prevalence, malaria death rate, and under-five mortality as vulnerability indicators, and have included physician density as a capacity-coping indicator. The World Risk Index (171 countries considered) presented by Birkmann and Welle, and the Integrated Research on Disaster Risk (IRDR) team [19], have combined susceptibility, lack of coping, and adaptive capacity within vulnerability. They considered a dependency ratio for susceptibility, physicians, and hospital beds ratio for coping capacity, and private and public medical expenditure for adaptive capacity. Table 2 below compares the health components considered in the two mentioned indexes and those included in this index. The INFORM model and the Word Risk Index were built with sophisticated calculations and variables from different aspects in risk assessments such as health-related components, economic status, political environment, and infrastructure. Yet, many important health vulnerability burdens such as non-communicable diseases were not included.

The study aims to advance the current disaster risk assessment to include health vulnerability, which will inevitably affect population vulnerability in times of crisis. Thus, the discussion here focused on health-related components. The index proposed in this study has included indicator(s) of seven important health components in disaster risk assessment. Specifically, although chronic diseases have been cited as the most important causes of mortality and morbidity [31], attention has yet to be placed on global disaster risk assessment. People living with chronic diseases usually highly rely on long-term medicine for disease management. Unstable medicine access during and after disasters may lead to preventable adverse health consequences for the affected individual and the community. Considering the increasing prevalence of chronic diseases globally, related factors are suggested to be included as a vulnerability indicators in estimating disaster risks.

Table 3 shows the top 10 countries with the highest vulnerability/lowest coping capacity obtained from the three indexes. Despite the lack of consideration of the socio-economic, political, and infrastructural aspects and the different health components considered in the proposed index, five out of the 10 countries also appeared in top 10 from the other two indexes. This suggested that the health dimension is a strong determinant for disaster risk vulnerability. It is of note that although South Sudan was shown to be the most vulnerable with least coping capacity in the INFORM model, due to the missing data for South Sudan in the dataset that was used in this study (WHO and the World Bank), South Sudan was not included in this analysis. Ukraine was the most vulnerable country in Europe according to this study. Its vulnerability was mainly due to the country's low vaccination rate, which was almost the lowest among all of the studied countries in the dataset. Since this study only accounted for health-related aspects calculating vulnerabilities, rather than other factors such as economic and political factors, Ukraine was found to be more vulnerable for disaster risk compared to the INFORM and the World Risk Indexes. The relatively higher coping capacity for European countries might reflect the better socio-economic status in these countries.

Vulnerability made substantial contributions to understandings and conceptualizations of disaster risk. When populations are exposed to natural disasters, vulnerable groups such as young children, older people, and people with mobility problems have more difficulties in evacuations, and might have a higher immediate risk of injuries. After extreme natural events, people might lose their homes and have to stay closely together in temporary shelters where hygiene and living conditions are usually compromised. In communities with low vaccination rates, outbreaks of infectious diseases might happen. Chronic diseases, as well as mental and psychological problems, also create health concerns and add extra stress to the healthcare system. Efficient medical services are important for handling immediate and indirect health needs in affected areas. Delayed or insufficient medical support to the affected people would increase fatality and morbidity. This could be due to the non-perfect healthcare system in local areas with poor coping capacity. Thus, this study proposed to include health vulnerability in estimating disaster risks. The results of this study have shown that populations with higher vulnerability were under higher overall risks than populations with lower vulnerability, given that they have comparable hazards and exposures. For example, both Japan and Bangladesh were prone to earthquakes (hazard), and were densely populated (exposure). However, after considering the vulnerability index proposed in this study, area near Bangladesh has a higher overall disaster risk than Japan.

Table 2. Health-related components considered in the Index For Risk Management (INFORM) model, the World Risk Index, and the index developed in this study.

Components	INFORM	World Risk Index	The Proposed Index
Infectious diseases	Tuberculosis prevalence		Tuberculosis prevalence
	Estimate % of adults (>15) living with HIV		
	Malaria death rate		
Chronic diseases			Age-standardized raised blood pressure
Maternal outcome	Maternal mortality		Maternal mortality
Children under five	Under-five mortality		Under five mortality
	Malnutrition in children under five		
Medical services and access	Physician ratio	Physicians ratio	Physicians ratio
		Hospital beds ratio	Hospital beds ratio
	Per capita expenditure on private and public health care	Public medical expenditure; private medical expenditure	
Immunization	Measles immunization coverage		Coverage of two the MCV1 and DTP3 vaccine
Dependency ratio		Proportion of population <15 years old and >65 years old	Proportion of population <15 years old and >65 years old

Table 3. The top 10 countries with the highest vulnerability/lowest coping capacity from the INFORM model, the World Risk Index, and the proposed index developed in this study.

Top 10 Countries/Regions with Highest Vulnerability/Capacity	INFORM		World Risk Index	The Proposed Index
	Coping Capacity	**Vulnerability**	**Vulnerability Including Susceptibility, Coping Capacities, and Adaptive Capacities**	**Vulnerability**
1	**South Sudan**	**South Sudan**	**Chad**	**Somalia**
2	**Somalia**	**Somalia**	Eritrea	**Central African Republic**
3	**Chad**	**Central African Republic**	Afghanistan	**Chad**
4	**Central African Republic**	**Democratic Republic of the Congo**	Haiti	Equatorial Guinea
5	**Democratic Republic of the Congo**	**Chad**	**Niger**	Nigeria
6	Yemen	Yemen	**Central African Republic**	**Guinea**
7	Guinea-Bissau	Syria	Liberia	**Sierra Leone**
8	Eritrea	Afghanistan	**Sierra Leone**	Mali
9	Liberia	Haiti	Mozambique	**Niger**
10	Togo	Sudan	**Guinea**	**Democratic Republic of the Congo**

The study has several limitations. Firstly, due to the study focus, vulnerability (including adaptive and coping capacity) related to other aspects such as sociodemographic and political aspects were not included for this specific model. Secondly, this study applied factor analysis in determining the underlying constructs of the selected predictors. It is important to highlight that factor analysis does not explain the cause of the convertibility [32]; the factors presented in this study were based on the understandings and experience in the field and the references considered. Despite the sample size that was used for this factor analysis being less than the common agreed size of 200 [32] due to the limited number of countries, it was larger than the suggested minimum size of 100 [32], which should provide considerable power for the analysis. Finally, the results presented were based on the 147 countries along the Belt and Road region; the reported vulnerability ranking is subject to change when different countries are considered.

Thirdly, this proposed index is highly driven by data availability and accuracy. Although the disability rate is another important health determinant in disasters that is advocated by WHO, due to the lack of data, disability was not included in this analysis. Similarly, this study can only include a few indicators as proxies for each health dimension due to the limitation of data. This study did not impute missing data due to simplicity and accuracy. Therefore, the number of missing data would be more than those used in the compared indexes. The accuracy of the results of this analysis was highly dependent on the accuracy of the open access data. Data from different organizations may not be consistent due to inconsistency in collection methods, study periods, calculations, imputation methods, or even data sources. Results should be read with caution.

In addition, although the use of all-hazard approach intended to include all disaster types for the hazard index, the health vulnerability index may face constrains in covering the whole disaster spectrum. For instance, physician density may be an important health indicator for coping capacity during disease outbreaks; however, it may be less relevant to injury risk and health vulnerability during and after tsunamis.

According to the WHO, disaster risk management involving health components can avoid or reduce relevant health impacts [33]. While disaster risk assessment is one of the important components of risk management, hazard, vulnerability and capacity are the three elements that were most commonly considered in disaster risk assessment [33]. Among various dimensions of human vulnerability, low sociodemographic status, female gender, large dependency ratio, chronic diseases and disability are risk factors for disaster-associated mortality and morbidity [33]. Some current risk assessment indexes indicated vulnerability or coping capacity by using sociodemographic factors such as age, poverty, ethnic minority and education level [34,35] while some of them also included health-related variables [18,19].

However, not many existing global based disaster risk assessment model considered underlying non-communicable diseases patterns. A country specific vulnerability index for wildfire from the Environmental Protection Agency, the United State, considered chronic diseases such as asthma, diabetes, hypertension and obesity [36]. This study suggests the inclusion of chronic disease in addition to the health-variables considered in current disaster risk assessment tools (World Risk Index, INFORM) and demonstrated how health-related vulnerability could be added into existing risk assessment tools using a relative simple statistical method and open access data. The results of this study could be served as a basis for future development of disaster risk assessment model or adding a health related component to the existing one.

Specifically, the BRI counties are undergoing rapid socio-economic development. Lifestyle changes and westernized diets may increase the prevalence of chronic diseases such as diabetes and cardiovascular diseases [22]. The index presented in this paper may provide a more comprehensive health-related disaster risk assessment tool which may of the Belt and Road Imitative countries. This would help in improving Health-EDRM capacity planning, resources distribution and arrangement for the regions.

5. Conclusions

This paper presents a health vulnerability index that aims to enhance disaster risk assessment for disaster risk reduction. The suggested health vulnerability index covers seven health vulnerability dimensions, including infectious disease, maternal mortality, under-five mortality, healthcare services, immunization, the dependency ratio, and chronic disease. This new index incorporated important health dimensions such as chronic diseases into the existing hazard-based disaster risk mapping approach.

Attention has to be paid specifically to the health vulnerability, which is associated with population living with chronic diseases. As more comprehensive health-related disaster risk assessments emerge, policy makers and program planners may engage in better resources and capacity planning, distribution, and arrangement to address the needs of Health-EDRM in the disaster-affected regions along the Belt and Road Initiative countries.

Author Contributions: Conceptualization, E.Y.Y.C.; Methodology, Z.H. and Q.Z.; Software, Q.Z.; Validation, Z.H. and H.C.Y.L.; Formal Analysis, Z.H.; Data Curation, Z.H., C.K.P.W.; Writing—Original Draft Preparation, E.Y.Y.C., Z.H. and H.C.Y.L.; Writing—Review & Editing, E.Y.Y.C., Z.H., H.C.Y.L., C.K.P.W. and Q.Z.; Project Administration, C.K.P.W.; Funding Acquisition, Z.H.

Funding: This research was funded by Global Health and Disaster Studies and Research Development Fund, CUHK, CLP/OUT//2017, OAL China, CUHK and International partnership program of Chinese Academy of Sciences (Grant No. 131551KYSB20160002).

Acknowledgments: The authors thank Prof. Peng Cui for his support and advice in this collaborating project and study outcome discussions.

Conflicts of Interest: The authors declare no conflict of interest

References

1. CRED & UNISDR. Economic Losses, Poverty & Disasters, 1998–2017. 2018. Available online: https://www.unisdr.org/files/61119_credeconomiclosses.pdf (accessed on 10 December 2018).
2. CRED. Natural disasters in 2017: Lower mortality, Higher Cost. 2018. Available online: https://cred.be/sites/default/files/CredCrunch50.pdf (accessed on 17 December 2018).
3. Guha-Sapir, D.; Hoyois, P.H.; Wallemacq, P.; Below, R. *Annual Disaster Statistical Review 2016: The Numbers and Trends*; Centre for Research on the Epidemiology of Disasters (CRED): Brussels, Belgium, 2017.
4. IPCC (Intergovernmental Panel on Climate Change). Climate Change 2014: Impacts, Adaptation, and Vulnerability. 2014. Available online: http://www.ipcc.ch/report/ar5/wg2/ (accessed on 11 December 2018).
5. UN (United Nations). Sendai Framework for Disaster Risk Reduction 2015–2030. 2015. Available online: https://www.unisdr.org/files/43291_sendaiframeworkfordrren.pdf (accessed on 14 December 2018).
6. Kron, W. Flood Risk = hazard• values• vulnerability. *Water Int.* **2005**, *30*, 58–68. [CrossRef]
7. UNISDR. *Terminology on Disaster Risk Reduction*; UNISDR: Geneva, Switzerland, 2009.
8. Chan, E.Y.Y.; Murray, V. What are the health research needs for the Sendai Framework? *Lancet.* **2017**, *390*, e35–e36. [CrossRef]
9. Brooks, N.; Adger, W.N.; Kelly, P.M. The determinants of vulnerability and adaptive capacity at the national level and the implications for adaptation. *Glob. Environ. Chang.* **2005**, *15*, 151–163. [CrossRef]
10. Cutter, S.L.; Carolina, S.; Boruff, B.J.; Carolina, S.; Shirley, W.L.; Carolina, S. Social Vulnerability to Environmental Hazards n. *Soc. Sci. Q.* **2003**, *84*, 242–261. [CrossRef]
11. UNDP (United Nations Development Programme). *Reducing Disaster Risk: A Challenge for Development*; United Nations Development Programme: New York, NY, USA, 2004.
12. Reid, C.E.; O'neill, M.S.; Gronlund, C.J.; Brines, S.J.; Brown, D.G.; Diez-Roux, A.V.; Schwartz, J. Mapping community determinants of heat vulnerability. *Environ. Health Perspect.* **2009**, *117*, 1730. [CrossRef] [PubMed]
13. Wolf, T.; McGregor, G. The development of a heat wave vulnerability index for London, United Kingdom. *Weather Clim. Extrem.* **2013**, *1*, 59–68. [CrossRef]

14. Zhu, Q.; Liu, T.; Lin, H.; Xiao, J.; Luo, Y.; Zeng, W.; Zeng, S.; Wei, Y.; Chu, C.; Baum, S.; et al. The spatial distribution of health vulnerability to heat waves in Guangdong Province, China. *Glob. Health Action* **2014**, *7*, 25051. [CrossRef] [PubMed]
15. Phung, D.; Rutherford, S.; Dwirahmadi, F.; Chu, C.; Do, C.M.; Nguyen, T.; Duong, N.C. The spatial distribution of vulnerability to the health impacts of flooding in the Mekong Delta, Vietnam. *Int. J. Biometeorol.* **2016**, *60*, 857–865. [CrossRef] [PubMed]
16. Pastrana, M.E.; Brito, R.L.; Nicolino, R.R.; de Oliveira, C.S.; Haddad, J.P. Spatial and statistical methodologies to determine the distribution of dengue in Brazilian municipalities and relate incidence with the health vulnerability index. *Spat. Spatio-Temporal Epidemiol.* **2014**, *11*, 143–151. [CrossRef] [PubMed]
17. Malik, S.M.; Awan, H.; Khan, N. Mapping vulnerability to climate change and its repercussions on human health in Pakistan. *Glob. Health* **2012**, *8*, 31. [CrossRef] [PubMed]
18. Inter-Agency Standing Committee (IASC) and the European Commission. Interpreting and Applying the INFORM Global Model. 2015. Available online: http://www.inform-index.org/LinkClick.aspx?fileticket=M-RXb0tKsjs%3d&tabid=101&portalid=0&mid=447 (accessed on 17 December 2018).
19. Welle, T.; Birkmann, J. The world risk index–an approach to assess risk and vulnerability on a global scale. *J. Extrem. Events* **2015**, *2*, 1550003. [CrossRef]
20. Chan, E.Y.Y. *Public Health Humanitarian Responses to Natural Disasters*; Routledge: London, UK, 2017.
21. NDRC (National Development and Reform Commission). Vision and Actions on Jointly Building Silk Road Economic Belt and 21st-Century Maritime Silk Road. 2015. Available online: http://http://en.ndrc.gov.cn/newsrelease/201503/t20150330_669367.html (accessed on 16 December 2018).
22. Hu, R.; Liu, R.; Hu, N. China's Belt and Road Initiative from a global health perspective. *Lancet Glob. Health.* **2017**, *5*, e752–e753. [CrossRef]
23. Lo, S.T.T.; Chan, E.Y.Y.; Chan, G.K.W.; Murray, V.; Ardalan, A.; Abrahams, J. Health Emergency and Disaster Management (H-EDRM): Developing the research field within the Sendai Framework paradigm. *Int. J. Disaster Risk Sci.* **2017**. [CrossRef]
24. Nardo, M.; Saisana, M.; Saltelli, A.; Tarantola, S.; Hoffman, A.; Giovannini, E. *Handbook on Constructing Composite Indicators*; OECD: Paris, France, 2008.
25. Everitt, B.; Hothorn, T. *An Introduction to Applied Multivariate Analysis with R*; Springer Science & Business Media: New York, NY, USA, 2011.
26. Kaiser, H.F. The varimax criterion for analytic rotation in factor analysis. *Psychometrika* **1958**, *23*, 187–200. [CrossRef]
27. Li, V.O.; Han, Y.; Lam, J.C.; Zhu, Y.; Bacon-Shone, J. Air pollution and environmental injustice: Are the socially deprived exposed to more PM 2.5 pollution in Hong Kong? *Environ. Sci. Policy.* **2018**, *80*, 53–61. [CrossRef]
28. UNEP/UNISDR. Global Risk Data Platform. 2013. Available online: https://preview.grid.unep.ch (accessed on 1 November 2018).
29. Shi, P.; Kasperson, R. *World Atlas of Natural Disaster Risk*; Springer: Heidelberg, Germany, 2015.
30. SEDAC (Socioeconomic Data and Applications Center). UN-Adjusted Population Density, v4. Available online: http://beta.sedac.ciesin.columbia.edu/data/set/gpw-v4-population-density-adjusted-to-2015-unwpp-country-totals/maps (accessed on 15 December 2018).
31. WHO (World Health Organization). Global Health Risks: Mortality and Burden of Disease Attributable to Selected Major Risks. 2009. Available online: https://www.who.int/healthinfo/global_burden_disease/GlobalHealthRisks_report_full.pdf (accessed on 17 December 2018).
32. Trninić, V.; Jelaska, I.; Štalec, J. Appropriateness and limitations of factor analysis methods utilized in psychology and kinesiology: Part, I.I. *Fizička Kultura*, 2013; 67, 1–7.
33. WHO (World Health Organization). Emergency Risk Management for Health—Overview. 2011. Available online: http://www.who.int/hac/techguidance/preparedness/risk_management_overview_17may2013.pdf?ua=1 (accessed on 10 December 2018).
34. Ciurean, R.L.; Schröter, D.; Glade, T. Conceptual frameworks of vulnerability assessments for natural disasters reduction. In *Approaches to Disaster Management*; IntechOpen: London, UK, 2013.

35. Matyas, D.; Pelling, M. *Disaster Vulnerability and Resilience: Theory, Modelling and Prospective*; Foresight: London, UK, 2012.
36. Rappold, A.G.; Reyes, J.; Pouliot, G.; Cascio, W.E.; Diaz-Sanchez, D. Community vulnerability to health impacts of wildland fire smoke exposure. *Environ. Sci. Technol.* **2017**, *51*, 6674–6682. [CrossRef] [PubMed]

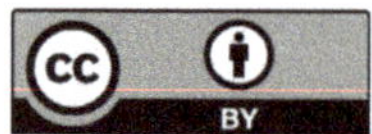

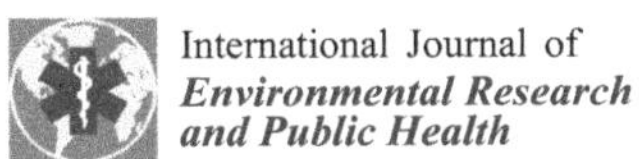
International Journal of
Environmental Research and Public Health

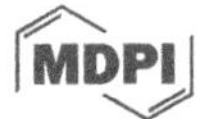

Article

From Science to Policy and Practice: A Critical Assessment of Knowledge Management before, during, and after Environmental Public Health Disasters

Mélissa Généreux [1,2,*], Marc Lafontaine [3] and Angela Eykelbosh [4]

1 Eastern Townships Integrated University Centre in Health and Social Services—Sherbrooke Hospital University Centre, Sherbrooke, QC J1G 1B1, Canada
2 Department of Community Health Sciences, Faculty of Medicine and Health Sciences, Université de Sherbrooke, Sherbrooke, QC J1H 5N4, Canada
3 Chemical Emergency Preparedness and Response Unit, Environmental Health Science and Research Bureau, Healthy Environments and Consumer Safety Branch, Health Canada, Ottawa, ON K1A 0K9, Canada; marc.lafontaine@canada.ca
4 National Collaborating Centre for Environmental Health, Vancouver, BC V5Z 4C2, Canada; angela.eykelbosh@bccdc.ca
* Correspondence: Melissa.genereux@usherbrooke.ca; Tel.: +1-819-829-3400 (ext. 45453); Fax: +1-819-564-5435

Received: 15 January 2019; Accepted: 11 February 2019; Published: 18 February 2019

Abstract: Canada regularly faces environmental public health (EPH) disasters. Given the importance of evidence-based, risk-informed decision-making, we aimed to critically assess the integration of EPH expertise and research into each phase of disaster management. In-depth interviews were conducted with 23 leaders in disaster management from Canada, the United States, the United Kingdom, and Australia, and were complemented by other qualitative methods. Three topics were examined: governance, knowledge creation/translation, and related barriers/needs. Data were analyzed through a four-step content analysis. Six critical success factors emerged from the analysis: blending the best of traditional and modern approaches; fostering community engagement; cultivating relationships; investing in preparedness and recovery; putting knowledge into practice; and ensuring sufficient human and financial resources. Several promising knowledge-to-action strategies were also identified, including mentorship programs, communities of practice, advisory groups, systematized learning, and comprehensive repositories of tools and resources. There is no single roadmap to incorporate EPH expertise and research into disaster management. Our findings suggest that preparation for and management of EPH disaster risks requires effective long-term collaboration between science, policy, and EPH practitioners at all levels in order to facilitate coordinated and timely deployment of multi-sectoral/jurisdictional resources when and where they are most needed.

Keywords: knowledge transfer; knowledge management; environmental public health; disaster risk management

---

1. Introduction

Canada, like many countries, increasingly faces emergencies and disasters that have public health impacts [1], including large-scale chemical incidents (e.g., the 2013 Lac-Mégantic train derailment) and natural disasters (e.g., the 2016 Fort McMurray wildfires). Such environmental public health (EPH) disasters may cause extensive environmental, human, and material losses, and may sometimes affect entire communities and/or necessitate evacuation and relocation. In addition to acute health risks, a large body of literature indicates that the population burden of psychopathology in the aftermath of EPH disasters is substantial and potentially of long duration [2–5]. EPH disasters may differ from other public health emergencies (e.g., Ebola outbreak, pandemic influenza), as most require both a short-term response (within hours), as well as a longer-term response (including monitoring, remediation and/or restoration efforts) that may stretch over years. And generate a need for multidisciplinary scientific expertise (chemistry, epidemiology, human health risk assessment, mental health, etc.). The increasing frequency and severity of EPH events is thought to be driven by the interactions of complex phenomena such as population and economic growth, land-use, resource scarcity, urbanization, and climate change, all of which are expected to continue into the foreseeable future.

The governance required to prepare for, respond to, and recover from a wide range of EPH disasters—natural or human-induced—is arguably the most complex and critical function of disaster management. Such EPH governance should serve to facilitate and strengthen capacity for risk assessment, surveillance, risk management, public communication, monitoring and evaluation, and mitigation and recovery activities. The components of EPH governance should, therefore, include not just policies, programs, and coordination structures, but should also address gathering and interpretation of relevant and up-to-date information with which to guide action [6].

1.1. Background

As the successor to the Hyogo Framework for Action 2005–2015: Building the Resilience of Nations and Communities to Disasters (HFA), the Sendai Framework for Disaster Risk Reduction 2015–2030 (Sendai Framework), adopted by 187 Member States at the Third United National World Conference on Disaster Risk Reduction, has shifted its emphasis from disaster management to disaster risk management [7]. With 35 explicit references to health, this people-centered framework encourages both risk reduction and resilience strengthening through an all-hazard, all-of-state and all-of-society approach [8]. Science should routinely be used to support disaster risk reduction [9] and, therefore, holds a key place in the Sendai Framework. Knowledge flowing from and to different stakeholders ensures that policy and practice are evidence-based and risk-informed (Figure 1; [10]).

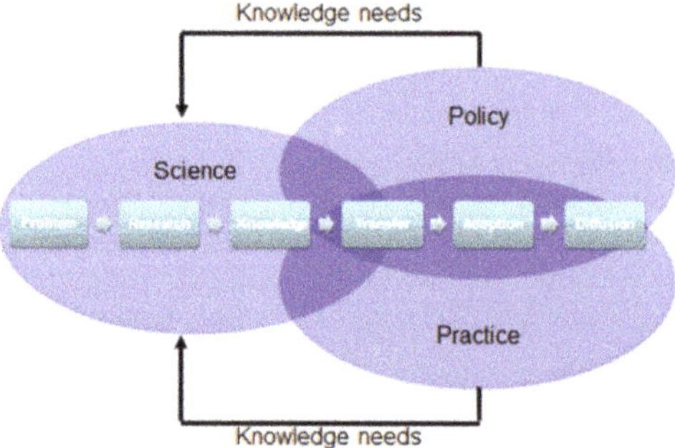

Figure 1. The science-policy-practice continuum (adapted from [10]).

1.2. Knowledge-to-Action (KTA) Process

Evidence-informed decision-making, in emergency management and in all other areas of public health, requires effective knowledge translation to turn research knowledge into action. The Canadian Institutes of Health Research (CIHR) have proposed a cyclical knowledge-to-action (KTA) process [11,12]. This process has been divided into various phases, from the identification of the problem to monitoring and sustaining the use of the available pertinent knowledge. The funnel, located at the heart of this cycle, represents knowledge creation. As it moves through the funnel, knowledge is refined and becomes more easily applicable to end-users. However, once created, knowledge needs to be translated into action. This cycle provides a framework for strategies in knowledge creation and translation.

Various types of knowledge may be utilized within KTA strategies in disaster settings. These include knowledge generated through science, as well as local (community-based) or indigenous knowledge [13]. Too often disaster management practitioners tend to focus on the former, ignoring the latter which is, nevertheless, of great value for disaster management, given local knowledge may provide contextual information not found in science-based information sources. For its part, scientific knowledge refers to primary literature (e.g., first-generation knowledge), knowledge synthesized from literature review (e.g., second-generation knowledge), and also to more user-friendly tools and resources, including decision aids, training modules, practice guidelines, lessons learned, and protocols (e.g., third-generation knowledge) [14]. Knowledge can also be classified as either tacit (i.e., understood or implied knowledge that exists without being stated) or explicit (i.e., formal or codified knowledge that is stated in detail) [15]. Such concepts build notably on the "knowledge creation spiral" theory within organizations, introduced by Nonaka and Takeuchi in 1995, which emphasizes on the importance of involving both the top and front-line employees in knowledge creation process [16]. By integrating top-down and bottom-up approaches, this system enables the creation, accumulation, and translation of tacit and explicit knowledge.

Effective KTA processes must also account for how knowledge is shared and transformed through sharing. Four processes transforming knowledge from one form to another have been identified, namely:

- Socialization;
- Externalization;
- Internalization; and
- Combination.

Socialization consists of sharing of individual tacit knowledge through collaborative methods, like meetings (tacit to tacit). Externalization refers to codifying the tacit knowledge into tools and resources (tacit to explicit). Internalization corresponds to learning by doing, through simulations or exercises (explicit to tacit). Finally, combination can be defined as the extraction and the combination of explicit knowledge, in order to organize it into various forms, such as repositories (explicit to explicit) [17].

1.3. Toward a National Framework

Canada has gained significant expertise and knowledge from recent EPH disasters, including the 2013 Lac-Mégantic train derailment, the 2016 Fort McMurray wildfires, and the 2016 Seaforth Channel diesel spill [18–21]. However, despite this growing expertise, two fundamental challenges remain. First, how can we improve knowledge generation (through research) before, during, and after disasters? Although disasters mobilize public health practitioners in a matter of hours, organizing scientific research efforts, and/or acquiring access to the knowledge generated may take weeks or months. Second, how can we improve dissemination and use of new and existing knowledge? These are especially complex challenges in Canada, in which knowledge-generating entities must cooperate across three levels of government, two official languages, and vast geographic distances. Rather than reinventing the wheel time and time again, how can we ensure that public health actors at all levels know what has been done elsewhere, how can we understand the uncertainties, and how can we integrate it in the face of a disaster?

Given the short time-frames and potentially high human costs that characterize EPH disasters, a national framework is urgently needed to facilitate and integrate knowledge creation and associated research into emergency response and recovery in Canada. Such a framework would allow public health professionals to systematize what has already been done, build on existing assets—such as expertise, evidence, guidelines, lessons learned, resources, training and protocols—and clarify what remains to be achieved through future collaborations.

Our aim was to determine how to better integrate EPH knowledge and assets in disaster settings in Canada [22], using the Sendai Framework as a template [23]. To that end, we conducted a critical assessment of knowledge management (i.e., providing the right information, in the right place, at the right time) before, during, and after EPH disasters in Canada. The following specific objectives were pursued to achieve this goal:

1. Describe various existing models of governance for disaster management, with a focus on the science-policy-practice interface;
2. Identify main resources available and challenges for knowledge management; and
3. Formulate recommendations toward the establishment of a national framework.

2. Materials and Methods

2.1. Design

This project draws heavily on the US National Institutes of Health (NIH) Disaster Research Response (DR2) Program. The DR2 Program is a national framework for research on the medical and public health aspects of disasters and public health emergencies [24,25] which offers data collection tools and resources, training and exercise materials, and research protocols, and facilitates networking between researchers and practitioners responding to environmental emergencies. This project was led in close collaboration with a national steering committee created in 2016, to oversee the development of a Canadian DR2 (CanDR2); the committee is co-chaired by Health Canada and the National Collaborating Centre for Environmental Health (NCCEH) and is composed of representatives from many Canadian and international agencies.

2.2. Sample Selection

Key informants (KIs) involved in preparedness for, response to, and recovery from EPH disasters, both at the local and national (i.e., provincial or federal) levels in Canada and other countries were invited to participate in this initiative.

The KIs identified were experienced emergency planners from health or non-health sectors, medical officers of health, knowledge transfer experts, or academics, who possessed expertise in the management of natural (e.g., floods, winter storms, heat waves, hurricanes, wildfires) or technological (e.g., chemical spills, train derailments) disasters.

At least one representative from each of the provinces of British Columbia, Alberta, Ontario, Québec, and the Atlantic Canada region was sought. These provinces or regions were selected based on their geographic location (dispersed across Canada), their experiences in facing EPH disasters, and the varying size and capacity of their public health workforce. In addition, KIs from the federal level in Canada were invited to participate in this initiative, as well as KIs from governmental or non-governmental organizations in other key English-speaking countries, including the United States, the United Kingdom, and Australia. While we emphasized the importance of diversity across KIs (at all levels, from governmental and non-governmental organizations, from health and non-health sectors), this diversity did not prevent our study from reaching data saturation (i.e., we obtained a sample large enough such that no new data were generated from additional participants).

An initial list of KIs was generated by the CanDR2 Steering Committee and invited to participate through an introductory email briefly describing the project. Nearly all invitees accepted, with a final sample of 23 KIs.

2.3. Data Collection Instrument and Methods

An interview guide containing mostly open-ended questions deemed to be relevant to our objectives was developed and endorsed by the members of the CanDR2 Steering Committee. Four overarching dimensions of the EPH response to disasters were explored, namely (1) governance, (2) knowledge creation, (3) knowledge translation, and (4) barriers and needs related to these processes [26]. The interview guide drew heavily on the World Health Organization (WHO)'s toolkit for assessing health system capacity for crisis management, more specifically on the governance and leadership function. This standardized toolkit is organized according to the six functions of the WHO health system framework. For the first function, that is effective leadership and governance, fourteen essential attributes are described, including programs on preparedness, and research and evidence base [6].

The interview process comprised two parts. In the first part of the interview, seven questions were used to broadly characterize the governance model/strategic framework in each of the jurisdictions under study, in order to obtain an overview of disaster management structures and coordination mechanisms. The second part of the interview specifically addressed knowledge creation (three questions) and knowledge translation processes (five questions). Existing barriers and factors conducive to strengthening of science-policy-practice interface and integration of knowledge into action were assessed throughout the interviews. A specific question on obstacles and strengths was also added at the end of the guide. Each interview lasted approximately 60 min. Interviews were conducted by the project leader in English (n = 16) or in French (n = 7), either on the telephone (n = 19) or face-to-face (n = 4), from April to July 2017.

2.4. Other Data Sources

In-depth interviews were complemented by other qualitative methods. The project leader was involved as the public health director or a medical adviser during three large-scale EPH disasters in Canada, namely the 2013 Lac-Mégantic train derailment, the 2016 Fort McMurray wildfires, and the 2017 Quebec flood. Furthermore, she attended 15 scientific fora (conferences, workshops, symposia, etc.) related to EPH disaster management from July 2016 to July 2017. Throughout these meetings and informal discussions with key international experts, additional explanations and good practices were documented. Field notes were taken after each scientific forum. Finally, a wide range of documents and websites suggested by KIs were consulted to deepen the understanding of laws, structure, policies, plans, procedures and programs identified during interviews.

2.5. Analysis

In order to carry out the analysis of the KIs' discourse and other data gathered, we conducted a four-step content analysis: (1) double-reading of transcripts, (2) data coding, (3) data processing, and (4) interpretation of data.

In Step 1, an initial (appropriation) reading of interviews and field notes was used to identify the main ideas characterizing each interview or event. The second (reading served to confirm and clarify these ideas. In Step 2, raw qualitative data were classified into an analysis grid, with a coding structure based on four dimensions established a priori: governance, knowledge creation, knowledge translation, and barriers and needs [26]. In the data processing Step 3, the analysis grid was used to draw out themes and subthemes from the coded transcripts. Data that were conceptually related to one another were first identified within each dimension. This set of data became sub-themes corresponding to ideas or concepts in relation with our subject. Examination of these sub-themes across all four pre-determined dimensions then led to their grouping into cross-cutting themes. The final Step 4 was interpretation of the coded and processed data in the context of our initial objectives [27].

2.6. Integrated Knowledge Translation

In accordance with the principle of integrated knowledge translation, as promoted by CIHR [28], members of the CanDR2 Steering Committee were involved in each step of the project. Early in the process, they contributed in identifying the problem and clarifying the aim of the project, they were invited to comment on the protocol and the interview guide, and they identified a list of potential KIs. Once data were gathered and analyzed, preliminary and final findings were presented and discussed with members of the CanDR2 Steering Committee on two occasions. Presentation of findings and recommendations to various stakeholders (e.g., organizations involved in disaster management in Canada) is also planned in the upcoming months.

3. Results

3.1. Description of the Data

Overall, 16 interviews were conducted among KIs from Canada (n = 16) and other jurisdictions (n = 7) (see Table 1). Fifteen KIs came from the public health or health sector, whereas the remaining KIs came from the municipal sector (n = 4), academia (n = 2), or non-governmental organizations (NGO; n = 2). The sample had balanced representation at the national and local levels, and of both genders. Two KIs represented the indigenous communities' perspective. Interestingly, many KIs had been involved in the management of EPH disasters, including the 2005 explosion and fire at the Buncefield oil storage depot (United Kingdom), the 2009 Black Saturday Bushfires in Victoria (Australia), the 2011 Alberta Slave Lake floods (Canada), the 2012 Neptune Technologies explosion (Canada), the 2013 Lac-Mégantic train derailment (Canada), the 2016 Fort McMurray wildfires (Canada), the 2016 Seaforth Channel diesel spill (Canada), Hurricane Matthew in 2016 (United States), the 2017 New Brunswick ice storm (Canada), the 2017 Quebec flood (Canada), the Flint water crisis (United States), as well as annual flooding in Ontario (Canada).

Table 1. Profiles of KIs interviewed in this study.

ID	Jurisdiction	Sector	Level	Gender
1	British Columbia	Health	National	F
2	British Columbia	Public Health	National	F
3	British Columbia	Public Health	Local	F
4	Alberta	Health	National	F
5	Alberta	Public Health	Local	M
6	Ontario	Health	National	M
7	Ontario	Public Health	Local	M
8	Québec	Municipal	Local	M
9	Québec	Municipal	Local	M
10	Québec	Municipal	Local	M
11	Québec	Academic	National	F
12	Atlantic	Public Health	Local	F
13	Canada	Public Health	National	F
14	Canada	Public Health	National	F
15	Canada	NGO	National	F
16	Canada	Public Health	National	M
17	United States	Public Health	National	F
18	United States	Academic	Local	M
19	United Kingdom	Public Health	National	F
20	United Kingdom	Public Health	National	F
21	United Kingdom	Municipal	Local	F
22	Australia	Public Health	Local	F
23	Australia	NGO	National	M

3.2. Emerging Themes: Critical Success Factors

Six cross-cutting themes, which are here identified as critical factors in successful disaster knowledge management, materialized from the data interpretation, with a range of sub-themes emerging in each category. These sub-themes, which represent the current situation and challenges, are further discussed below.

3.2.1. Blending the Best of Traditional and Modern Approaches

The data revealed that, in Canada and other developed countries, disaster management is well structured at all levels and that, overall, public health authorities are involved in these institutional arrangements. Most structures rely on the incident command system (ICS) for coordinating disaster responses, consider all phases of the disaster management continuum (mitigation, preparedness, response, and recovery) and are supported by laws, policies, plans, and procedures. Routine surveillance and epidemiological investigations are fairly well integrated during the response phase, as are conferences, meetings, training activities, and exercises during the preparedness phase. In short, the above traditional approaches are adequately implemented.

More modern all-hazard approaches [29,30] as promoted in many key documents, including the Sendai Framework [7], are currently integrated into disaster management preparedness and response in some jurisdictions. However, for most KIs in Canada and elsewhere, the Sendai Framework is not known or not a priority. Some KIs nevertheless expressed their desire for a major paradigm shift: "Requirements are based on old emergency management approaches and principles, we need governance from a different perspective" (KI#6). Others emphasized the importance of better understanding the potential risks: "It is important to be involved in risk assessment before a disaster strikes, to better manage risks altogether, as proposed in the Sendai Framework" (KI#9). An observation made at the Fifth Regional Platform for Disaster Risk Reduction in the Americas [31], which was also noted by one KI, is the poor representation of local-level participants of some major countries at this meeting: "Those involved don't share with lower levels, it's the opposite than [sic] what's proposed in the framework" (KI#18). This suggests that even if we are on the right track in implementing modern approaches, additional efforts are required to fully achieve this goal.

3.2.2. Fostering Community Engagement

The importance of identifying and leveraging existing assets or resources at the community level, including local health agencies, and working with existing capacities were strongly valued among KIs. Furthermore, it was indicated that local knowledge should be given consideration in the same manner as scientific knowledge: "We need to hear more from the community, it's really important" (KI#15). However, it was broadly acknowledged that communities typically remain poorly engaged in disaster management and that strategies to foster community engagement while maintaining the efficiency of disaster response and research are yet to be developed [32]. The interviewees indicated that ideally such strategies would provide a mixture of top-down and bottom-up approaches, and mobilize local knowledge and expertise before, during, and after a disaster.

Although leveraging local capacity was recognized as important, KIs also noted that building capacity in small municipalities, rural and Indigenous communities remains a challenge, and that support is required from higher-level governmental and academic institutions. For example, one KI (who has previously responded to a fuel spill) noted that more detailed technical guidance is needed to support local risk assessment: "What kind of environmental and biospecimen sample should be taken? What's needed? How often? What parameters? What detection limits? What should be the benchmarks (or appropriate end-points)?" (KI#3). Developing this type of technical guidance is often beyond the capacity of those responding to the crisis at hand, as such work requires time, research, and multidisciplinary expertise.

3.2.3. Cultivating Relationships

Many of the successes identified by KIs relied on individual leadership (or "champions") and strong interpersonal connections. Beyond structures, plans, and procedures, formal or informal relationships and networks have been identified by the majority of KIs as the most promising avenue to strengthen knowledge management capacities in disaster settings. Indeed, many KIs emphasized the need for breaking down silos between sectors (e.g., first responders vs. public health), practitioners and academics, French-speaking and English-speaking provinces, local and national levels, and even within public health organizations [33]. For example, KI#16 noted that "First Nations communities can ask for support, but this depends a lot on relationships previously built with governmental agencies". As noted by KI#9, "Strong links must be established right from the start between public health and first responders to establish a risk assessment and management strategy." Because public health authorities are well connected with universities in many jurisdictions, it may be possible to build bridges with academics to bring additional expertise to affected communities.

Some KIs mentioned that an overlap exists between academic and public health expertise in the context of EPH disasters, in that both may offer expertise in epidemiology, toxicology, surveillance, risk, and exposure assessment, etc. These two essential partners, therefore, need to clarify their respective roles, in order to unite their efforts and act in a synergistic manner. Building such functional partnerships may unlock latent resiliency, especially if accomplished before a disaster strikes. As expressed by one KI, "We need to connect the dots. We need to better know each other before an event; it is too late to learn during the crisis" (KI#10). Indeed, the power of these "connected dots" was apparent during the response to the 2017 Quebec floods. Within 24 h, an international network of renowned organizations including the US Centers for Disease Control and Prevention (CDC), Public Heath England (PHE), and WHO were bringing concrete support to Quebec public health authorities. This pre-established network permitted rapid access to validated materials, including the Community Assessment for Public Health Emergency Response (CASPER) toolkit in the US [34] and a protocol and questionnaires from the National Study of Flooding and Health in the UK [35].

3.2.4. Investing in Preparedness and Recovery

Although the four phases of disaster management are usually considered in disaster management structures, our data suggested local efforts are (by necessity) oriented toward the short-term. Our interviews suggested that Canadian EPH practitioners, particularly those at the local level, are struggling with one crisis activation after another; some organizations contacted during this study report remaining in near continual response mode in recent years. Consequently, little energy can be allocated to preparedness and recovery. Recovery is perhaps the most difficult task because of the accumulating burden on EPH professionals, including emotional load, fatigue, cumulative workload, and organizational factors, including less effective coordination structure and gradually weakening political commitment. According to one respondent, "we could probably do more between disasters, it is all about prioritization" (KI#5). As a result of this "disaster hangover", long-term monitoring of physical and mental health issues is not routinely carried out, despite the fact that those issues probably have the most significant impact on populations [36].

Another critical area that is typically overlooked in the post-disaster landscape is the identification and sharing of problems and lessons learned. Once the disaster is over, teams are asked to return to their regular tasks as quickly as possible, such that "Practitioners don't have enough time to think, to learn, to gain knowledge" (KI#11). As reported by many KIs, subsequent crises arise and similar problems are again encountered. For example, during the 2017 ice storm in New Brunswick (NB), one KI observed that public health was not as prepared as it could be, noting that "We always have to reinvent the wheel" (KI#12). This strongly expressed desire to improve learning from past events was the most consistent finding across KIs interviewed.

3.2.5. Putting Knowledge into Practice

The interviewees reported the science-policy-practice interface before, during, and after EPH disasters is not as robust as it could be, at either the local or national level in Canada, or in the other countries considered. Several interviewees from local organizations, within and outside the health sector, mentioned working infrequently with researchers due to the demands of day-to-day operations. The lack of systematic mechanisms to incorporate research and expertise into disaster management was also noted. The first challenge identified was "making sure that we are asking the right questions to inform and to learn from a given event" (KI#2). While accessing local data (e.g., environmental monitoring, epidemiological investigations, victim registries, response information, and after action reports) is essential to generate knowledge, as suggested by some KIs, such sharing can be sensitive for partners involved in disaster response, including first responders, local authorities, and non-governmental organizations. Various cultural backgrounds, lack of clarity in respective roles and responsibilities, privacy issues, security clearance, fear of being judged, not having the mandate, and competition might explain this phenomenon. The search of those responsible and/or the causes after disasters is negatively perceived in many countries, which may become a growing obstacle to learning from previous experiences.

Once knowledge is generated, this newly developed evidence has to be transferred from experts and researchers to inform policies and practices. In the aftermath of the Fort McMurray wildfires, "an evaluation of the psychosocial response and recovery was conducted through focus groups and interviews to identify further needs and current gaps" (KI#4). These findings emphasize the importance of having trained, dedicated staff who are tasked with taking on these "additional" data collection and knowledge translation activities.

Another issue commonly reported is the need to adapt scientific knowledge to local context, to make it clear and concise. Ideally, more user-friendly tools and resources would be produced (i.e., third-generation knowledge): "There is a lot of knowledge, amazing amount of information, really good evidence. The challenge is having the time to make it digestible" (KI#15). The same issue has been raised regarding the Sendai Framework, which is much better known among academics than practitioners. Although "it is important, it is not clear how it will materialize" (KI#13). Finally, many local organizations are trying to develop a resource repository, but few have a comprehensive one yet. For example, although the current Canadian Disaster Database (https://www.publicsafety.gc.ca/cnt/rsrcs/cndn-dsstr-dtbs/index-en.aspx) facilitates learning by identifying events geographically and by types, Canada does not currently have a central repository to share resources (tools, reports, etc.) and connect seekers to the experts involved.

3.2.6. Ensuring Sufficient Human and Financial Resources

Unsurprisingly, a recurring theme related to human and financial capacities. With few exceptions, disaster risk management and capacity-building activities are not prioritized, leading to insufficient funding and resources. According to many KIs, having trained, dedicated staff, either in local authorities or in specialized branches at the national level, could certainly help. Local emergency planners or coordinators have been found to play central roles in Canada and elsewhere. Although more focused on acute care than public health, Health Emergency Management BC (HEMBC) has been providing expertise, education, tools, and support since 2004 in BC, being "in charge of strategic planning, priority setting, networking, and performance measures" (KI#1). Another issue raised pertains to disaster research funding, which can be very complex. The first weeks following a disaster offer a window of opportunity that should be exploited, as political commitment and willingness to support research and long-term monitoring activities rapidly decrease thereafter. To secure funds, some KIs proposed that "disaster research should be seen as a national priority, with disaster-specific funding opportunities" (KI#11). Canada does not currently have an expedited research funding or ethical review process in place to address the immediate aftermath of disasters. For example,

CIHR offered $2 million in health research funding after the Fort McMurray wildfires, but this grant competition did not start until October 2016 (i.e., a few months after the fires).

3.3. Promising Knowledge-to-Action Strategies

Throughout the multiple data sources examined, we discovered a wide range of effective solutions already adopted by many countries worldwide to promote the integration of current knowledge into emergency preparedness, response, and recovery. The objective of this project was not to undertake an exhaustive inventory of these solutions, but rather to draw attention to strategies that might be adaptable to the Canadian context. For each country surveyed, the most promising strategies have been categorized according to the four types of KTA processes identified by Rhem [17] (i.e., socialization, externalization, internalization, combination; see Table 2). Few, if any, innovative strategies were found with respect to the internalization process, which refers to learning by doing (e.g., drills or exercises). By contrast, a plethora of socialization strategies have been identified. These strategies, all more creative than the internalization strategies, have two common denominators. First, they draw on human capital. Second, whether they are deployed before, during, or after an EPH disaster, they all promote more effective interplay of science, policy, and practice.

Table 2. Examples of promising KTA strategies.

Socialization	Externalization	Combination
	Canada	
Opportunities for professional growth from mentorships at Canadian Red Cross	Report on lessons learned by the community after the 2016 Seaforth channel spill	User-friendly Sharepoint® with resources and tools shared on an ongoing basis in Alberta
Lessons learned from Slave Lake and Lac-Mégantic integrated into the mental health recovery plan in Fort McMurray	Book on the Lac-Mégantic tragedy sharing lessons learned by health and community networks	Environmental public health response and recovery toolkit in Alberta
Multisectoral debriefing after Neptune Technologie explosion that led to a better response in Lac-Mégantic	Mapping of responsibilities/accountabilities following recommendations at Canadian Red Cross	Emergency preparedness and response working group in NB to facilitate access to documents and resources
During 2017 Quebec floods, meeting with a city previously affected by a major flood to learn from past experiences		
During 2017 Quebec floods, visit of an expert on the ground to share his knowledge		
Provincial symposium organized by HEMBC		
	United States	
Local emergency planning committees (federal mandate)	Rapid Needs Assessment facilitated by CASPER toolkit	Lessons learned database at FEMA
Phone call organized by CDC between 4 states affected after Hurricane Matthew	Central office for all after-action reports at CDC (problems and corrections)	Disaster Lit®: 12,000 records (grey literature) related to public health disasters at NLM

Table 2. *Cont.*

Socialization	Externalization	Combination
Midwest Consortium for Hazardous Waste Worker Training		NIH DR2 Program: Repository of surveys, questionnaires, protocols, guidance, forms
Environmental Justice Summit organized in Flint (Michigan)		
Disaster epidemiology community of practice		
Disaster information specialists at NLM		
	United Kingdom	
Newcastle conference on psychosocial impacts of emergencies	Overview and Scrutiny Committee in Newcastle following after-action reports	Mapping of the Sendai Framework implementation: resources, projects, all sectors
Local resilience forums		
PHE Centre for Radiation, Chemical and Environmental Hazards		
UK Alliance for Disaster Research		
	Australia	
Expert advisory panel/group activated by Chief Public Health Officer	Lessons from the community after 2009 Victoria bushfires	
Mentoring network at the Australian Red Cross		
	The Netherlands	
Expert Group Health Research and Care after Disasters and Environmental Crises		
	Global	
WHO Thematic Platform for Health Emergency and Disaster Risk Management Research Group	International Federation of Red Cross Psychosocial Center website: a lot of very useful resources	Global Public Health Intelligence Network (GPHIN): a web-based early-warning tool
UNISDR Scientific and Technical Advisory Group		Evidence Aid: reliable, up-to-date evidence on interventions in the context of emergencies
WHO collaborating center on chemical incidents		Weekly updates from the PHE Global Hazards Weekly Bulletin

Mentorship programs among employees and/or community members appear well established in the Canadian and Australian Red Cross organizations. For example, a mayor of a city previously devastated by a bushfire could in turn support another mayor currently facing a similar situation by sharing tools and lessons learned. Moreover, in the Netherlands and New South Wales (Australia), expert advisory groups can be activated to assist health authorities dealing with complex issues raised by environmental public health emergencies; depending on the situation, various types of expertise (e.g., environmental health, mental health, epidemiology, toxicology) can be mobilized within these jurisdictions to rapidly provide an overview of current scientific knowledge that might inform decision-making [37].

Various networks or communities of practice, both at national and international levels, have been put in place to better incorporate scientific and/or local knowledge into practice. An example of this is the WHO Thematic Platform for Health Emergency and Disaster Risk Management Research Group, a growing international network of policy-makers, practitioners, and researchers [38]. This initiative, recently underscored at the Global Platform in Cancun in May 2017 [39], is a good example of how the various stakeholders in disaster planning and management can all work together more effectively. An additional benefit of this global network whose members span all time zones is that the group can collectively support the response to a disaster occurring anywhere in the world at any time.

Externalization and combination processes were less frequently reported than socialization. However, two communities have released or are about to release reports on lessons learned after 2009 Victoria (Australia) bushfires [40] and the 2016 Seaforth Channel (Canada) diesel spill for public review and as learning resources.

Various approaches combining KTA processes have been developed. The USA has some of the most promising strategies, including "Lessons Learned Information Sharing", a database set up by the Federal Emergency Management Agency (FEMA), and a comprehensive repository easily available on the National Library Medicine (NLM) website called Disaster Lit®. Through the latter, the NIH has put together 12,000 records of hand-picked documents related to public health disasters from the grey literature, including factsheets, guidelines, assessment tools, training material, reports, web pages, and web sites [41]. Another example is Evidence Aid, an initiative that aims to improve access to evidence on disaster-related health interventions, actions, and policies [42].

The city of Newcastle (UK) has demonstrated an exceptional degree of commitment to emergency/disaster preparedness and response. The city has hired three emergency planners who are fully dedicated to disaster management. Their work is undertaken in a multiagency space (including public health), with joint risk assessment and planning and a community risk register that drives the action plan. After every incident or exercise, a structured debrief is organized, as is often the case in many other jurisdictions; however, in Newcastle such information is also presented as a report to the city council and the "Overview and Scrutiny Committee" (led by the opposition), which together look at all of the council actions. According to KI#21, giving politicians ownership of the report makes the whole process open, transparent, and accountable. Local engagement and leadership has also led to the incorporation of other KTA strategies, including the recent organization of a conference entitled "Psychosocial Impacts of Emergencies" [43]. This event aimed to bring together people from multiple levels and different agencies to foster collaboration, promote community engagement, and raise awareness of the current gaps in disaster risk management.

4. Discussion

Authors translating knowledge to action by closing gaps between knowledge and practice is an iterative, dynamic, and complex process [12]. This project aimed to identify factors influencing this process, and explore solutions to promote the bridge between science, policy, and practice for disaster management. Our results corroborate and expand upon the published literature. Several studies have previously identified similar factors that may limit knowledge translation in disaster preparedness and response, including gaps in basic knowledge, such as the lack of long-term observational and interventional research [44–46], challenges in systematically collating and delivering lessons learned from events, and difficulties in creating and sustaining effective community engagement [47–50]. And as with other studies [15], we also found several factors facilitating the uptake of knowledge, including the importance that knowledge is tailored to local contexts and made actionable. Overall, our interview results support the promotion of interactions between researchers, experts, and users from all sectors to produce, disseminate, and make use of knowledge for the purpose of improving disaster preparedness and management [51–53].

More specifically, five recommendations emerged from the interviews with KIs and field observations:

(1) Community of practice: A pan-Canadian community of practice involving emergency managers, public health practitioners, academics, local champions, Red Cross professionals, and any other stakeholders interested in EPH disasters, should be hosted within a trusted organization to support disaster preparedness. Within this community of practice, local initiatives could be shared and general consensus or understanding could be achieved regarding best practices in disaster response (e.g., risk assessment) and recovery (e.g., long-term monitoring). This would also be the ideal setting for the development of standardized tools for disaster health research as a basis for further action.
(2) Roster of experts: Linked to the above community of practice, a roster of Canadian experts (e.g., researchers, toxicologists, epidemiologists, environmental health, occupational health, and mental health experts) should be created to support disaster response and recovery. We anticipate that this network could be called upon as needed to form scientific advisory groups to assist local authorities dealing with EPH disasters in both the short- and long-term. Such an initiative could also increase collaboration and sharing of expertise between researchers and EPH personnel in the field. Drawing on existing models (such as DR2), it would also lead to the identification of relevant research questions and the development of a research agenda that fits operational objectives [24,37,54].
(3) Knowledge generation: A systematic mechanism to promote retention of learning from past events is required. All types of knowledge gained responding to previous disasters should be valued, whether this is first-, second-, or third-generation scientific knowledge, or local knowledge such as success stories, pilot initiatives, and lessons learned from the field [13]. As part of recovery operations, emergency managers and EPH practitioners should take the time to learn from their experiences and contribute to establishing a solid foundation upon which to can build national capacities. Debriefs should involve multiple sectors and seek the input from members of the community [55]. Standardized templates for after-action reports and a tracking system for correctable issues should be made available. Their use should be legislated after any exercise or real event in order to identify lessons, and most importantly to learn from them locally. The storage of completed templates in a central location (publicly available) would facilitate access to local knowledge and foster vertical and horizontal knowledge translation.
(4) Knowledge transfer: There is an urgent need in Canada (and elsewhere) to gather and synthesize disaster-related knowledge, and to transfer it to other communities, ideally using same central space (i.e., a virtual repository) identified in item (3) above. This knowledge might take the form of research findings, research protocols, practice guidelines, data collection tools and resources, training and exercises materials, lessons learned, etc. Such a virtual repository could be developed de novo, but Canadian documents could also be identified and shared through the extensive repository of tools and resources available from the US (i.e., Disaster Lit®, an NLM resource guide). Moreover, Canadian representatives should be appointed to the NLM Disaster Information Specialist Program, which supports the provision of disaster-related health information resources to the disaster workforce through a network of information professionals and librarians.
(5) Guidance on Sendai Framework: Guidance for a better integration of the Sendai Framework into health emergency management in the Canadian context should be developed. Such guidance would be particularly helpful for a growing number of stakeholders wishing a paradigm shift from disaster management to disaster risk management.

It is hoped our findings and recommendations will contribute to the identification and implementation of concrete solutions that foster the creation and the use of knowledge before, during, and after EPH disasters. Based on the challenges and successes identified during our interviews, we believe that there is no single roadmap to incorporate EPH expertise and research into disaster management. However, one thing is certain: these solutions should be developed not only during but also (or primarily) before and after disasters. The search for solutions should be based on the assumption that various types of knowledge translation processes are necessary [16].

Their complementary nature should be exploited in such a way as to develop a pan-Canadian framework that is adaptable to the needs of each province and territory, and other levels of government or sectors.

Strengths and Limitations

This project is, to the best of our knowledge, the first to critically assess capacity for knowledge management in EPH disaster settings in Canada. Our diverse sample of KIs represented a wide range of Canadian perspectives: rural and urban, indigenous and non-indigenous, anglophone and francophone, and from the east coast to west coast. This sample was further complemented by respondents from other countries to capture perceptions, ideas, and experiences on a broader basis. The measuring instrument (i.e., the interview guide) was based upon a standardized toolkit developed by the WHO to assess capacities for crisis management [6]. Furthermore, examination of qualitative data followed a rigorous protocol that helped to increase the internal validity of the data collected for coding purposes. Finally, a steering committee composed of knowledge users from various backgrounds accompanied the entire process, from the identification of the problem to the validation of potential solutions.

There are inherent limitations to a qualitative approach based primarily on KI interviews. First, the sample size was limited to 23 KIs. Our interviews also gathered opinions and ideas that may have been influenced by many factors including past experiences, recall bias, social desirability, and hidden agendas. In order to minimize the effect of those factors, we used additional sources of information to complement the interview data. Our design has therefore facilitated triangulation of findings and improved both reliability and validity.

5. Conclusions

Generally speaking, critical success factors for public health action include good governance, development of strong and sound partnerships, dedicated capacity and resources, and use of evidence to inform actions. Good governance is perhaps the single most important factor influencing the effectiveness of emergency preparedness, response and recovery. Beyond structures and plans, it is necessary to cultivate relationships and share responsibility for ensuring the safety, health, and well-being of affected communities, while respecting the local culture, capacity, and autonomy. Preparation for and management of EPH disaster risks requires effective long-term collaboration between science, policy, and EPH practitioners at all levels in order to facilitate coordinated and timely deployment of multi-sectoral/jurisdictional resources when and where they are most needed.

Author Contributions: Conceptualization: M.G., M.L., A.E.; methodology: M.G., M.L., A.E.; software: N/A.; validation: N/A.; formal analysis: N/A.; investigation: N/A.; resources: N/A.; data curation: N/A.; writing—original draft preparation: M.G., M.L., A.E.; writing—review and editing: M.G., M.L., A.E.; supervision, N/A.; project administration: co-authors.; funding acquisition: N/A.

Funding: This research received no external funding.

Conflicts of Interest: The authors declare no conflict of interest.

References

1. Canadian Disaster Network on Disaster Risk Reduction. *Eighth Annual National Roundtable on Disaster Risk Reduction*; Public Safety Canada: Halifax, NS, Canada, 2017.
2. Galea, S.; Nandi, A.; Vlahov, D. The epidemiology of post-traumatic stress disorder after disasters. *Epidemiol. Rev.* **2005**, *27*, 78–91. [CrossRef] [PubMed]
3. Goldmann, E.; Galea, S. Mental health consequences of disasters. *Annu. Rev. Public Health* **2014**, *35*, 169–183. [CrossRef] [PubMed]
4. Neria, Y.; Nandi, A.; Galea, S. Post-traumatic stress disorder following disasters: A systematic review. *Psychol. Med.* **2008**, *38*, 467–480. [CrossRef] [PubMed]

5. Warsini, S.; West, C.; Dip, E.G.; Mills, J.; Usher, K. The psychosocial impact of natural disaster among adult survivors. An integrative review. *Issues Mental Health Nurs.* **2014**, *35*, 420–436. [CrossRef] [PubMed]
6. World Health Organization. *Strengthening Health-system Emergency Preparedness: Toolkit for Assessing Health-system Capacity for Crisis Management*; WHO: Copenhagen, Denmark, 2012.
7. United Nations Office for Disaster Risk Reduction. *Sendai Framework for Disaster Risk Reduction 2015–2030. United Nations Office for Disaster Risk Reduction*; United Nations: Geneva, Switzerland, 2015.
8. Aitsi-Selmi, A.; Murray, V. The Sendai framework: Disaster risk reduction through a health lens. *Bull. World Health Organ.* **2015**, *93*, 362. [CrossRef] [PubMed]
9. Southgate, R.J.; Roth, C.; Schneider, J.; Shi, P.; Onishi, T.; Wenger, D.; Amman, W.; Ogallo, L.; Beddington, J.; Murray, V. Using Science for Disaster Risk Reduction. UNISDR. 2013. Available online: www.preventionweb.net/go/scitech (accessed on 15 January 2019).
10. Spiekermann, R.; Kienberger, S.; Norton, J.; Briones, F.; Weichselgartner, J. The Disaster-Knowledge Matrix—Reframing and evaluating the knowledge challenges in disaster risk reduction. *Int. J. Disaster Risk Reduct.* **2015**, *13*, 96–108. [CrossRef]
11. Graham, I.D.; Logan, J.; Harrison, M.B.; Straus, S.E.; Tetroe, J.; Caswell, W.; Robinson, N. Lost in knowledge translation: Time for a map? *J. Contin. Educ. Health Prof.* **2006**, *26*, 13–24. [CrossRef]
12. Straus, S.E.; Tetroe, J.; Graham, I. Defining knowledge translation. *Can. Med. Assoc. J.* **2009**, *181*, 165–168. [CrossRef]
13. Mercer, J.; Kelman, I.; Taranis, L.; Suchet-Pearson, S. Framework for integrating indigenous and scientific knowledge for disaster risk reduction. *Disaster* **2010**, *34*, 214–239. [CrossRef]
14. Brouwers, M.; Stacey, D.; O'Connor, A. Knowledge creation: Synthesis, tools and products. *Can. Med. Assoc. J.* **2009**, *182*, 68–72. [CrossRef]
15. Seneviratne, K.; Baldry, D.; Pathirage, C. Disaster knowledge factors in managing disasters successfully. *Int. J. Strateg Prop. M.* **2010**, *14*, 376–390. [CrossRef]
16. Nonaka, I.; Takeuchi, H. *The Knowledge Creating Company*; Oxford University Press: Oxford, UK, 1995.
17. Rhem, A.J. "Sound the Alarm!": Knowledge management in emergency and disaster preparedness. In *Knowledge Management in Practice*; Taylor and Francis Group: Abingdon, UK, 2017.
18. Eykelbosh, E.; Kosatky, T. Oil spills: Treating patients, counselling communities. *B. C. Med. J.* **2017**, *59*, 61–64.
19. Généreux, M.; Petit, G.; Maltais, D.; Roy, M.; Simard, R.; Boivin, S.; Shultz, J.M.; Pinsonneault, L. The public health response during and after the Lac-Mégantic train derailment tragedy: A. case study. *Disaster Health* **2015**, *2*, 1–8. [CrossRef] [PubMed]
20. Géreux, M.; Petit, G.; Lac-Mégantic Community Outreach Team; O'Sullivan, T. Public health approach to supporting resilience in Lac-Mégantic: The EnRiCH Framework. In *Health 2020 Priority Area Four: Creating Supportive Environments and Resilient Communities. A Compendium of Inspirational Examples*; Erio, Z., Ed.; World Health Organization: Geneva, Switzerland, 2018; pp. 156–162.
21. Généreux, M.; Petit, G.; Roy, M.; Maltais, D.; O'Sullivan, T. The "Lac-Mégantic tragedy" seen through the lens of The EnRiCH Community Resilience Framework for High-Risk Population. *Can. J. Public Health* **2018**, *109*, 261–267. [CrossRef] [PubMed]
22. *CIHR Best Brain Exchange Report: Integrating Environmental Health Research into Chemical Emergency/Disaster Management. CIHR*; The Science, Knowledge Translation & Ethics Branch; Public Safety Canada: Ottawa, ON, Canada, 2016.
23. Wahlström, M. New Sendai framework strengthens focus on reducing disaster risk. *Int. J. Disaster Risk Sci.* **2015**, *6*, 200–201. [CrossRef]
24. Miller, A.; Yeskey, K.; Garantziotis, S.; Arnesen, S.; Bennett, A.; O'Fallon, L.; Thompson, C.; Reinlib, L.; Masten, S.; Remington, J.; et al. Integrating health research into disaster response: The new NIH disaster research response program. *Int. J. Environ. Res. Public Health* **2016**, *13*, 676. [CrossRef]
25. National Institute of Health. NIH Disaster Research Response (DR2). 2017. Available online: https://dr2.nlm.nih.gov/ (accessed on 15 January 2019).
26. Andreani, J.C.; Conchon, F. Fiabilité et validité des enquêtes qualitatives: Un état de l'art en marketing. *Revue Française du Marketing* **2005**, *201*, 5–21. (In French)
27. Feldman, M.S. *Strategies for Interpreting Qualitative Data*; Sage Publications: Thousand Oaks, CA, USA, 1994.
28. Canadian Institutes of Health Research. *Guide to Knowledge Translation Planning at CIHR: Integrated and End-of-Grant Approaches*; Canadian Institutes of Health Research: Ottawa, ON, Canada, 2012.

29. Federal Emergency Management Agency. *National Preparedness Goal*, 2nd ed.; US Department of Homeland Security: Washington, DC, USA, 2015.
30. Public Safety Canada. *An Emergency Management Framework for Canada*, 2nd ed.; Emergency Management Policy Directorate; Public Safety Canada: Ottawa, ON, Canada, 2011.
31. Government of Canada. 5th Regional Platform for Disaster Risk Reduction in the Americas. 2017. Available online: http://eird.org/rp17/ (accessed on 15 January 2019).
32. Lichtveld, M.; Kennedy, S.; Krouse, R.Z.; Grimsley, F.; El-Dahr, J.; Bordelon, K.; Sterling, Y.; White, L.; Barlow, N.; DeGruy, S.; et al. From design to dissemination: Implementing community-based participatory research in post-disaster communities. *Am. J. Public Health* **2016**, *106*, 1235–1242. [CrossRef]
33. Généreux, M.; Pinsonneault, L.; Roy, M. Fostering partnerships between public health functions within health and social services organizations: A perspective from the province of Quebec (Canada). *J. Prev. Med. Care* **2016**, *1*, 23–27. [CrossRef]
34. Centers for Disease Control and Prevention. *Community Assessment for Public Health Emergency Response (CASPER) Toolkit*, 2nd ed.; CDC: Atlanta, GA, USA, 2012.
35. Waite, T.D.; Chaintarli, K.; Beck, C.R.; Bone, A.; Amlôt, R.; Kovats, S.; Reacher, M.; Armstrong, B.; Leonardi, G.; Rubin, J.; Oliver, I. The English national cohort study of flooding and health: Cross-sectional analysis of mental health outcomes at year one. *BMC Public Health* **2017**, *17*, 129. [CrossRef]
36. Géreux, M.; Maltais, D. Three years after the tragedy: How the Le Granit community is coping. In *Bulletin d'information de la direction de santé publique de l'Estrie*; Vision Santé publique: Sherbrooke, QC, Canada, 2017.
37. Alting, D.; Duckers, M.L.; Yzermans, J. The expert group health research and care after disasters and environmental crises: An analysis of research questions formulated by Dutch health authorities for the expert group between 2006 and 2016. *Prehosp. Disaster Med.* **2017**, *32*, S197. [CrossRef]
38. Lo, S.T.T.; Chan, E.Y.Y.; Chan, G.K.W.; Murray, V.; Abrahams, J.; Ardalan, A.; Kayano, R.; Wai Yau, J.C. Health emergency and disaster risk management (Health-EDRM): Developing the research field within the Sendai Framework paradigm. *Int. J. Disaster Risk Sci.* **2017**, *8*, 145–149. [CrossRef]
39. WHO. *WHO statement to the 2017 global platform for disaster risk reduction*; WHO: Geneva, Switzerland, 2017.
40. McAllan, C.; McAllan, V.; McEntee, K.; Gale, B.; Taylor, D.; Wood, J.; Thompson, T.; Elder, J.; Mutsaers, K.; Leeson, W.; et al. Lessons Learned by Community Recovery Committees of the 2009 Victorian Bushfires Advice We offer to Communities Impacted by Disaster. Available online: https://www.redcross.org.au/getmedia/7f796fb7-958f-4174-98da-00b6e0182856/Lessons-Learned-by-Community-Recovery-Committees-of-the-2009-Victorian-Bushfires-v1-0.pdf.aspx (accessed on 15 January 2019).
41. Norton, E. A toolkit for disaster preparedness & response information. *World Association for Disaster and Emergency Medicine Webinar*. 2017. Available online: https://wadem.org/wp-content/uploads/2017/02/toolkit-nlm-2-23-17-norton.pdf (accessed on 11 February 2019).
42. Gerdin, M.; Clarke, M.; Allen, C.; Kayabu, B.; Summerskill, W.; Devane, D.; MacLachlan, M.; Spiegel, P.; Ghosh, A.; Zachariah, R.; et al. Optimal evidence in difficult settings: Improving health interventions and decision making in disasters. *Plos Med.* **2014**, *11*, e1001632. [CrossRef] [PubMed]
43. Newcastle City Council. Psychosocial Impacts of Emergencies. 2017. Available online: http://www.fuse.ac.uk/media/sites/researchwebsites/fuse/eventdocs/Psychological%20impacts%20of%20emergencies.pdf (accessed on 15 January 2019).
44. Birnbaum, M.L.; Daily, E.K.; O'Rourke, A.P. Research and evaluations of the health aspects of disasters, Part VII: The Relief/Recovery Framework. *Prehosp. Disaster Med.* **2016**, *31*, 195–210. [CrossRef] [PubMed]
45. Chan, E.Y.Y.; Murray, V. What are the health research needs for the Sendai Framework? *Lancet* **2017**, *390*, E35–E36. [CrossRef]
46. Tsutsumi, A.; Takashi, I.; Ito, A.; Thronicroft, G.; Patel, V.; Minas, H. Mental health mainstreamed in new UN disaster framework. *Lancet Psychiatr.* **2015**, *2*, 679–680. [CrossRef]
47. Gamboa-Maldonado, T.; Marshak, H.H.; Sinclair, R.; Montgomery, S.; Dyjack, D.T. Building capacity for community disaster preparedness: A call for collaboration between public environmental health and emergency preparedness and response programs. *J. Environ. Health.* **2012**, *75*, 24–29.
48. Jong, S.V.Z. *Let's Talk Oil Spill Risk. Lessons Learned from Coastal Communities in British Columbia, Canada*; Routledge: Kentuck, AL, USA, 2016.

49. Leadbeater, A. Community leadership in disaster recovery: A case study. *Aust. J. Emerg. Manag.* **2013**, *28*, 41–47.
50. Svendsen, E.R.; Whittle, N.; Wright, L.; McKeown, R.E.; Sprayberry, K.; Heim, M.; Caldwell, J.J.; Gibson, J.; Vena, J. GRACE: Public health recovery methods following an environmental disaster. *Int. Arch. Occup. Environ. Health* **2010**, *65*, 77–85. [CrossRef]
51. Dar, O.; Buckley, E.J.; Rokadiya, S.; Huda, Q.; Abrahams, J. Integrating health into disaster risk reduction strategies: Key considerations for success. *Am. J. Public Health* **2014**, *104*, 1811–1816. [CrossRef]
52. Lurie, N.; Manolio, T.; Patterson, A.P.; Collins, F.; Frieden, T. Research as a part of public health emergency response. *N. Engl. J. Med.* **2013**, *368*, 1251–1255. [CrossRef] [PubMed]
53. Yeskey, K.; Miller, A. Science unpreparedness. *Disaster Med. Public Health Prep.* **2015**, *9*, 444–445. [CrossRef] [PubMed]
54. Decker, J.A.; Kiefer, M.; Reissman, D.B. A decision process for determining whether to conduct responder health research following disasters. *Am. J. Disaster Med.* **2013**, *8*, 25–33. [CrossRef] [PubMed]
55. Gibson, T.; Wisner, B. "Let's talk about you ... ": Opening space for local experience, action and learning in disaster risk reduction. *Disaster Prev. Manag. Int. J.* **2016**, *25*, 664–684. [CrossRef]

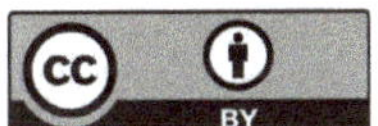

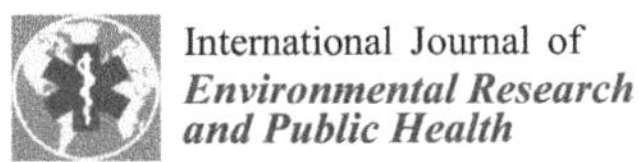

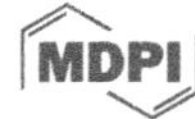

Article

Is Urban Household Emergency Preparedness Associated with Short-Term Impact Reduction after a Super Typhoon in Subtropical City?

Emily Ying Yang Chan [1,2,*], **Asta Yi Tao Man** [1], **Holly Ching Yu Lam** [1], **Gloria Kwong Wai Chan** [1], **Brian J. Hall** [3] **and Kevin Kei Ching Hung** [4]

1 Collaborating Centre for Oxford University and CUHK for Disaster and Medical Humanitarian Response (CCOUC), The Chinese University of Hong Kong, Hong Kong, China; asta.man@cuhk.edu.hk (A.Y.T.M.); hollylam@cuhk.edu.hk (H.C.Y.L.); gloria.chan@cuhk.edu.hk (G.K.W.C.)
2 Nuffield Department of Medicine, University of Oxford, Oxford OX37BN, UK
3 Global and Community Mental Health Research Group, Faculty of Social Sciences, University of Macau, Macao, China; brianhall@um.edu.mo
4 Accident & Emergency Academic Unit, The Chinese University of Hong Kong, Prince of Wales Hospital, Hong Kong, China; kevin.hung@cuhk.edu.hk
* Correspondence: emily.chan@cuhk.edu.hk; Tel.: +852-2252-8411

Received: 31 January 2019; Accepted: 14 February 2019; Published: 19 February 2019

Abstract: Climate change-related extreme events are increasing in frequency and severity. Understanding household emergency preparedness capacity in Health-Emergency and Disaster Risk Management (Health-EDRM) for at risk urban communities is limited. The main objective of the study is to explore the association among risk perception, household preparedness, and the self-reported short-term impacts of Typhoons for urban residents. A population-based, cross-sectional telephone survey using random digit-dialling was conducted among Hong Kong adults within 2 weeks following 2018 Typhoon Mangkhut, the most intense typhoon that affected Hong Kong, a subtropical city, in thirty years. Among the 521 respondents, 93.9% and 74.3% reported some form of emergency preparedness and typhoon-specific preparedness measure (TSPM) against Mangkhut, respectively. Respondents who perceived a higher risk at home during typhoons and had practiced routine emergency preparedness measures (during nonemergency periods) were more likely to undertake TSPM. Of the respondents, 33.4% reported some form of impact (11.1% were household-specific) by Typhoon Mangkhut. Practicing TSPM was not associated with the reduction of short-term household impacts. Current preparedness measures may be insufficient to address the impact of super typhoons. Strategies for health-EDRM for urban residents will be needed to cope with increasing climate change-related extreme events.

Keywords: typhoon; hurricane; cyclone; strong wind levels; natural disaster; Health-EDRM; household preparedness; urban; climate change related extreme events; subtropical city

---

1. Introduction

Typhoons, also known as cyclones or hurricanes depending on its location and strength, are the most common natural hazard in the Asia Pacific and Southeast Asia region [1]. Doocy et al. highlighted although the global hurricane/typhoon-related mortality trends have decreased in the past seventy years, severe typhoons have increased in frequency in the last decade. Hong Kong, a densely populated subtropical metropolis in Southern China, has on average 5–6 annual typhoons [2]. Between 1980–2010, only two T10 typhoons, the highest Tropical Cyclone Warning Signal, occurred, yet three happened in one decade (2012, 2017, and 2018) [2]. Since 2018, the last typhoon-related death was recorded in 1999; between 129 and 458 people were injured in the last three T10 typhoons. These climate-related events have brought on landslides, torrential rain, and flooding which led to cascading impacts on the city. With climate change, more severe typhoons are expected, and the coping capacity of typhoon-prone densely populated urban cities needs to be explored in order to plan for effective disaster risk reduction strategies.

Health-emergency and disaster risk management (Health-EDRM) encompasses the systematic analysis and management of health risks through the reduction and mitigation of hazards and vulnerability in all stages of the disaster management cycle. Preventive measures to mitigate disaster-related health risks are needed, which includes assessing the individual, household, and community's capacity for food security, clean water and sanitation, and injury prevention [3–5]. Health-EDRM research in Asia suggests that despite high knowledge about typhoons, people have a low self-perception of the associated health risks and many do not adhere to government warnings [6–8].

Recent studies in Hong Kong, a subtropical city, for urban disaster and emergency preparedness found just over 75% of residents had some form of household emergency preparedness items (first-aid kit, basic aid supplies, emergency food and drinking water, basic medication, and/or a fire extinguishing equipment) [9]. Other studies in the same city indicated 69% of residents had not taken any precautions when a severe weather warning was announced [10], and in a subsequent study, 82.3% did not perceive Hong Kong to be a city susceptible to disasters [11]. Few relayed the correct responses to a typhoon warning signal, and they did not have adequate first-aid knowledge [12]. Notably, how personal risk perceptions and routine emergency preparedness might be associated with household preparedness in extreme meteorological events have yet to be studied in Asia.

Typhoon Mangkhut, which swept across the Philippines, Hong Kong, and Macao in September 2018, was the second most intense storm which battered Hong Kong since recording began in 1946 and was the most intense storm in the past three decades [13]. The typhoon, which landed in September, had wind speeds reaching 161 km/h in Hong Kong and was classified as a T10; only sixteen of such Tropical Cyclone Warning Signals have been hoisted in over seventy years [2,14]. It is equivalent to a category two Hurricane according to the Saffir–Simpson Hurricane Wind Scale, comparable to the 2018 Hurricane Katia which left parts of Mexico in disarray [15]. The Philippines reported over 100 deaths; while in Hong Kong, there were no fatalities, over 450 people were injured [16,17]. The objectives of this paper are (1) to examine the household preparedness measures conducted, the responsive activities undertaken, and the short-term impacts experienced by the Hong Kong community during Typhoon Mangkhut; (2) to identify the associating sociodemographic factors of preparedness, response, and impact; and (3) to explore the associations between risk perceptions, preparedness, responses, impacts, and attitudes for future preparation. The findings will bridge the current knowledge gaps associated with urban Health-EDRM for climate change related extreme events in Asia.

2. Materials and Methods

A cross-sectional study, population-based, household telephone survey using random digit dialling, was conducted just over two weeks after Typhoon Mangkhut's landing in September 2018. The "last birthday method" was used to ensure randomization at the household level. The interviewer would seek the household member whose birthday was the closest to the interview date to ensure the respondent was randomly selected within the family unit. Hong Kong residents who understood Cantonese and were 18 years old or above were interviewed. Verbal informed consent was obtained at the start of each interview, and ethics approval was sought from the Survey and Behavioural Research Committee at The Chinese University of Hong Kong (SBRE-18-075).

A multiple choice-based survey was used to collect self-reported information: (a) sociodemographic information, (b) the floor lived on, (c) risk perception toward typhoons, (d) routine household preparedness, (e) household preparedness measures for Typhoon Mangkhut, (f) activities conducted during the typhoon period (whether they had left home when a typhoon signal T8 or higher was hoisted, (g) whether they had paid attention to the weather conditions and the source of the information, and (h) the short-term impact brought on by Mangkhut. Other impacts reported but not included in the multiple-choice options were recorded separately in text format. Short-term impact refers to any impact occurring from the time when Typhoon Mangkhut approached Hong Kong to the date of interview (from immediate to two weeks after landfall). Respondents were also asked to comment on the information provided by the Hong Kong Government regarding Typhoon Mangkhut and their willingness to prepare for future typhoons.

For the routine household preparedness measures, general preparedness actions enquired included if basic supplies may be available for injury and wound management, possession of medication to manage existing health conditions, and any other measures to maintain a general state of health (Table 1). For the household preparedness measures for Typhoon Mangkhut, it included the combination of the routine measures mentioned above and the typhoon-specific preparedness measures (TSPM). Specifically, TSPM included (1) retrieving/storage of outdoor items that could be blown away, (2) applying anti-leaking or anti-seeping measures, and (3) taping windows (Table 1).

Statistical analyses were performed using IBM SPSS, version 24. Descriptive chi-square (or X^2) tests and multivariable logistic regression were performed to identify the associations among typhoon preparedness, typhoon risk perception, and sociodemographic factors. Covariates were selected for the multivariable model based on the chi-square tests ($p < 0.10$). All odds ratios (OR) present in this paper were adjusted odds ratios from the multivariable models.

Table 1. The uptake rate of preparedness activities applied on usual days and for Typhoon Mangkhut.

Types of Household Preparedness Measures (n = 521)	Health-EDRM Implications	Routine Emergency Preparedness	Typhoon Mangkhut Preparedness
General emergency preparedness measures			
Food Supply	To ensure food security and to maintain proper nutritional intake	432 (82.9%)	355 (68.1%)
Drinking water	To have clean water for sanitation, hydration, and food preparation	255 (48.9%)	197 (37.8%)
Basic medication (e.g., pain relievers)	To deal with acute clinical symptoms related to pains and fever	488 (93.7%)	242 (46.4%)
Long term medication (2 weeks)	To sustain treatment plan(s) and the continuous management of chronic diseases	279 (53.6%)	148 (28.4%)
Backup light source	To provide visual aid to prevent injuries such as falling	417 (80.0%)	281 (53.9%)
Backup electrical source	To elongate the functionality of electronical appliances such as medical equipment or cooking apparatuses	109 (20.9%)	98 (18.8%)
First-aid kit	For the immediate treatment and mitigation of emergencies and accidents	288 (55.3%)	-
Basic first-aid supplies, e.g., Band-Aids and ace bandages	For the treatment and mitigation of minor injuries	496 (95.2%)	-
Fire extinguishing equipment	To control the fire hazard and to prevent fire-related injuries	63 (12.1%)	-
Typhoon-specific preparedness measures (TSPM)			
Taped windows	To reduce shattered glass pieces for injury prevention	-	268 (51.4%)
Collect or tied down items that can be blown away (e.g., flower pots)	To reduce the risk of blunt force trauma from objects carried by the storm	-	273 (52.4%)
Anti-flooding, leaking, and seeping measures	To reduce injury risks related to slippery surfaces and allergies or airborne toxins related to mould and fungi	-	195 (37.4%)

Health-EDRM: Health-Emergency and Disaster Risk Management.

3. Results

Data collection was completed within 16 days (17 September 2018 to 2 October 2018) after the landfall on 16 September 2018. The final sample size constituted to 521 valid respondents (response rate was 31.6% among valid telephone numbers called), and the study sample comprised of 57.6% women, 41.7% aged below 45, just over 50.0% that attained a post-secondary education, and 42.0% that had a monthly household income of over $40,000 HKD (Table 2). The study sample was comparable to the 2016 Hong Kong Census for gender and residential district, and consisted of slightly more middle-aged adults (Table 2).

Table 2. The descriptive statistics about demographics, perception, preparedness, and impact.

Demographics	Sampled Respondents (n = 521)		HK 2016 Population by Census Data (n = 6,506,130)		Sample vs. Census p-Value [a]
	n	%	n	%	
Gender					
Male	221	42.4%	2,947,073	45.3%	0.202 [b]
Female	300	57.6%	3,559,057	54.7%	
Age					
18–24	63	12.1%	785,981	12.1%	0.005 *
25–44	154	29.6%	2,228,566	34.3%	
45–64	224	41.5%	2,328,430	35.8%	
≥65	80	15.4%	1,163,153	17.9%	
Area of residence					
Hong Kong Island	102	19.6%	1,120,143	17.2%	0.219
Kowloon	164	31.5%	1,987,380	30.6%	
New Territories	254	48.8%	3,397,499	52.2%	
Education attainment					
Primary and below	56	10.7%	1,673,431	25.7%	<0.001 *
Secondary	195	37.4%	2,841,510	43.7%	
Post-secondary	265	50.9%	1,991,189	30.6%	
Marital status					
Single	212	40.7%	2,708,709	41.6%	0.695 [b]
Married	309	59.3%	3,797,421	58.4%	
Income					
<2000–9999	45	9.4%	480,117	19.2%	<0.001 *
10,000–19,999	73	15.2%	547,784	21.8%	
20,000–39,999	160	33.4%	699,450	27.8%	
≥40,000	201	42.0%	782,383	31.2%	
Perceived home to be at high risk during typhoons (n = 520)					
Yes	49	9.4%	-	-	-
No	471	90.4%	-	-	-
Impact from Typhoon Mangkhut (n = 521)					
Yes	174	33.4%	-	-	-
No	347	66.6%	-	-	-
Practiced at least 1 typhoon-specific preparedness (n = 521)					
Yes	387	74.3%	-	-	-
No	134	25.7%	-	-	-
Went out when typhoon signal was T8 or above (n = 520)					
Yes	83	16.0%	-	-	-
No	437	84.0%	-	-	-

[a] The χ^2 test was used to measure the overall difference between this survey and the 2016 Hong Kong Population Census data. A p-value < 0.05 indicates a significant difference. [b] The χ^2 test with continuity correction was used. * $p < 0.05$.

3.1. Risk Perception and Preparedness Activities

Of the 521 respondents, 9.4% perceived their home to be at high risk of danger during typhoons. For preparedness efforts during nonemergency periods, the most commonly reported routine preparedness measures included the procession of basic first-aid supplies, e.g., Band-Aid's and ace bandages (95.2%); basic medication, e.g., pain killers (93.7%); and food supply (82.9%) (Table 1). Specifically for Typhoon Mangkhut, the three most frequently reported routine preparedness measures undertaken (out of six) included having extra food supplies (68.1%), a backup light source (54%), and having basic medication (46.4%). When examining TSPM for Typhoon Mangkhut, 74.3% of respondents practiced at least one (i.e., retrieved/stored outdoor items that could be blown away, applied anti-leaking or anti-seeping measures, or taped windows). Of note, 6.1% of the respondents reported undertaking no preparedness measure at all for Typhoon Mangkhut.

No significant associations were found between sociodemographic factors and a high typhoon risk perception ($p > 0.20$) both before and after adjusting for the height of the residential location. Results of univariable analyses (Table 3) showed a significant association between practicing at least one TSPM and education ($p < 0.001$), age group ($p < 0.001$), and perceived risk ($p = 0.023$). The association was sustained in the multivariable analyses for education (secondary vs. post-secondary, OR = 0.48; 95% CI = 0.03–0.77), age group (25–44 vs. 65+, OR = 2.80; 95% CI = 1.39–5.65), and high typhoon risk perception (vs. low perception, OR = 2.63; 95% CI = 1.07–650). Routine household preparedness was also found to be associated with practicing at least one TSPM. Of those nine routine measures, four measures were significantly associated with practicing at least one TSPM after adjusting for gender, age, education, and risk perception. They were having had a first-aid kit (OR = 1.79; 95% CI = 1.18–2.73), food supply (OR = 1.80; 95% CI = 1.08–3.03), fire extinguishing equipment (OR = 3.13; 95% CI = 1.36–7.20), and a backup light source (OR = 1.69; 95% CI = 1.03–2.77) (Table A1).

Table 3. The association of demographics with practiced typhoon-specific preparedness measures (TSPM) and risk perception.

Characteristics		Practiced at Least 1 Typhoon-Specific Preparedness Measure (TSPM) ^				
		χ^2 Test; n = 521 *			Logistic Regression; n = 515	
		Yes	No	p-Value	OR (95% CI)	p-Value
Gender	Male	161 (41.6%)	60 (44.8%)	0.522	1	
	Female	226 (58.4%)	74 (55.2%)		1.16 (0.76–1.77)	0.493
Age	18–24	50 (12.9%)	13 (9.7%)	<0.001	1.75 (0.75–4.07)	0.193
	25–44	131 (33.9%)	23 (17.2%)		2.80 (1.39–5.65)	0.004
	45–64	158 (40.8%)	66 (49.3%)		1.43 (0.81–2.53)	0.219
	≥65	48 (12.4%)	32 (23.9%)		1	
Education attainment (n = 516)	Primary and below	37 (9.6%)	19 (14.4%)	<0.001	0.59 (0.29–1.22)	0.156
	Secondary	127 (33.1%)	68 (51.5%)		0.48 (0.30–0.77)	0.003
	Post-secondary	220 (57.3%)	45 (34.1%)		1	
Income (n = 479)	<2000–9999	27 (7.6%)	18 (14.8%)	0.110	-	-
	10,000–19,999	55 (15.4%)	18 (14.8%)		-	-
	20,000–39,999	119 (33.3%)	41 (33.6%)		-	-
	≥40,000	156 (43.7%)	45 (36.9%)		-	-
Perceived home to be at high risk during typhoons (n = 520)	Yes	43 (11.1%)	6 (4.5%)	0.023	2.63 (1.07–6.50)	0.036
	No	343 (88.9%)	128 (95.5%)		1	

^ Retrieved/stored outdoor items that could be blown away, applied anti-leaking or anti-seeping measures, or taped windows. * The sample size was 521 unless stated otherwise due to missing data.

3.2. Responsive Activities Undertaken during the Typhoon

The three main routes of seeking weather-related information about Typhoon Mangkhut was television (52.6%), mobile apps (24.6%), and internet-based websites (14.2%). With the exception of website usage, which had no special association with gender, women were more likely to use any of the information channels mentioned above than men (p = 0.002). Most respondents (87.9%) felt the Hong Kong Government provided enough information for respondents to prepare and respond to Typhoon Mangkhut. Of public safety concern, 16.0% of respondents reported leaving their homes when the storm was at its height of strength (i.e. the warning signal was T8 or above). Among those who left their home, 74.7% reported such behaviour was for non-occupational and nonemergency related reasons (such as going out for meals and to cinemas). Adjusted for gender and age, men (OR = 1.98; 95% CI = 1.22–3.22) and younger groups (18–24 vs. $\geq$65; OR = 3.40; 95% CI = 1.29–8.93) were found more likely to go out for nonemergency and non-occupational purposes when the warning signal was T8 or above.

3.3. Impact of the Typhoon

Of all the respondents, 33.4% reported experiencing short-term impacts resulted from the typhoon. The most common impacts included road or traffic blockages which prevented respondents from going to work or school after landfall (70.7%), power outages (14.9%), and home damages during the typhoon (13.8%); less than 6% reported financial loss (of any form, such as cancelled trips and business losses), item loss, and injury. Specifically for household impacts, 11.1% reported being affected, which cited household damages, the loss of property, and power outages as the most common impacts. Our study sample showed 4 (0.77%) respondents reported injuries, which were related to slipping and wounds from broken glass.

Among the 74.3% who had practiced at least one TSPM for Typhoon Mangkhut, 37.2% reported short-term impacts (12.9% specific to household impacts) by the typhoon. The univariable analysis found respondents who did at least one TSPM were associated with a higher risk of having a household impact due to Typhoon Mangkhut (p = 0.027) (Table 4). This association, however, became statistically nonsignificant after adjusting for the perceived risk of typhoons.

3.4. Experiences and Future Preparedness

Half of respondents (49.9%) indicated they would prepare for future typhoons. Multivariable analysis indicated that respondents who had applied at least one TSPM against Typhoon Mangkhut (OR = 3.07; 95% CI = 1.93–4.91), who were of the female gender (OR = 1.75; 95% CI = 1.18–2.58), and who reported household impact from Typhoon Mangkhut (OR = 2.11; 95% CI = 1.08–4.12) were more likely to prepare for future typhoons (Table 5).

Table 4. The associating factors of typhoon household impact.

Characteristics		Household Impact due to Typhoon Mangkhut				
		χ^2 Test; n = 521 *			Logistic Regression; n = 515	
		Yes	No	p-Value	OR (95% CI)	p-Value
Gender	Male	19 (32.8%)	202 (43.6%)	0.114	-	-
	Female	39 (67.2)	261 (56.4%)		-	-
Age	18–24	8 (13.8%)	55 (11.9%)	0.132	-	-
	25–44	23 (39.7%)	131 (28.3%)		-	-
	45–64	23 (39.7%)	201 (43.4%)		-	-
	≥65	4 (6.9%)	76 (16.4%)		-	-
Education attainment (n = 516)	Primary and below	3 (5.5%)	53 (11.5%)	0.184	-	-
	Secondary	18 (32.7%)	177 (38.4%)		-	-
	Post-secondary	34 (61.8%)	231 (50.1%)		-	-
Income (n = 479)	<2000–9999	3 (5.8%)	42 (9.8%)	0.533	-	-
	10,000–19,999	6 (11.5%)	67 (15.7%)		-	-
	20,000–39,999	21 (40.4%)	139 (32.6%)		-	-
	≥40,000	22 (42.3%)	179 (41.9%)		-	-
Floor levels	<6	18 (31.6%)	91 (19.7%)	0.185	-	-
	6–15	20 (35.1%)	166 (36.0%)		-	-
	16–25	11 (19.3%)	113 (24.5%)		-	-
	≥26	8 (14.0%)	91 (19.7%)		-	-
Perceived home to be at high risk during typhoons	Yes	17 (29.3%)	32 (6.9%)	<0.001	5.16 (2.63–10.14)	<0.001
	No	41 (70.7%)	430 (93.1%)		1	
Practiced at least one typhoon specific preparedness measure	Yes	50 (86.2%)	337 (72.8%)	0.027	2.02 (0.92–4.45)	0.080
	No	8 (13.8%)	126 (27.2%)		1	

* The sample size was 521 unless stated otherwise due to missing data.

Table 5. The multivariable logistic regression for willingness to prepare for future typhoons.

Characteristics		Willingness to Practice Future Preparedness for Typhoons				
		χ^2 test; $n = 521$ *			Logistic Regression; $n = 515$	
		Yes	No	*p*-Value	OR (95% CI)	*p*-Value
Gender	Male	94 (36.2%)	127 (48.7%)	0.004	1	
	Female	166 (63.8%)	134 (51.3%)		1.75 (1.18–2.58)	0.005
Age	18–24	33 (12.7%)	30 (11.5%)	0.116	-	-
	25–44	88 (33.8%)	66 (25.3%)		-	-
	45–64	100 (38.5%)	124 (47.5%)		-	-
	≥65	39 (15.0%)	41 (15.7%)		-	-
Education attainment ($n = 516$)	Primary and below	31 (12.1%)	25 (9.7%)	0.057	1.32 (0.63–2.77)	0.471
	Secondary	84 (32.7%)	111 (42.9%)		0.65 (0.41–1.03)	0.064
	Post-secondary	142 (55.3%)	123 (47.5%)		1	
Income ($n = 479$)	<2000–9999	22 (9.0%)	23 (9.8%)	0.096	1.36 (0.64–2.88)	0.428
	10,000–19,999	47 (19.3%)	26 (11.1%)		2.29 (1.21–4.34)	0.011
	20,000–39,999	76 (31.1%)	84 (35.7%)		1.03 (0.65–1.64)	0.891
	≥40,000	99 (40.6%)	102 (43.4%)		1	
Perceived home to be at high risk during typhoons	Yes	33 (12.7%)	16 (6.2%)	0.011	1.43 (0.71–2.90)	0.319
	No	227 (87.3%)	244 (93.8%)		1	
Practiced at least one typhoon specific preparedness measure	Yes	222 (85.4%)	165 (63.2%)	<0.001	3.07 (1.93–4.91)	<0.001
	No	38 (14.6%)	96 (36.8%)		1	
Household impacted by Typhoon Mangkhut	Yes	40 (15.4%)	18 (6.9%)	0.002	2.11 (1.08–4.12)	0.028
	No	220 (84.6%)	243 (93.1%)		1	

* The sample size was 521 unless stated otherwise due to missing data.

4. Discussion

The current study aims to explore the preparedness measures applied, the response activities conducted, and the impact experienced by urban residents when Typhoon Mangkhut landed in Hong Kong. The association among preparedness and response activities, impact, and willingness for future preparedness, along with their associating factors were also evaluated. More than 90.0% of respondents took up at least one preparedness measure against Typhoon Mangkhut, while more than 70.0% had applied at least one TSPM. People with a higher educational level, with a younger age, with a higher risk perception, and who practiced routine household preparedness were associated with a higher TSPM uptake. All respondents reported checking the weather information during the typhoon. The most commonly used information acquisition routes were television broadcast and mobile apps. However, during the typhoon, around 16.0% of respondents went out, and about three quarters of them were out for nonemergency or non-occupational reasons. About one-third of respondents reported some form of impact, and about 11% reported specific household impacts from Typhoon Mangkhut. Among those who had applied at least one TSPM, 12.9% reported household impacts. This study showed a higher risk perception was associated with more willingness to practice TSPM. Practicing TSPM was, however, not associated with the risk of household impacts.

4.1. Preparedness

Consistent with previous studies [18], this study found that a higher educational level, a higher risk perception, more routine emergency preparedness, and previous experience of impact were positively associated with people who engage in disaster preparedness. Studies from China [6], Japan [19], and the Philippines [20] have also reported positive links between risk perception and willingness to mitigate typhoon-related risks. The study from the Philippines showed experiencing previous impacts from typhoon disasters and a higher educational level was associated with better perception of preparedness against typhoons [20], similar to the associations found in Japan [19]. This current study also found people who engaged certain routine preparedness measures, such as having a first-aid kit and backup light source, were 1–3 times more likely to prepare for Typhoon Mangkhut. Studies about hurricanes in the United States did not find sociodemographic factors, such as education and age, as associating factors of having disaster supplies (e.g., food supplies, a first-aid kit, and a backup light source) [21]. This reflects the consistency in emergency preparedness for general disaster risk and disaster-specific risk in the community, which may be reinforced by the higher awareness and risk perception among this group.

Of note, compared to a study in Hong Kong (2012), the proportion of routine household preparedness has decreased in five years from 75.1% to 70.6% (practicing at least three out of five measures: having a first-aid kit, basic aid supplies, emergency food and drinking water, basic medication, and fire extinguishing equipment) [9]. Although the pattern difference was not of statistical significance (comparison of proportions: $p = 0.06$), the decrease suggested disaster risk awareness should be reinforced in the community for enhancing public health emergency preparedness with the face of more challenging meteorological conditions associated with climate change [22]. Inconsistent with another study which found 69.0% of people did not prepare during a severe weather warning, this study reported only 6.1% of respondents did not do any preparedness measures for Typhoon Mangkhut [10]. Besides the different sample methods adopted, the contrasting results may be due to a preference of Hong Kong residents to prepare for typhoons over other extreme weather events such as rainstorms, landslides, and thunderstorms, all of which are also categorized under severe weather warnings.

4.2. During the Typhoon

In spite of the Hong Kong Government's Weather Services warning to stay indoors until winds were reduced to moderate severity, 16.0% of respondents had reported to have ventured outside when the storm was the strongest and most of them were out for nonemergency reasons. Although this figure is much lower in comparison to a previous local study (where 20.6% of respondents said that they would be "staying in a safe place until the T8 Tropical Cyclone Warning had passed" [12]), it may indicate the community regarded the Typhoon Mangkhut more seriously than previous typhoons. More efforts should be invested to prevent people from venturing outside for nonessential and unnecessary reasons. Leaving or travelling between shelters during strong winds may result in higher risks of injuries due to an increase length of exposure to hazards, e.g., flying objects [23]. This could also add an extra burden to the emergency response system and may even delay rescue for people with more pertinent needs.

Compared to other Chinese community [6], our urban community was more attentive to typhoon signals (100% vs. 54.8% in Zhejiang). Television was the most commonly used channel of communication for weather information in the community, which was on par with previous studies on information acquisition in Hong Kong about temperature events, infectious disease, and other disasters [12,24–26], in rural Zhejiang, China [6] and in the Philippines [20]. Despite the increase in use of mobile devices and apps, television still remains as the most commonly used channel for typhoon signals in both urban and rural communities.

4.3. Health Impacts

Official report indicated that no deaths and 450 injuries were directly resulted from the 2018 Typhoon Mangkhut in Hong Kong, yet this study found an injury rate of 0.77% among all respondents. If the event-specific injury rate was applied to the population of 7 million in Hong Kong (Table 2), there might be more than 50,000 unreported injury cases of varying severity. Although this is a crude estimation, the potential health impacts and the possible allocation of resources involved should be noted and considered for future disaster action plans. Most literature report injury figures based on public hospital records which may not include cases that did not seek professional medical assistance; the types of injury and other related disaggregate information also tend to be unavailable. Typhoon Hato in 2017, also categorized as a T10, killed at least ten people and caused 240 injuries in Macao [27]. In the west coastal cities of Japan, including Osaka and Kyoto, at least 11 deaths and 400 injuries have been reported due to Jebi in 2018, the strongest storm in Japan for 25 years [28], and in New York City, 43 deaths were reported caused by hurricane Sandy in 2012 [23]. The results of this study infer the injury figures reported in Macao [27], Japan [28] and New York City [23] might be underestimated as less severe cases which did not required hospitalizations though could cause public health problems might not be reported.

Currently, there are not many studies reporting the short-term health impacts of climate change-related storms on urban cities, especially for those with densely packed high-rise buildings like Hong Kong. This is important as the disaster impacts faced by the cities with and without high-rise buildings can vary drastically. For example, drowning due to flooding is one of the major health risks during storms [23], but it is less commonly reported in cities with densely packed high-rise buildings. A study found climate change has increased the intensity of typhoons in the East and Southeast Asia in the past few decades [22]. Coastal Asian cities in Korea, Japan, China, and Taiwan will become more vulnerable [22]. Coastal megacities such as Tokyo, Osaka, and Shanghai will be under an even higher risk due to the large and highly dense population. This study showed that injuries, mainly caused by falls, were the major health risks during the strong typhoon in Hong Kong. More evidence about the specific health risks during storms for high-rise building cities is needed.

4.4. What is the Gap Found in this Study

The biggest gap identified in this study is the effectiveness of the study TSPM in reducing storm-related impacts. This level of household preparedness may not be enough or appropriate for super typhoons as those who applied at least one TSPM were not associated with a lower risk of household impacts during the typhoon. This goes against the common understanding that appropriate preparedness should be able to reduce adverse effects during unfavourable events. Most of the household impacts reported, such as household damages and the suspension of the electricity or water supply, were uncommon typhoon impacts experienced in Hong Kong and are hardly preventable through applying the household protective measures mentioned in this study, such as taping windows. Other severe impacts were also reported from local media such as dizziness from swaying high-rise buildings, injuries from falling air conditioners, and the battering of construction sites where an elevator shaft had collapsed [29,30]. This further questions whether the current typhoon preparedness measures provide enough protection for super typhoons like Typhoon Mangkhut. Furthermore, there were disaster response and recovery measures which could not be addressed by individuals. One of the most common issues is road blocks, which in extreme events directly hinders relief efforts [31,32], but less is known about how it affects the daily routine of local residents, also referred to as secondary stressors [33]. The Hong Kong government reported 46,500 fallen trees that blocked major roads and several overhead rail lines [16]. Other unexpected health risks that arose included falling glass from twenty-story-high windows, of which mitigation efforts require more than just from homeowners but also input of various expertise from architecture and civil engineering.

4.5. Limitations

The cross-sectional nature of this study meant the inferences are limited to associations and the causation cannot be attributed. In addition, the landline telephone survey study design naturally excluded households without a landline; and in Hong Kong, residential landline penetration reported a decreasing rate from 102.6% in 2013 to 89.0% in 2018 [34]. Moreover, reporting bias may occur as as preparedness activities were self-reported and could not be validated. The current study also lacked the household location precision in Hong Kong and could not ascertain whether they were objectively at greater risk to assess the accuracy of the self-reported risk perceptions. The greater proportion of higher educated and higher income respondents might have also biased the results. Also, risk perceptions may have been biased based on the exposure to Typhoon Mangkhut, which may overestimate the association between typhoon exposure and risk perceptions. This study also only focused on the short-term impacts of the typhoon; the long-term impacts, such as psychiatric morbidity [35], and economic impact from the typhoon could not be included. Yet, despite the limitations, telephone surveys still offer the best opportunity to obtain quick overviews of various health and acute emergency impact status of the community [9,36]. As the survey was conducted just over two weeks following Typhoon Mangkhut, it may also reduced recall bias.

4.6. Implications

With climate change, more frequent and more intense typhoons may affect the Southeast Asian regions [22,37]. Residents, as well as the government and other stakeholders, should be aware of the potential risks arising from climate change-related disasters and should be prepared for new challenges. Effective protective measures should also be identified, evaluated, and applied to minimize avoidable risk, especially for densely populated high-rise building cities. More proactive Health-EDRM measures, such as having windows checked and repaired before typhoon seasons, should be considered and promoted. Our results indicated that the practice of routine emergency preparedness, risk perception, and education level were associated with a higher uptake rate of protective measures against typhoons. This suggests increasing the awareness and educational promotion, in particular targeting people with a lower educational level. Relevant stakeholders should also help encourage community preparedness and evidence for future policy-level disaster preparedness plans [11]. Research with long-term follow up on trends and community perception and behaviour changes will be important to ensure relevant, appropriate, and effective household protective measures against future extreme weather events.

5. Conclusions

The results of this cross-sectional telephone survey study suggested that even the high uptake of TSPM might not be effective in preventing related adverse impacts in the face of a super typhoon. Effective protective measures should be identified, evaluated, and applied to cope with the possibility of more intense typhoons and other unprecedented risks. Low urban risk perception and the fact that a considerable proportion of respondents venturing out during strong winds found in this study further urges the need to raise the awareness and preparedness practices among the community against typhoons and strong wind events. Education level and risk perception were found associated with the uptake of the TSPM; hence, educational promotion is suggested to raise awareness and to encourage the community to be better prepared. This is of timely importance since climate-related natural disasters are expected to increase in frequency and severity due to the effects of climate change [22]. The commonplace and prevalence of disasters, no matter the scale, should not inhibit emergency and disaster contingency plans from being updated or further adapted by the latest scientific evidence.

Author Contributions: Conceptualization, E.Y.Y.C.; methodology, E.Y.Y.C. and H.C.Y.L.; validation, H.C.Y.L.; formal analysis, A.Y.T.M.; investigation, A.Y.T.M. E.Y.Y.C., H.C.Y.L., G.K.W.C., B.J.H. and K.K.C.H.; data curation, A.Y.T.M. and H.C.Y.L.; writing—original draft preparation, A.Y.T.M., E.Y.Y.C. and H.C.Y.L.; writing—review and editing, A.Y.T.M. E.Y.Y.C., H.C.Y.L., G.K.W.C., B.J.H. and K.K.C.H.; visualization, A.Y.T.M.; supervision, E.Y.Y.C.; funding acquisition, E.Y.Y.C.

Funding: This research was jointly funded by the CCOUC development fund of The Chinese University of Hong Kong and the Hong Kong Jockey Club for the establishment of the Hong Kong Jockey Club Disaster Preparedness and Response Institute.

Conflicts of Interest: The authors declare no conflict of interest.

Appendix A

Table A1. Association of practicing at least 1 typhoon-specific preparedness measure (TSPM) and routine household preparedness measures.

Multivariable Logistic Regression—Practiced at Least 1 Typhoon-Specific Preparedness (n = 515)					
Variables					
Routine Household Preparedness	**First-Aid Kit**	**Food Supply**	**Basic Medicine**	**Fire Extinguishing Equipment**	**Back Up Light Source**
Yes	1.79 (1.18–2.73) **	1.80 (1.08–3.03) *	1.69 (0.75–3.65)	3.13 (1.36–7.20) **	1.69 (1.03–2.77) *
No	1	1	1	1	1
Education					
Primary	0.65 (0.31–1.35)	0.65 (0.31–1.35)	0.62 (0.30–1.29)	0.62 (0.30–1.28)	0.58 (0.28–1.19)
Secondary	0.51 (0.31–0.82) **	0.48 (0.30–0.78) **	0.48 (0.30–0.78) **	0.47 (0.29–0.77) **	0.49 (0.30–0.79) **
Post-secondary	1	1	1	1	1
Gender					
Male	1	1	1	1	1
Female	1.14 (0.75–1.75)	1.11 (0.72–1.71)	1.16 (0.76–1.78)	1.20 (0.78–1.85)	1.16 (0.76–1.78)
Age					
18–24	1.60 (0.69–3.75)	1.63 (0.70–3.80)	1.70 (0.73–3.97)	1.73 (0.74–4.04)	1.70 (0.73–3.96)
25–44	2.61 (1.28–5.30) **	2.69 (1.33–5.46) **	2.69 (1.33–5.46) **	2.79 (1.38–5.66) **	2.89 (1.43–5.87) **
45–64	1.33 (0.75–2.37)	1.43 (0.81–2.54)	1.40 (0.79–2.48)	1.37 (0.77–2.43)	1.49 (0.84–2.64)
65+	1	1	1	1	1
Perceived home to be at high risk during typhoons					
Yes	2.67 (1.08–6.60) **	2.82 (1.14–7.00) *	2.65 (1.08–6.55) *	2.65 (1.07–6.55) *	2.49 (1.01–6.15) *
No	1	1	1	1	1

* $p < 0.05$. ** $p < 0.01$.

References

1. Doocy, S.; Dick, A.; Daniels, A.; Kirsch, T.D.; Hopkins, J. The Human Impact of Tropical Cyclones: A Historical Review of Events 1980-2009 and Systematic Literature Review Citation Abstract Authors. *PLOS Curr. Disasters* **2013**, *1*, 1–25. [CrossRef]
2. The Hong Kong Observatory HKO Warnings/Signals Database. Available online: http://www.weather.gov.hk/wxinfo/climat/warndb/warndb1_e.shtml (accessed on 12 November 2018).
3. Lo, S.T.T.; Chan, E.Y.Y.; Chan, G.K.W.; Murray, V.; Abrahams, J.; Ardalan, A.; Kayano, R.; Yau, J.C.W. Health Emergency and Disaster Risk Management (Health-EDRM): Developing the Research Field within the Sendai Framework Paradigm. *Int. J. Disaster Risk Sci.* **2017**, *8*, 145–149. [CrossRef]
4. World Health Organization. *Emergency Risk Management for Health Emergency Risk Management for Health Fact Sheets*; World Health Organization: Geneva, Switzerland, 2013.
5. Chan, E.Y.Y.; Murray, V. What are the health research needs for the Sendai Framework? *Lancet* **2017**, *390*, e35–e36. [CrossRef]
6. Zhang, W.; Wang, W.; Lin, J.; Zhang, Y.; Shang, X.; Wang, X.; Huang, M.; Liu, S.; Ma, W. Perception, knowledge and behaviors related to typhoon: A cross sectional study among rural residents in Zhejiang, China. *Int. J. Environ. Res. Public Health* **2017**, *14*, 492. [CrossRef] [PubMed]
7. Jiang, L.-P.; Yao, L.; Bond, E.F.; Wang, Y.-L.; Huang, L.-Q. Risk perceptions and preparedness of typhoon disaster on coastal inhabitants in China. *Am. J. Disaster Med.* **2011**, *6*, 119–126. [CrossRef] [PubMed]
8. Chan, E.Y.Y.; Man, A.Y.T.; Lam, H.C.Y. Scientific evidence on natural disasters and health emergency and disaster risk management in Asian rural-based area. *Br. Med. Bull.* **2019**. [CrossRef]
9. Chan, E.Y.Y.; Yue, J.; Lee, P.; Wang, S.S. Socio-demographic predictors for urban community disaster health risk perception and household based preparedness in a Chinese urban city. *PLoS Curr.* **2016**, *8*, 1–11. [CrossRef]
10. Wong, T.F.; Yan, Y.Y. Perceptions of severe weather warnings in Hong Kong. *Meteorol. Appl.* **2002**, *9*, 377–382. [CrossRef]
11. Chan, E.Y.Y.; Yeung, M.P.; Lo, S.T. *Hong Kong's Emergency and Disaster Response System Policy Brief*; The Hong Kong Jockey Club Charities Trust: Hong Kong, China, 2015.
12. Lam, R.P.K.; Leung, L.P.; Balsari, S.; Hsiao, K.H.; Newnham, E.; Patrick, K.; Pham, P.; Leaning, J. Urban disaster preparedness of Hong Kong residents: A territory-wide survey. *Int. J. Disaster Risk Reduct.* **2017**, *23*, 62–69. [CrossRef]
13. Choy, C.; Wu, M. Observatory's Blog: A Wake up Call from Mangkhut. Available online: http://www.hko.gov.hk/blog/en/archives/00000216.htm (accessed on 7 January 2019).
14. The Hong Kong Observatory The Weather of September 2018. Available online: https://www.weather.gov.hk/wxinfo/pastwx/mws2018/mws201809.htm (accessed on 12 November 2018).
15. Avila, L.A. Hurricane Katia, National Hurricane Center Tropical Cyclone Report. Available online: https://www.nhc.noaa.gov/data/tcr/AL132017_Katia.pdf (accessed on 12 November 2018).
16. Hong Kong Legislative Council. *The Government's Preparations, Emergency Response and Recovery Efforts Arising from Super Typhoon Mangkhut*; Hong Kong Legislative Council: Hong Kong, China, 2018.
17. World Health Organization. *Update: Typhoon Ompong (Mankghut) as of 27 September 2018, 2:00 PM*; World Health Organization: Geneva, Switzerland, 2018 27 September.
18. Kohn, S.; Eaton, J.L.; Feroz, S.; Bainbridge, A.A.; Hoolachan, J.; Barnett, D.J. Personal disaster preparedness: An integrative review of the literature. *Disaster Med. Public Health Prep.* **2012**, *6*, 217–231. [CrossRef]
19. Nozawa, M.; Watanabe, T.; Katada, N.; Minami, H.; Yamamoto, A. Residents' awareness and behaviour regarding typhoon evacuation advice in Hyogo Prefecture, Japan. *Int. Nurs. Rev.* **2008**, *55*, 20–26. [CrossRef] [PubMed]
20. Bollettino, V.; Alcayna, T.; Enriquez, K.; Vinck, P. *Perceptions of Disaster Resilience and Preparedness in the Philippines*; Harvard University: Cambridge, MA, USA, 2018.
21. Cherniack, E.P.; Sandals, L.; Brooks, L.; Mintzer, M.J. Trial of a survey instrument to establish the hurricane preparedness of and medical impact on a vulnerable, older population. *Prehosp. Disaster Med.* **2008**, *23*, 242–249.
22. Mei, W.; Xie, S. Intensification of landfalling typhoons over the northwest Pacific since the late 1970s. *Nat. Geosci.* **2016**, *9*. [CrossRef]

23. Lane, K.; Charles-guzman, K.; Wheeler, K.; Abid, Z.; Graber, N.; Matte, T. Health Effects of Coastal Storms and Flooding in Urban Areas: A Review and Vulnerability Assessment. *J. Environ. Public Health* **2013**, *2013*, 13. [CrossRef]
24. Chan, E.Y.Y.; Huang, Z.; Ka, C.; Mark, M. Weather Information Acquisition and Health Significance during Extreme Cold Weather in a Subtropical City: A Cross-sectional Survey in Hong Kong. *Int. J. Disaster Risk Sci.* **2017**, *8*, 134–144. [CrossRef]
25. Tam, G.; Huang, Z.; Chan, E. Household Preparedness and Preferred Communication Channels in Public Health Emergencies: A Cross-Sectional Survey of Residents in an Asian Developed Urban City. *Int. J. Environ. Res. Public Health* **2018**, *15*, 1598. [CrossRef] [PubMed]
26. Loke, A.Y.; Lai, C.K.Y.; Fung, O.W.M. At-home disaster preparedness of elderly people in Hong Kong. *Geriatr. Gerontol. Int.* **2012**, *12*, 524–531. [CrossRef] [PubMed]
27. The Hong Kong Observatory Super Typhoon Hato 20 to 24 August 2017. Available online: http://www.weather.gov.hk/informtc/hato17/report.htm (accessed on 10 October 2018).
28. Kyodo Typhoon Jebi, Most Powerful to Hit Japan in 25 Years, Leaves Trail of Destruction in Kansai Region. Available online: https://www.japantimes.co.jp/news/2018/09/04/national/strong-typhoon-poised-make-landfall-shikoku-kii-peninsula-afternoon/ (accessed on 12 January 2019).
29. Cheng, K. Video: Construction Elevator Shaft Falls From Building as Typhoon Mangkhut Rips through Hong Kong | Hong Kong Free Press HKFP. Available online: https://www.hongkongfp.com/2018/09/16/video-crane-falls-housing-development-project-tai-kok-tsui-super-typhoon-mangkhut/ (accessed on 14 November 2018).
30. Cheung, J.; Hui, S. Monstrous Mangkhut: Super Typhoon Leaves More Than 200 Injured and Paralyzes Transport as It Pummels Hong Kong With Record-Breaking Winds—The Standard. Available online: http://www.thestandard.com.hk/section-news.php?id=200244&sid=11 (accessed on 13 November 2018).
31. Eisenman, D.P.; Cordasco, K.M.; Asch, S.; Golden, J.F.; Glik, D. Disaster planning and risk communication with vulnerable communities: lessons from Hurricane Katrina. *Am. J. Public Health* **2007**, *97* (Suppl. 1), S109–S115. [CrossRef]
32. Sahin, H.; Kara, Y.; Karasan, O.E. Debris removal during disaster response: A case for Turkey. *Socioecon. Plann. Sci.* **2016**, *53*, 49–59. [CrossRef]
33. Lock, S.; Rubin, G.J.; Murray, V.; Rogers, M.B.; Amlôt, R.; Williams, R. Secondary Stressors and Extreme Events and Disasters: A Systematic Review of Primary Resesearch from 2010–2011. *PLoS Curr.* **2015**, *4*, 1–17. [CrossRef] [PubMed]
34. Office of the Communications Authority Key Communications Statistics. Available online: https://www.ofca.gov.hk/en/data_statistics/data_statistics/key_stat/ (accessed on 15 January 2019).
35. Hall, B.J.; Xiong, Y.X.; Yip, P.S.Y.; Lao, C.K.; Shi, W.; Elvo, K.L.; Chang, K.; Wang, L.; Lam, A.I.F.; Hall, B.J.; et al. The association between disaster exposure and media use on post-traumatic stress disorder following Typhoon Hato in Macao, China The association between disaster exposure and media use on post-traumatic. *Eur. J. Psychotraumatol.* **2019**, *10*. [CrossRef] [PubMed]
36. Lau, J.T.F.; Griffiths, S.; Choi, K.C.; Tsui, H.Y. Widespread public misconception in the early phase of the H1N1 influenza epidemic. *J. Infect.* **2009**, *59*, 122–127. [CrossRef] [PubMed]
37. Chang, C.H. Preparedness and storm hazards in a global warming world: Lessons from Southeast Asia. *Nat. Hazards* **2011**, *56*, 667–679. [CrossRef]

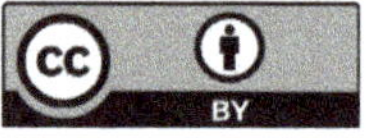

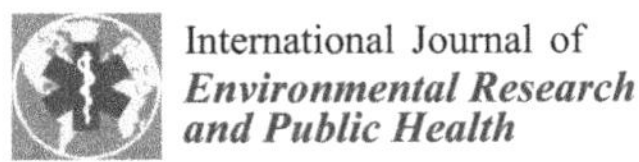
International Journal of
Environmental Research and Public Health

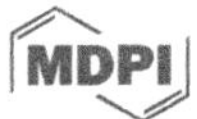

Communication

Research Methods and Ethics in Health Emergency and Disaster Risk Management: The Result of the Kobe Expert Meeting

Myo Nyein Aung [1], Virginia Murray [2,*] and Ryoma Kayano [3]

1 Advanced Health Science Institute and Faculty of International Liberal Arts, Juntendo University, Hongo 2-1-1, Bunkyo-ku, Tokyo 113-8421, Japan; myo@juntendo.ac.jp
2 Head of Global Disaster Risk Reduction, Public Health England, Wellington House, 133-155, Waterloo Road, London SE1 8UG, UK
3 World Health Organization Centre for Health Development, 1-5-1 Wakinohama-kaigandori, Chuo-ku, Kobe 651-0073, Japan; kayanor@who.int
* Correspondence: Virginia.Murray@phe.gov.uk; Tel.: +44-(0)-797-074-7849

Received: 31 January 2019; Accepted: 27 February 2019; Published: 3 March 2019

Abstract: In October 2018, at Asia Pacific Conference for Disaster Medicine (APCDM), an expert meeting to identify key research needs was organized by the World Health Organization (WHO) Centre for Health Development (WHO Kobe Centre (WKC)), convening the leading experts from Asia Pacific region, WHO, WHO Thematic Platform for Health Emergency and Disaster Risk Management (Health-EDRM) Research Network (TPRN), World Association for Disaster and Emergency Medicine (WADEM), in collaboration with Asia Pacific Conference for Disaster Medicine (APCDM) and Japan International Cooperation Agency (JICA). International experts, who were pre-informed about the meeting, contributed experience-based priority issues in Health-EDRM research, ethics, and scientific publication. Two moderators, experienced in multi-disciplinary research interacted with discussants to transcribe practical issues into related methodological and ethical issues. Each issue was addressed in order to progress research and scientific evidence in Health-EDRM. Further analysis of interactive dialogues revealed priorities for action, proposed mechanism to address these and identified recommendations. Thematic discussion uncovered five priority areas: (1) the need to harmonize Health-EDRM research with universal terms and, definitions via a glossary; (2) mechanisms to facilitate and speed up ethical review process; (3) increased community participation and stakeholder involvement in generating research ideas and in assessing impact evaluation; (4) development of reference materials such as possible consensus statements; and (5) the urgent need for a research methods resource textbook for Health-EDRM addressing these issues.

Keywords: health emergency and disaster risk management (Health-EDRM); Sendai Framework for Disaster Risk Reduction; WHO Thematic Platform for Health-EDRM; research methods; ethics; glossary

1. Introduction

At the Asia Pacific Conference for Disaster Medicine (APCDM) [1], October 2018, an expert meeting to identify key research needs in major research areas was organized by the World Health Organization (WHO) Centre for Health Development (WHO Kobe Centre (WKC), convening the leading experts from Asia Pacific region, WHO, WHO Thematic Platform for Health Emergency and Disaster Risk Management (Health-EDRM) Research Network (TPRN), World Association for Disaster and Emergency Medicine (WADEM). An expert meeting was conducted along with aseries of progresses in scientific aspects of the implementation of the 2015 Sendai Framework on Disaster

Risk Reduction (SFDRR) [2], the resulting document of the Third UN World Conference on Disaster Risk Reduction (WCDRR), included the establishment of TPRN [3,4] and following journal papers on recommended Health-EDRM research activities [5,6]. Through the expert meeting and related review of literature and existing projects and activities, key research needs in five major Health-EDRM research areas were identified.

The Health-EDRM Network identified one major area of work that is important to address was clarity in relevant 'Research Methods and Ethics'. The broad intersection of health and disaster risk reduction has resulted in an area of work now known as Health-EDRM which encompasses emergency and disaster medicine, disaster risk reduction, community health resilience, health system resilience, and impact of changing climate on health. Public health response during and after disasters has traditionally been focused on protecting populations from immediate threats [7]. Health-EDRM research involves the systematic analysis and management of health risks in emergencies and disasters by reducing the health risks and vulnerability. The complexity of undertaking research in disasters, and complying with ethical standards for these research, is critical but often much more difficult to ensure. This paper summarizes the outcome of the discussions and the proposed actions needed to support the delivery of Health-EDRM research.

2. Material and Methods

Prior to the meeting a range of international experts contributed experience-based priority issues in Health-EDRM research, ethics and scientific publication. It is of note that even in 1997, Stallings was able to state that " ... *it is the context of research not the methods that makes disaster research unique*" [8]. The lead discussant, the rapporteur, and the other experts who participated to the discussion primarily aimed to identify priorities in scientific evidence on Research Methods and Ethics in Health Emergency and Disaster Risk Management Research focused on questions and issues to fill these gaps. In addition to identifying knowledge gaps, experts also aimed to assess knowledge-to-practice gaps in order to better integrate current expertise and research in this area into each phase of disaster risk management. Following a preliminary literature review and expert consultations, a series of questions that were thought to be very important to address for building better understanding of research methods and ethics in Health-EDRM included

(a) What are the definitions of research methods and technical terms for Health-EDRM?
(b) How can impact evaluation methods for intervention and qualitative—quantitative mixed methods be standardized?
(c) How can the publication process for Health-EDRM research become more systematic and effective?

Those participated in discussion were leading experts in Health-EDRM as well as country experts in disaster and emergency, and came from multiple disciplines such as public health, emergency medicine, nursing, and health care management. They discussed major issues in Health-EDRM research from practitioner viewpoints and different regional perspectives. Each issue was addressed by active discussion of participants with the aim of addressing priorities and actions on how to progress research and scientific evidence in Health DRM. Interactive dialogues noted simultaneously into minutes of discussion were further analyzed by the moderators into the gaps, proposed mechanism to overcome the gaps and to provide a summary of recommendations.

3. Results and Discussion

Experts from different parts of the globe participated in this thematic group discussion. The findings from this discussion were wide ranging. It was noted that research findings from disaster research is not easily translated into different contexts of the many countries around the world, and there were challenges and difficulties in implementing practices in addressing national health system, cultural and religious issues before, during, and after interventions. These issues were difficult to address without more complete and systematic evidence to inform Health-EDRM policy and practice. Although translating research findings into policy is the ambition of many researchers and practitioners in order to develop evidence-based policies, there are issues of how much researchers can communicate with policy makers in comparison to the opportunities to facilitate policy makers' uptake of research findings. A key strategy to overcome this barrier is stakeholders' involvement and community participation since the development of research ideas in designing phase of the research project. For example, research in disaster affected area might recruit participants who were disasters casualties and there should be rules and regulation especially listing ethical 'don't's such as providing food as an incentive for participation in the research. For instance, food is sometimes used as incentive for the participation in the research, in some context. However, in the disaster and emergency situation, food is the basic need provided as the humanitarian aid regardless of participation in the research. Thus, if food is used as incentives for research recruiting such persons, it might be forcing someone to participate in the research, in the fear that they cannot receive food supply. Therefore, it is not appropriate to use food as incentives in Health-EDRM research.

Thematic discussion in the meeting uncovered five priority areas: (1) the need to harmonize Health-EDRM research with universal terms and definitions via a glossary; (2) mechanisms to facilitate and speed up ethical review process; (3) development of reference materials such as possible consensus statements; (4) increased community participation and stakeholder involvement in generating research ideas and in assessing impact evaluation; and (5) and the urgent need for a textbook for Health-EDRM research addressing these and other issues. Discussions also agreed that there was a need to harmonize definitions in Health-EDRM research with universal terms, and the development of a glossary of definitions. Such a glossary could promote common understanding and common usage of concepts, terms, and aims for Health-EDRM. If undertaken by WHO, the glossary might have the additional advantage of being translated into the WHO official languages. Even though the United Nations Office for Disaster Risk Reduction (UNISDR) convened an Open-ended Intergovernmental Expert Working Group (OIEWG) to report on indicators with recommended terminology relating to disaster risk reduction, which was delivered in 2016 [9], and adopted by the UN General Assembly on 2 February 2017 and updated the 2009 UNISDR Terminology on Disaster Risk Reduction [10]; however, not all the necessary Health-EDRM terms were included in these or other terminologies.

The need to find mechanisms to facilitate and speed up ethical review process was addressed and the need to quicken the review process for disaster research ethics was noted as being complex and very dynamic. A basic requirement was to agree on methodological terms and should reflect research undertaken in the spectrum of disaster chronology such from preparedness and risk reduction, to emergency management, and to post disaster rehabilitation. One key suggestion was the requirement to reduce the review time for ethical approval with, wherever possible, with pre-agreed ethical approval. As Chan et al. (2019) pointed out their recent Lancet editorial that "research stakeholders have a responsibility to protect the interests of communities involved in research, achieving this is rarely straightforward in emergencies" [11]. From the discussion that it would require international consensus among the professionals and researchers, possibly using as good practice models the CONSORT (Consolidated Standards of Reporting Trials) statement for randomized controlled trials [12,13] and STROBE (STrengthening the Reporting of OBservational studies in Epidemiology) statement for cohort studies [14,15]. Additional models of good practice such as the Guidance for Managing Ethical Issues in Infectious Disease Outbreaks [16] and the Health Emergency and Disaster Risk Management fact sheet on ETHICS [17] were thought to be practical and helpful examples. More data on these topics to address Health-EDRM were considered to be of importance. Once a research proposal can fit in a standardized check list, the ethical committee should be able to agree the research proposed via an expedited channel.

Such activities could be part of the development of reference materials such as possible consensus statements. Such consensus statement provide a checklist of methodology details which allows researcher to check the proposal themselves. Ethical committee can quickly assessthe quality assurance and safety through the list, speeding up the approval. Therefore, it is very essential step to develop a consensus for disaster research.

The call for increased community participation and stakeholder involvement in generating research ideas and in assessing impact evaluation was considered and the need to listen to the voice of the affected and their community leaders and local representatives is increasingly critical. However, relatively few Health-EDRM reports on community participation and stakeholder involvement in generating research ideas were shared in the discussion. There are examples of where research to address stakeholder involvement in health research, such as the recent report from Kapiriri (2018) [18], but it is not from emergency or disaster research. Very little has been published definitively on this area.

Much more is described in the quest of methodological rigour for impact evaluation. The experts brain-stormed how can impact evaluation apply quantitative methods in additional to commonly applied case-studies in disaster research.

Impact evaluation is usually applied to see how a research programme works well in a particular setting. It is a term understood readily by multiple stakeholders whereas it dictates how to measure the outcome an intervention in basic research methodology. There are many methodological tools to measure how an intervention brought about changes in comparison to pre-existing situation or in comparison to naïve control group. A proposed intervention should be tested by efficacy and effectiveness trials before it comes into the guidelines and practice. It was considered that the synthesis of evidence would be primarily through the process of systematic reviewing and, if appropriate, modelling and cost effectiveness decision analysis [19]. The efficacy depends on how the intervention is planned to measure (design), how accurate are the measurement tools (validity and reliability) whereas the effectiveness will inform how robust is the intervention in the real world setting. Furthermore, the scalability of intervention will be challenged by the economic, social, and political context and the resource need. It would be important to follow process recommended where possible by organisations and their reports of activities that are already engaged in working in this area such as WHO [20,21], UK Medical Research Council [22], Organisation for Economic Co-operation and Development [23], and the Humanitarian Policy Group at the Overseas Development Institute and its Good Practice Review [24] with its chapter on Monitoring and Evaluation [25,26].

Diverse research methods from case studies, natural experiment designs and randomized controlled trials can be applied in impact monitoring and evaluation. For example, clinical epidemiology is a discipline to determine clinical outcomes applying tools of epidemiology. Likewise, epidemiological tools can be selected to match where and how they would be applied in Health-EDRM research but are often less easy to monitor and evaluate as they are used in more difficult environments. Through the synergy of Health-EDRM experts and the discussion on research methods, designs, and tools, it might be possible to encourage selection and use of more appropriate mechanisms. Events to gather such multidisciplinary professionals such as international workshops are important opportunity to generate the list of strategic research methodology tools. Relatively few resources for disaster risk reduction and management research methods have been identified and some excellent examples are cited below [27–32]. However most of these do not specifically address the full range of Health-EDRM research domains. Therefore, it is considered that there is relatively little currently that reflects the wide needs of Health-EDRM researchers, practitioners, and policy makers. Therefore, a text book linked to a website for easy updating is needed and such a resource could be tentatively entitled "research methods for health emergency and disaster risk management". This would be a rewarding endeavor and would be beneficial to the establishment of the WHO Thematic Platform for Health Emergency and Disaster Risk Management Research Network.

4. Conclusions

It is hoped this paper on key issues in research methods and ethics in health emergency and disaster risk management will contribute to the identification and implementation of concrete solutions that foster the creation and the use of knowledge for research and ethics building resilience before, during, and after disasters. In the discussion, issues were raised on potential gap areas in the disaster research methodology: impact evaluations; Consensus on the definitions; development of common research statements like the CONSORT or STROBE for disaster research; how research findings in disaster research can be translated into different contexts of the many countries around the world; and the need to develop the textbook in disaster research methodology to help guide international researchers.

As for other major Health-EDRM research areas, research and ethics requires collaboration between experts, decision-makers, practitioners, and communities in order to facilitate coordinated response when and where it is most needed. It is critical a text book is created to provide a reference which would be fundamental and global contribution to the establishment of the WHO Thematic Platform for Health Emergency and Disaster Risk Management Research Network.

Author Contributions: Conceptualization, R.K. and V.M.; Methodology, M.N.A. and V.M.; Writing—Original Draft Preparation, M.N.A. and V.M.; Writing—Review & Editing, V.M., M.N.A. and R.K.; Project Administration, R.K.

Funding: This research received no external funding.

Acknowledgments: The authors thank all the meeting participants who contributed to achieving the results (alphabetical order of their last name): Jonathan Abrahams (WHO), Francis Archer (Monash University, Australia), Sarah Louise Barber (WHO), Emily YY Chan (The Chinese University of Hong Kong, China), Shinichi Egawa (Tohoku University, Japan), Paul Farrell (WADEM), Teodoro Herbosa (University of the Philippines, Philippines), Sonoe Mashino (University of Hyogo, Japan), Toshiyuki Ojima (Hamamatsu University School of Medicine, Japan), Philip Schluter (University of Canterbury, New Zealand), Shiori Usami (Kumamoto University, Japan).

Conflicts of Interest: The authors declare no conflict of interest.

References

1. Asian Pacific Conference for Disaster Medicine. 2018. Available online: http://www.apcdm2018.org/index.html (accessed on 28 January 2019).
2. Sendai Framework for Disaster Risk Reduction 2015–2030. Available online: https://www.unisdr.org/we/inform/publications/43291 (accessed on 28 January 2019).
3. World Health Organization. WHO Thematic Platform for Health Emergency and Disaster Risk Management. Available online: http://www.who.int/hac/techguidance/preparedness/WHO-Thematic-Platform-Health-EDRM-Terms-Reference-2018.pdf?ua=1 (accessed on 28 January 2019).
4. World Health Organization. WHO Thematic Platform for Health Emergency and Disaster Risk Management Research Network. Available online: http://www.who.int/hac/techguidance/preparedness/WHO-Thematic-Platform-Health-EDRM-Research-Network-2018.pdf?ua=1 (accessed on 3 March 2019).
5. Chan, E.Y.Y.; Murray, V. What are the health research needs for the Sendai Framework. *Lancet* **2017**, *390*, e35–e36. Available online: https://www.thelancet.com/journals/lancet/article/PIIS0140-6736(17)31670-7/fulltext (accessed on 28 January 2019). [CrossRef]
6. Lo, S.T.T.; Chan, E.Y.Y.; Chan, G.K.W.; Murray, V.; Abrahams, J.; Ardalan, A.; Kayano, R.; Yau, J.C.W. Health Emergency and Disaster Risk Management (Health-EDRM): Developing the Research Field within the Sendai Framework Paradigm. *Int. J. Disaster Risk Sci.* **2017**, *8*, 145–149. [CrossRef]
7. Aitsi-Selmi, A.; Murray, V. The Sendai framework: Disaster risk reduction through a health lens. *Bull. World Health Organ.* **2015**, *93*, 362. Available online: https://www.who.int/bulletin/volumes/93/6/15-157362.pdf (accessed on 1 January 2019). [CrossRef] [PubMed]
8. Stallings, R.A. Methods of Disaster Research: Unique or Not? *Int. J. Mass Emerg. Disasters March* **1997**, *15*, 7–19. Available online: http://ijmed.org/articles/408/download/ (accessed on 1 January 2019).
9. United Nations General Assembly. Report of the Open-Ended Intergovernmental Expert Working Group on Indicators and Terminology Relating to Disaster Risk Reduction A/71/644. 2016. Available online: https://www.preventionweb.net/files/50683_oiewgreportenglish.pdf (accessed on 3 March 2019).
10. United Nations International Strategy for Disaster Reduction (UNISDR). UNISDR Terminology on Disaster Risk Reduction. 2009. Available online: https://www.unisdr.org/files/7817_UNISDRTerminologyEnglish.pdf (accessed on 1 January 2019).

11. Chan, E.Y.; Wright, K.; Parker, M. Health-emergency disaster risk management and research ethics. *Lancet* **2019**, *393*, 112–113. [CrossRef]
12. Schulz, K.F.; Altman, D.G.; Moher, D. CONSORT 2010 statement: Updated guidelines for reporting parallel group randomised trials. *BMJ* **2010**, *340*, c332. [CrossRef] [PubMed]
13. CONSORT Website: Consolidated Standards of Reporting Trials and Encompasses Various Initiatives Developed by the CONSORT Group to Alleviate the Problems Arising from Inadequate Reporting of Randomized Controlled Trials. Available online: http://www.consort-statement.org/ (accessed on 29 January 2019).
14. Vandenbroucke, J.P.; von Elm, E.; Altman, D.G.; Gotzsche, P.C.; Mulrow, C.D.; Pocock, S.J.; Poole, C.; Schlesselman, J.J.; Egger, M. Strengthening the Reporting of Observational Studies in Epidemiology (STROBE): Explanation and elaboration. *Int. J. Surg.* **2014**, *12*, 1500–1524. [CrossRef] [PubMed]
15. STROBE Website: Strengthening the Reporting of Observational Studies in Epidemiology (STROBE) Statement: Guidelines for Reporting Observational Studies. 2014. Available online: https://www.strobe-statement.org/index.php?id=strobe-home (accessed on 29 January 2019).
16. World Health Organization. WHO Guidelines on Ethical Issues in Public Health Surveillance. 2017. Available online: http://apps.who.int/iris/bitstream/10665/255721/1/9789241512657-eng.pdf (accessed on 20 January 2019).
17. World Health Organization; Public Health England. Health Emergency and Disaster Risk Management ETHICS. 2017. Available online: https://www.who.int/hac/techguidance/preparedness/risk-management-ethics-december2017.pdf?ua=1 (accessed on 20 January 2019).
18. Kapiriri, L. Stakeholder involvement in health research priority setting in low income countries: The case of Zambia. *Res. Involv. Engagem.* **2018**, *4*, 41. [CrossRef] [PubMed]
19. National Institute for Health and Care Excellence (NICE). Research Recommendations Interim Process and Methods Guide. 2015. Available online: https://www.nice.org.uk/Media/Default/About/what-we-do/Research-and-development/Research-Recommendation-Process-and-Methods-Guide-2015.pdf (accessed on 29 January 2019).
20. World Health Organization. The WHO Strategy on Research for Health. 2012. Available online: https://www.who.int/phi/WHO_Strategy_on_research_for_health.pdf (accessed on 3 March 2019).
21. World Health Organization. *Monitoring and Evaluating Digital Health Interventions: A Practical Guide to Conducting Research and Assessment*; World Health Organization: Geneva, Switzerland, 2016; Available online: https://apps.who.int/iris/bitstream/handle/10665/252183/?sequence=1 (accessed on 1 January 2019).
22. Medical Research Council. Developing and Evaluating Complex Interventions. 2019. Available online: https://mrc.ukri.org/documents/pdf/complex-interventions-guidance/ (accessed on 20 January 2019).
23. Organisation for Economic Co-operation and Development (OECD). Outline of Principles of Impact Evaluation. 2006. Available online: http://www.oecd.org/dac/evaluation/dcdndep/37671602.pdf (accessed on 20 January 2019).
24. Twigg, J. Disaster Risk Reduction Good Practice Review. Humanitarian Policy Group, Overseas Development Institute, 2015. Available online: https://goodpracticereview.org/wp-content/uploads/2015/10/GPR-9-web-string-1.pdf (accessed on 20 January 2019).
25. Twigg, J. Disaster Risk Reduction Good Practice Review. Chapter 18 Monitoring and Evaluation, Humanitarian Policy Group, Overseas Development Institute, 2015. Available online: https://goodpracticereview.org/wp-content/uploads/2015/10/GPR_9_Chapter_18.pdf (accessed on 20 January 2019).
26. World Health Organization. *WHO Evaluation Practice Handbook*; World Health Organization: Geneva, Switzerland, 2013; ISBN 978-92-4-154868-7. Available online: https://apps.who.int/iris/bitstream/handle/10665/96311/9789241548687_eng.pdf?sequence= (accessed on 20 January 2019).
27. Rodríguez, H.; Donner, W.; Trainor, J.E. (Eds.) *Handbook of Disaster Research*, 2nd ed.; Springer: New York, NY, USA, 2018; Available online: https://www.springer.com/gb/book/9783319632537 (accessed on 1 January 2019).
28. Oliver-Smith, A.; Alcántara-Ayala, I.; Burton, I.; Lavell, A. *Forensic Investigations of Disasters (FORIN): A Conceptual Framework and Guide to Research*; IRDR FORIN Publication: Beijing, China, 2016.
29. Stallings, R.A. Methods of Disaster Research. Xlibris, 2003. Available online: https://www.xlibris.com/bookstore/bookdetail.aspx?bookid=SKU-0016862003 (accessed on 1 January 2019).

30. Phillips, B.D. *Qualitative Disaster Research*; Oxford University Press: Oxford, UK, 2014; Available online: https://global.oup.com/academic/product/qualitative-disaster-research-9780199796175?cc=gb&lang=en& (accessed on 29 January 2019).
31. Norris, F.; Galea, S.; Friedman, M.; Watson, P. *Methods for Disaster Mental Health Research*; Guildford Press: New, York, NY, USA, 2006; Available online: https://zodml.org/sites/default/files/Methods_for_Disaster_Mental_Health_Research.pdf (accessed on 29 January 2019).
32. Oakes, J.M.; Kaufman, J.S. (Eds.) *Methods in Social Epidemiology*; John Wiley & Sons: Hoboken, NJ, USA, 2017; Volume 16.

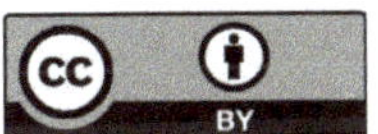

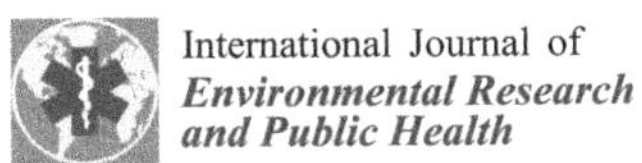

International Journal of
Environmental Research and Public Health

MDPI

Communication

Health Data Collection Before, During and After Emergencies and Disasters—The Result of the Kobe Expert Meeting

Tatsuhiko Kubo [1,*], Alisa Yanasan [2], Teodoro Herbosa [3], Nilesh Buddh [4], Ferdinal Fernando [5] and Ryoma Kayano [6]

1 Department of Environmental Epidemiology, Institute of Industrial Ecological Sciences, University of Occupational and Environmental Health, Kitakyushu 807-8555, Japan
2 Ministry of Public Health, Nonthaburi 11000, Thailand; yanasan.a@gmail.com
3 UP College of Medicine, University of the Philippines Manila, Manila 1000, Philippines; tjherbosa@up.edu.ph
4 WHO Regional Office for South-East Asia, New Delhi 110002, India; buddhan@who.int
5 The ASEAN Secretariat, Jakarta 12110, Indonesia; ferdinal.fernando@asean.org
6 World Health Organization Centre for Health Development, Kobe 651-0073, Japan; kayanor@who.int
* Correspondence: kubo@med.uoeh-u.ac.jp; Tel.: +81-93-603-1611

Received: 31 January 2019; Accepted: 4 March 2019; Published: 12 March 2019

Abstract: In October 2018, the World Health Organization (WHO) convened a meeting to identify key research needs, bringing together leading experts from WHO, WHO Thematic Platform for Health Emergency and Disaster Risk Management (Health-EDRM) Research Network (TPRN), World Association for Disaster and Emergency Medicine (WADEM), the Japan International Cooperation Agency (JICA), and delegates to the Asia Pacific Conference for Disaster Medicine (APCDM) 2018. The meeting identified key research needs in five major research areas for Health-EDRM. One of the five major research areas was "Health data collection during emergency and disaster". Experts for this research area highlighted WHO Emergency Medical Team Minimum Data Set (EMT MDS), a standardized medical data collection method during and after disasters, as an example of substantial progress, with knowledge gaps and challenges in implementation in some regions and countries (i.e., information collection methodology in medical facilities of affected local areas, seamless and practical connection between acute phase data collection and post-acute phase local surveillance). The discussion on this research area also identified key research needs in standardization of broader health-related data to inform effective Health EDRM (i.e., community vulnerabilities, hospital functional status, infrastructure, lifelines and health workforce).

Keywords: health emergency and disaster risk management (H-EDRM); Sendai Framework for Disaster Risk Reduction; WHO Thematic Platform for H-EDRM; Emergency Medical Team; Emergency Medical Team Minimum Data Set; epidemiology; Public Health Surveillance

1. Introduction

In October 2018 at the Asia Pacific Conference for Disaster Medicine (APCDM) 2018 [1], an expert meeting to identify key research needs in major research areas was organized by the World Health Organization (WHO) Centre for Health Development (WHO Kobe Centre (WKC)), convening the leading experts from the Asia Pacific region, WHO, WHO Thematic Platform for Health Emergency and Disaster Risk Management (Health-EDRM) Research Network (TPRN), World Association for Disaster and Emergency Medicine (WADEM). The expert meeting was conducted, along with progress in the scientific aspect of the implementation of the Sendai Framework on Disaster Risk Reduction 2015–2030 [2], the resulting document of the 3rd UN World Conference on Disaster Risk Reduction

(WCDRR), including establishment of TPRN, and following journal papers on recommended H-EDRM research activities [3–6]. Through the expert meeting and related review of literature and existing projects and activities, key research gaps in five major H-EDRM research areas were identified.

"Health Data collection before, during and after emergencies and disasters" is one of the five proposed major H-EDRM research areas. To conduct effective and timely health support in disaster relief and recovery activities, accurate and comprehensive health-related data is essential. Relief activities not based on relevant and accurate data could lead to negative impacts on recovery, related to the "do no harm" principle of Mary B. Anderson [7]. There have been a number of challenges in data collection in affected areas such as safe access to affected areas, preparing resources for data collection, obtaining informed consent from disaster victims, and fragmentation in data collecting and reporting methodology among different relief teams. All of these challenges cause a significant lack of scientific evidence in Health EDRM, especially the research with quantitative health data. For example, a MEDLINE search with MESH term "Disaster Medicine/statistics and numerical data" hit only 14 articles [8], which indicates a strong requirement of improvement in research and development of related methodology and tools for health data collection during and after disasters.

2. Material and Methods

The expert discussion of this research theme primarily aimed to identify recommended contents and source of health data to be collected, with reviewing the current available tools, methods and background systems and regulations in disaster relief activities. For the follow up of the expert meeting, a supplementary literature review and online discussion among the experts were conducted.

3. Results

Through the expert meeting based on a preliminary literature review, follow up online discussion, and a supplementary literature review, the experts developed the two research questions to be addressed, below. The greater details of the background of the proposed questions are described below.

(a) What are the national and regional challenges inhibiting implementation of the WHO standardized medical data collection systems during and after emergencies and disasters?

(b) What is the broader health-related data needed to inform effective Health-EDRM, i.e., community vulnerabilities, hospital functional status, infrastructure, lifelines and health workforce?

Firstly, the experts highlighted some key points for effective and practical data collection and utilization, including the "keep it simple" concept, which recommends simple and concise data, timely data collection for basic statistics in the manner to support operation, effective connection between collected data and ongoing response activities (i.e., recommendation to include geographical information).

Secondly, the current tools, methods and background systems and regulations in disaster relief were reviewed. A disaster is defined as a situation or event which overwhelms local capacity, necessitating a request for national or international level of assistance [9]. Although local health facilities are expected to function as a fundamental resource for disaster response, previous events revealed that local facilities often lose their functionally in major disasters. In a major disaster, a surge of affected patients further overwhelmed the damaged local capacities. To support local capacities by fulfilling the supply gaps, Emergency Medical Teams (EMTs), defined as a "groups of health professionals and supporting staff providing health care specifically to disaster- and health emergency-affected populations" are deployed to affected area [10]. To register as an EMT, verified by WHO, the team needs to meet EMT minimum standards, prepare resources for their activities by themselves, and regularly report their activities and status during their relief activities [11]. This nature of EMT supports the rationale for EMT to take a fundamental role for health data collection during and after disasters in collaboration with local capacities and under the agreement of affected countries. As EMTs can be deployed from different countries and organizations, the standardization of the data collection and reporting system has been a great challenge. Responding to this challenge, in 2017 EMT Minimum Data Set (MDS), a standardized medical data set to be collected and reported by EMT, was developed [12]. The fact that MDS became available was evaluated as an example of significant progress in health data collection by all of the experts who participated in the meeting.

Following the consensus on the improvement in health data collection by the development of MDS, the experts focused on the gaps and research needs for further comprehensive data collection to inform timely and effective disaster response and recovery. The expert meeting, and a following supplementary literature review, concluded that there is no internationally agreed or standardized methodology for public health data collection during and after a disaster, which indicates the substantial quality gaps between countries in post-acute phase health data collection and following response. The source and available tools and methods for health data collection are listed in Table 1.

Table 1. Source and available tools or methods for health data collection during and after emergencies and disasters.

Source of Data (Reporter)	Acute Phase	Post-Acute Phase
Emergency Medical Team (EMT)	WHO EMT Minimum Data Set (MDS)	(Demobilization)
Local Facilities (i.e., Hospitals)	(Often difficult to function to collect data)	Local surveillance
Public Health Sector	(No international consensus)	Local surveillance

Based on the proposed list of sources and tools for health data collection, several research priorities were identified. First, regarding the acute phase data collection, although WHO EMT MDS is available, some countries are not ready to implement it and need capacity-building and training to adapt their national system to meet international reporting standards. Experts supported research to analyze the best practices of and lessons from the implementation of MDS, for future effective capacity development in different countries.

Second, regarding data collection by and from local facilities, given the damaged capacity of local facilities during the acute phase, research on effective information collection and sharing systems through the collaboration between local facilities and EMTs is worth conducting. To address this research priority, including broader public health and environmental concerns (i.e., infrastructure, lifelines, hospital functional status, and health workforce available in communities) should be considered.

Third, in connection with the above-mentioned broader data collection, because there is no internationally agreed or standardized tool or method, research on setting up essential public health data for disaster response is expected to be conducted. The development process of WHO EMT MDS would inform the establishment of the broader data set.

Fourth, the experts also emphasized the critical knowledge gaps in an effective and harmonized transition from the acute phase, often relying on EMT activities to the post-acute phase relying on local capacities. Research on the seamless and effective connection of activities in those two phases is required.

4. Discussion

This expert discussion highlighted the needs and priorities in health data collection with a focus on on-site relief activities and medical support. To address the identified research needs for more comprehensive data for disaster response and recovery, inclusion of experts from other sectors such as United Nations International Strategy for Disaster Reduction, the World Bank and United Nations Development Programme will be the key. While the focus of this expert meeting was on post-disaster health data collection, understandably proper collection of baseline data before the disaster is essential to conduct efficient health emergency management.

In the Asia Pacific Region there are ongoing efforts to implement MDS, including the establishment and implementation of Surveillance in Post Extreme Emergencies and Disasters (SPEED) in the

Philippines, and the Japanese version of SPEED (J-SPEED). Those two data collection systems have already been used for large scale data collection. For example, in Japan, the health data of 8089 patients in the Kumamoto Earthquake in 2016, 3620 patients in the West Japan Heavy Rain in 2018 and 591 patients in the Hokkaido Earthquake in 2018 were collected through the J-SPEED system, and are being analyzed quantitatively. This experience supports the practical utility of WHO EMT MDS. To maximize the impact of the data collection during and after a disaster, usually health data registration is required as the preparedness before disasters. Strengthening the health system, including capacity building for disaster response, is also the key for successful data collection. More implementation research on practical adaptation of international standards is also required, as countries which still need support for capacity building face the requirement of partial implementation of the MDS to address their ongoing health challenges in disasters.

5. Conclusions

The expert meeting on "Health data collection before, during and after emergencies and disasters" provided a clear view on the sources and currently available tools for health data collection during and after emergencies and disasters, and therefore required research activities for further improvement for comprehensive health data collection for effective, timely and seamless interventions in disaster response and recovery. More implementation research should be conducted.

Author Contributions: Conceptualization, T.K., R.K.; Methodology, T.K., A.Y.; Writing—Original Draft Preparation, T.K.; Writing—Review & Editing, A.Y., T.H., N.B., F.F., R.K.; Project Administration, T.K.

Funding: This research received no external funding.

Acknowledgments: The opinions contained in the paper are those of its authors and, except where specifically stated, are not intended to represent the official policies or positions of the WHO. The authors thank all the meeting participants who contributed to achieving the results: Paul Farrell (WADEM), Shuichi Ikeda (Project for Strengthening the ASEAN Regional Capacity on Disaster Health Management (ARCH Project), JICA), Tatruro Kai (Saiseikai Senri Hospital, Japan), Yasushi Nakajima (ARCH Project, JICA), Yosuke Takada (Okayama University, Japan), Nobuyo Tsuboyama-Kasaoka (National Institute of Health and Nutrition, Japan).

Conflicts of Interest: The authors declare no conflict of interest.

References

1. Asian Pacific Conference for Disaster Medicine 2018. Available online: http://www.apcdm2018.org/index.html (accessed on 15 January 2019).
2. Sendai Framework for Disaster Risk Reduction 2015–2030. Available online: https://www.unisdr.org/we/inform/publications/43291 (accessed on 15 January 2019).
3. WHO Thematic Platform for Health Emergency and Disaster Risk Management. Available online: http://www.who.int/hac/techguidance/preparedness/WHO-Thematic-Platform-Health-EDRM-Terms-Reference-2018.pdf?ua=1 (accessed on 15 January 2019).
4. WHO Thematic Platform for Health Emergency and Disaster Risk Management Research Network. Available online: http://www.who.int/hac/techguidance/preparedness/WHO-Thematic-Platform-Health-EDRM-Research-Network-2018.pdf?ua=1 (accessed on 15 January 2019).
5. Chan, E.Y.Y.; Murray, V. What are the health research needs for the Sendai Framework. *Lancet* **2017**, *390*, e35–e36. [CrossRef]
6. Lo, S.T.T.; Chan, E.Y.Y.; Chan, G.K.W.; Murray, V.; Abrahams, J.; Ardalan, A.; Kayano, R.; Yau, J.C.W. Health Emergency and Disaster Risk Management (Health-EDRM): Developing the Research Field within the Sendai Framework Paradigm. *Int. J. Disaster Risk Sci.* **2017**, *8*, 145–149. [CrossRef]
7. Anderson, M.B. *Do No Harm: How aid Can Support Peace or War*; Lynne Rienner Publishers: Boulder, CO, USA, 1999; p. 161.
8. Kubo, T. Disaster Medical Record/J-SPEED—Towards national implementation and international sharing of lessons learned from the Great East Japan Earthquake and the Kumamoto earthquake. *Prehosp. Care* **2018**, *31*, 64–68.

9. World Health Organization. *Definitions: Emergencies. Humanitarian Health Action*; World Health Organization: Geneva, Switzerland, 2018; Available online: http://www.who.int/hac/about/definitions/en/ (accessed on 17 April 2016).
10. World Health Organization. Emergency Medical Team. Available online: http://www.who.int/hac/techguidance/preparedness/emergency_medical_teams/en/ (accessed on 15 January 2019).
11. World Health Organization. *Classification and Minimum Standards for Foreign Medical Teams in Sudden Onset of Disasters*; World Health Organization: Geneva, Switzerland, 2013.
12. Emergency Medical Team Minimum Data Set Working Group. *Minimum Data Set for Reporting by Emergency Medical Teams*; World Health Organization: Geneva, Switzerland, 2017.

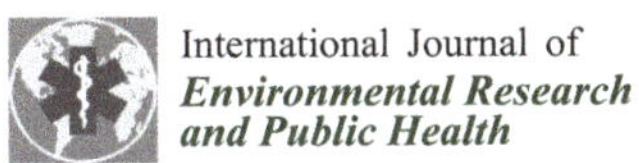
International Journal of
Environmental Research and Public Health

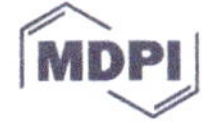

Article

Planning of a Health Emergency Disaster Risk Management Programme for a Chinese Ethnic Minority Community

Greta Tam [1], Emily Ying Yang Chan [2,3,4,*] and Sida Liu [2]

1. Jockey Club School of Public Health and Primary Care, the Chinese University of Hong Kong, Hong Kong, China; gretatam@cuhk.edu.hk
2. Collaborating Centre for Oxford University and CUHK for Disaster and Medical Humanitarian Response (CCOUC), the Jockey Club School of Public Health and Primary Care, the Chinese University of Hong Kong, Hong Kong, China; liusida2008@gmail.com
3. Nuffield Department of Medicine, University of Oxford, Oxford OX3 7BN, UK
4. FXB Center of Health and Human Rights, Harvard University, Boston, MA 02115, USA

* Correspondence: emily.chan@cuhk.edu.hk; Tel.: +852-2252-8850

Received: 30 January 2019; Accepted: 6 March 2019; Published: 22 March 2019

Abstract: Rural populations living in poverty are the most vulnerable to disaster. Despite this increased risk of recurrent disaster, previous disaster experience is not a good predictor for disaster preparedness in these populations. This was evidenced on 31 August 2012, when a major flood occurred in Sichuan, China. A health needs assessment carried out in December 2012 showed that residents of Hongyan village, a Yi-minority community in Sichuan lacked disaster preparedness. This indicated that measures were necessary to improve Health Emergency Disaster Risk Management (Health-EDRM) in the community. Nutbeam's planning model for health promotion was used to guide the development of a Health-EDRM programme at Hongyan Village, Liangshan Yi Autonomous Prefecture, Sichuan. Relevant information was obtained from sources such as literature review, household surveys and stakeholder interviews. A team of stakeholders conducted an interactive workshop to train villagers on disaster preparedness in March 2014. Disaster kits and equipment for Oral Rehydration Solution preparation were handed out to villagers.

Keywords: ethnic minority; China; Health-EDRM

---

1. Introduction

1.1. Disaster Health Preparedness in the Rural Poor Areas in China

Globally, 75% of people living below the poverty line of US $1.07/day live in rural areas. Despite economic growth in developing countries, the resulting benefits are not spread evenly. Poverty is becoming increasingly ruralized in China, Eastern Europe and Central Asia. Rural populations living in poverty are the most vulnerable to disaster. Climate change increasingly exposes rural areas to weather-related shocks and stresses (e.g., drought and repeated flooding) [1]. Meanwhile, poverty causes decreased disaster resilience due to lack of access to services (e.g., health care and education) and infrastructure (e.g., water and sanitation) [2]. Despite the increased risk of recurrent disaster among the rural poor, previous disaster experience is not a good predictor for disaster preparedness in these populations [3–5].

1.2. Building Disaster Health Resilient Communities

In 2015, the UN General Assembly endorsed the Sendai Framework for Disaster Risk Reduction. Priorities for Action included understanding disaster risk and enhancing disaster preparedness [6].

This built upon the previous Hyogo Framework for Action (2005–2015), which included as one of its priorities "use knowledge, innovation and education to build a culture of safety and resilience at all levels" [7].

Resilience is "the ability of a system, community or society exposed to hazards to resist, absorb, accommodate, adapt to, transform and recover from the effects of a hazard in a timely and efficient manner, including through the preservation and restoration of its essential basic structures and functions through risk management" [8]. The United Nations and Red Cross have advocated community-based disaster preparedness programmes to build disaster resilient communities [9,10]. This approach combines integrated programming and cooperation with local communities. Integrated programming ensures a holistic approach: elements from different sectors (e.g., health and hygiene education and disaster preparedness) are combined into one programme. Consulting local villagers ensures that interventions are tailored to specific community needs. Although efforts have been made to implement Health-EDRM programmes globally [9–11], Asia is still disproportionately affected by disasters: China, Indonesia, Philippines and India are among the top five countries most prone to natural disasters and Asia accounts for 90.1% of disaster victims [12].

1.3. Local Epidemiological and Demographic Data of Hongyan Village, Liangshan Yi Autonomous Prefecture, China

In the last decade, China has experienced the most natural disasters in the world [12]. Under the effects of climate change, there has been an increase of weather-related disasters by 69% globally in the last decade, with floods becoming increasingly frequent in China. Many remote villages in China have limited health and hygiene awareness and disaster preparedness, due to the low education level and lack of information. In addition, many lack basic sanitation infrastructures, such as proper latrines and access to basic medical care. Consequently, there is a risk of poor sanitation after a flood, as surface and groundwater are contaminated by effluent from latrines [10].

Hongyan village is one of 169 villages in Xide county, under the jurisdiction of Liangshan Yi Autonomous Prefecture, in the southern area of Sichuan province. Hongyan village is 5 km from the closest township, Lianghekou. Figure 1 shows a location map for the case area. It is composed of 4 sub-groups, with 218 households and 826 residents. The villagers live on the bank of Sunshui River, in a mountainous landscape with poor road conditions. Liangshan has the largest community of Yi ethnic minority group in China. Yi ethnic groups live mostly in rural and mountainous areas in Sichuan, Yunnan, Guizhou and Guangxi. Education levels are low in Yi ethnic groups and they speak their own language [13,14].

A major flood occurred on 31st August 2012 at Xide County, causing great damage: 218,000 residents were affected, 13,300 houses collapsed, and 29,000 houses were seriously damaged, while 1 death and 2 missing people were reported. Flooding also damaged the infrastructure, including roads, water supply, telephone and broadcasting. The county was therefore temporarily isolated from external information and assistance. In 2012, the Collaboration Centre for Oxford University and CUHK for Disaster and Medical Humanitarian Response (CCOUC) was invited by Wu Zhi Qiao Charitable Foundation to perform a health needs assessment and health intervention in Hongyan village.

This study aimed to identify and use relevant data to plan a Health-EDRM programme for Yi-minority community in Sichuan Province, China.

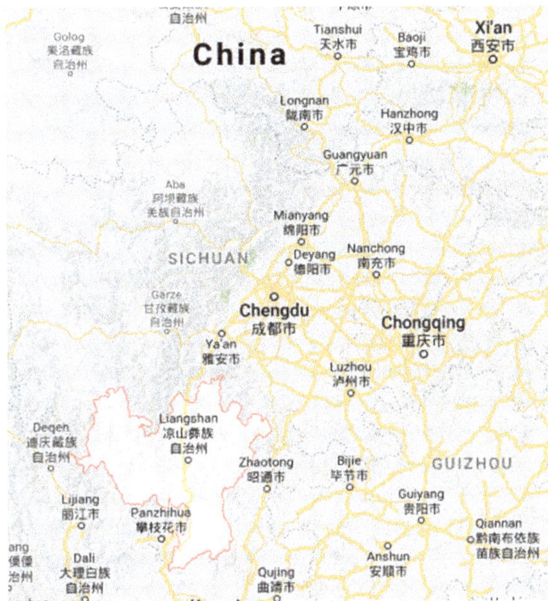

Figure 1. Geographical location of Sichuan Province and Liangshan Yi Autonomous Prefecture.

2. Materials and Methods

2.1. Planning Framework and Data Collection

Nutbeam's model for health promotion was employed for planning the health promotion programme (Figure 2). The model was created with the intention to help systematically link relevant research and theory to the practicalities of programme implementation and evaluation. The model was separated into three parts: (i) problem definition; (ii) solution generation; and (iii) capacity building. Problem definition aims to clarify what and who are the targets of the health-EDRM programme. Solution generation aims to determine how and when change could be achieved in the target population. Capacity building aims to create the best conditions for the health-EDRM programme through the assessment of resources (such as financial and human resources) to ensure the programme objectives are a good fit for the available resources. These 3 planning stages require unique information and are summarized in Table 1.

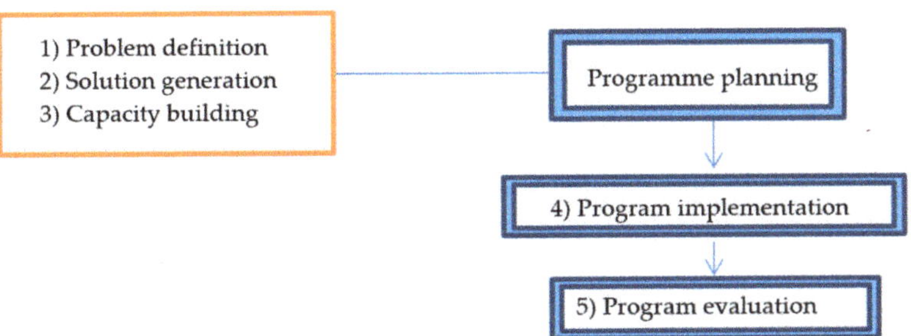

Figure 2. Three planning steps within Nutbeam's model for health promotion.

Table 1. Summary of information needed and sources for each planning stage.

Planning Stage	Information Needed	Source	Section
Problem definition	Local epidemiological and demographic data to determine the size and nature of the problem	Literature review	1.3
	Community needs and perceived priorities	Household survey Focus group	3.1
	Determinants of lack of disaster preparedness	Literature review Household survey	3.2
Solution generation	Theories and intervention models	Literature review	3.3
	Evidence from past programmes and practitioners	Discussion with stakeholders	3.3
Capacity building	Mobilizing resources, training and infrastructure development, raising public and political awareness	Discussion with stakeholders	3.4

2.2. Information for Health Planning

2.2.1. Literature Review

The literature review identified epidemiological data and relevant past studies. This aided description of the local situation and people, their behaviour, and any predictors for lack of disaster preparedness. In addition, this provided evidence for choosing the most appropriate theory and intervention model to improve Health-EDRM. MEDLINE, Embase and Google were searched for academic and grey literature, and titles were screened for relevance. To review the literature on local epidemiological and demographic data, the keywords "China" and "disaster" were used. Articles and websites were limited to those published between 2011 and 2016. To review the literature on the determinants of disaster preparedness, the keywords "severity", "diarrhoea", "treatment" and "household disaster preparedness" were used. To review the literature for the solution generation stage, the keywords "theory", "disaster preparedness" and "disaster risk communication" were used. Articles were limited to systematic reviews.

2.2.2. Household Survey

With limited information published about health status of people in the Liang Shan area, CCOUC conducted a field-based health needs assessment in Hongyan village of Xide county, Liangshan, Sichuan in December 2012. Cross-sectional household surveys were carried out to assess health status, health service availability and utilization of healthcare. A follow-up trip was conducted in March 2014. Cross-sectional household surveys were administered, covering demographics, health and access to health care, as well as knowledge, attitudes and practices of Health-EDRM. The surveys were administered face-to-face. For the 2012 survey, households were recruited using snowball sampling, and the last birthday method was used to recruit a participant within the household. The resulting sample size was 54. 52% were male and 48% female. The mean age of respondents was 43.6 years, with a maximum of 77 years and a minimum of 18 years. All were people of Yi ethnicity except one, who identified as a person of Miao ethnicity. 98% were local farmers and 2% worked as labour workers. 67.9% were illiterate, 11.3% received no formal education while 13.2% and 7.6% received primary and secondary education respectively. For the 2014 survey, all participants of the health-EDRM programme were recruited. The resulting sample size was 100. The respondent profile is reported in another paper [15].

2.2.3. Focus Group

One female and one male focus group (each consisting of 6–8 villagers) were studied. Participants were recruited using snowball sampling. Participants were asked what they would do if they felt sick, any barriers they encountered towards seeking healthcare, how they prepared for disasters, and what their response was during the previous flood. Focus groups were semi-structured. Ethics approval was obtained from the Joint Chinese University of Hong Kong—New Territories East Cluster Clinical Research Ethics Committee (ref no. 2016.334).

2.2.4. Discussion with Stakeholders

The sectors and stakeholders involved, and their roles and expertise, are summarized in Table 2.

Table 2. Stakeholders and their roles.

Sector	Stakeholders	Roles	Expertise
Public health, medicine	Collaborating Centre for Oxford and CUHK for Disaster and Medical Humanitarian Response (CCOUC)	-Recruit volunteers -Co-ordinate stakeholders -Carry out the health needs assessment -Plan, implement and evaluate the program	-Multi-disciplinary (members include doctors and public health professionals) -Health needs assessment -Planning, implementing and evaluating program
Architecture/housing	Wu Zhi Qiao (WZQ) Foundation, Department of Architecture, Chinese University of Hong Kong (CUHK)	-Assessing the need for a sustainable development project (e.g., building bridges, schools and housing)	-Access to the community, local knowledge (WZQ previously conducted exploration mission on 20–22 October 2012.
Local stakeholders	Local village representatives [1]	-Liaise with other stakeholders on behalf of local villagers -Facilitate programme planning, implementation and evaluation	-Access to the community, local knowledge
Programme volunteers	Students from CUHK	-Human resources	-Manpower

[1] A semi-structured interview was conducted with the village head regarding disaster preparedness. His opinion was also sought regarding the feasibility of proposed interventions.

A participatory research approach was used. The only external stakeholders were from the Architecture/housing sector: WZQ and the Department of Architecture, CUHK. The study team was composed of CCOUC staff and students from CUHK. Data analysis was also conducted by the study team.

2.3. Data Analysis

Articles and websites were screened for relevance to the information needed for the literature review. Data synthesis was by exploration of the application of the data to the planned health-EDRM programme in a narrative summary. Survey data were double entered and cleaned by trained staff. Descriptive statistics were generated using SPSS version 21.0. Focus group discussions were taped and transcribed into verbatim. A member of the health needs assessment team and the first author (G.T.) reviewed the transcript and carried out thematic analysis independently. G.T. compared the two sets of thematic analyses. Since the analysis carried out by the team member was for the purpose of writing a trip report, while the author's purpose was to summarize research according to the research framework, the author selected the final themes that were relevant to this study.

Data from the different sources were integrated according to common themes for each category of information needed into narrative summaries.

3. Results

3.1. Problem Definition: Community Needs and Perceived Priorities

Table 3 presents the community needs and perceived priorities in Hongyan village. The results suggest that gastrointestinal problems are common, especially during flood. Poverty and lack of infrastructure result in inadequate health care access, disaster prevention and response systems. Villagers lack empowerment to protect their family's health and safety during a disaster.

Table 3. The community needs and perceived priorities in Hongyan village.

Theme	Results	Source of Information #
Health needs	General health: -53.7% had good health status, but 43.5% complained of deteriorating health compared to 5 years ago. Diseases requiring long-term medication: -Gastrointestinal symptoms were most frequently reported (16.7%), followed by arthritis (6.2%) and respiratory complaints (2%) -38.9% reported experiencing diarrhoea in the last 3 months	-Survey
Healthcare access	-No village doctor was available in Hongyan village. No local emergency service is available: The closest ambulance station is in Xide county, with a response time of 1 h. -For health visits, 51.8% went to the township clinic, 20.4% went to the hospital, while 3.7% preferred to buy over-the-counter medicine -Many villagers only seek medical consultation when they cannot withstand discomfort, due to the cost of medical care. -50% had avoided medical care in the past 3 months as they were unable to afford it.	-Focus group -Survey -Focus group -Survey
Health needs during a disaster	-Only 38.9% of villagers thought they had the ability to protect their family's health and safety during a disaster -In the 2012 flood, 31.5% reported falling sick. Of those, the most common complaint was gastrointestinal symptoms (37.5%).	-Survey
Disaster preparation and response	-To prepare for disasters, regular exercises were held to demonstrate the route of evacuation. No other disaster preparation was done, due to lack of knowledge and financial support. -68.5% of respondents had no preparation before flooding. -The only warning system used mobile phones, which did not work during disasters, due to serious damage to communication infrastructure. During the 2012 flood, most villagers moved higher up the mountain to avoid landslides and house collapse. They stayed in temporary shelters for an average of 62 days.	-Focus group -Survey -Focus group

Household survey and focus groups conducted in 2012.

3.2. Problem Definition: Determinants of Lack of Disaster Preparedness

Literature review and survey of villagers provided information on patterns of gaps in lack of disaster preparedness in Hongyan village, which were used to design a tailored Health-EDRM programme. The following themes were identified:

3.2.1. Theme 1: Knowledge of Consequences and Treatment of Diarrhoea

Yoder et al. reported that in the home setting in developing countries, if diarrhoea was perceived as serious, treatment was more likely to be given [16]. In our survey, although most knew severe diarrhoea resulted in dehydration, fewer respondents realized the potential extent of severity. Only 17.6% of respondents had heard of Oral Rehydration Solution (ORS). This suggests Hongyan villagers lack knowledge regarding the potential severity of diarrhoea and its treatment. The further lack of knowledge of how to make ORS suggests that administering ORS is rarely put into practice in Hongyan village.

3.2.2. Theme 2: Knowledge, Attitude and Practice towards Use of Disaster Kit

CDC reported that household disaster preparedness (such as owning a disaster kit) was associated with disaster preparedness knowledge and attitudes [17]. In our survey, although 53.7% thought it necessary to prepare a disaster kit and 42.6% would consider preparing a disaster kit, only 24% already had a disaster kit and 16.7% knew how to prepare a disaster kit. This suggests that villagers were willing to prepare a disaster kit, but were hindered by lack of knowledge. Even if they possessed a disaster kit, the contents may be inadequate.

3.3. Solution Generation

3.3.1. Choice of Health Promotion Model and Intervention Strategy

A systematic review of the application of behavioural theories to health-EDRM reported that the Health Belief Model (HBM) was one of the most commonly applied models [18]. Under this model, five beliefs are required for an individual to exhibit behaviour change:

1. That they are susceptible to the problem.
2. That the problem could result in potentially severe consequences.
3. That course of action can reduce risks.
4. That benefits of action outweigh barriers
5. Self-efficacy [19].

Studies have shown that perception of susceptibility, severity, benefits and barriers influence predicted preparedness for disease outbreaks [20–22] and disaster (e.g., possessing a disaster kit) [23]. In planning this health promotion programme, the content followed the Health Belief Model constructs.

A systematic review of intervention studies of disaster risk communication reported that interventions with community involvement improved disaster preparedness [24]. This included community participation approach (training villagers in disaster preparedness) [25] and small group discussions with health promoters [26]. In addition, interventions using games led to increased knowledge of disasters [27–29]. In this programme, we planned to include villagers in an interactive intervention using a combination of posters, hands-on demonstration and games.

3.3.2. Experience from Past Programmes and Practitioners Applied to the Intervention

Since February 2009, CCOUC has been conducting health needs assessments and health interventions in disaster-prone rural poor villages in China. Based on past experience, it was decided a half-day interactive workshops would be useful to be conducted in the village.

The workshop was conducted by eight students: Four conducted the ORS intervention and four conducted the disaster kit intervention. Teams were comprised of medical and public health students, enabling sharing different skills and knowledge. 100 villagers participated. The village chief was consulted regarding the best time and location, as we wanted to include as many villagers as possible, for the greatest impact. The location's capacity was fully utilized, as it could accommodate 100 people. Since villagers spoke the local language, translators were recruited to facilitate communication.

The purpose of this workshop was to impart knowledge of the importance of ORS and disaster kits, as well as providing a hands-on demonstration to provide the necessary tools for self-empowerment: In the event of a disaster with poor access to external aid, villagers would still be able to take preliminary measures to improve their situation.

The ORS intervention consisted of using a poster to illustrate the consequences of gastroenteritis and components of ORS. Villagers were invited to demonstrate ORS preparation methods. In the end, standard teaspoons and 150 mL cups were given as souvenirs to solve the problem of differing spoons and cups in households. The disaster intervention used a poster to illustrate the importance and contents of a disaster kit. Visitors played a game of identifying disaster kit contents. In the end, disaster kits were given out, and Polaroid photos were taken of family members, to aid identification during disasters.

3.4. Capacity Building

3.4.1. Mobilizing Human, Material and Financial Resources

Our team consisted of CCOUC staff (doctors, nurses and public health practitioners) and students (with medical and public health background). CCOUC previously conducted health needs assessment and interventions in Sichuan, Gansu and Guangxi villages. CCOUC staffs were, therefore, experienced health educators. They also organized the logistics of the trip (accommodation, meals and transport). The students had mixed experience backgrounds; some had attended previous trips while others had not. Meetings involving all team members were held before the trip to evaluate poster designs and intervention plans. In this way, more experienced team members trained those who were new. Students designed and printed posters and flyers. CCOUC staff prepared ORS souvenirs (teaspoons and plastic cups), disaster kit (lighter, penknife, medication box, thermal blanket, whistle, torch and bag), and Polaroid cameras.

The intervention was held in an open space outside the village chief's house, as this was the biggest space available and convenient for villagers. Table 4 shows a typical example of financial resources required for the health-EDRM programme. The estimated budget in 2014 had a slight cost inflation compared to 2012, in order to take into account possible cost inflation over the years

Table 4. Example of typical items and equipment to conduct field based activities in China (as of 2012).

Category	Item	Cost (USD) in 2012	Estimated Budget (USD) for 2014
Manpower for background survey and focus group (2012 trip)	Air-tickets and road transportation costs for 10 team members	7987	
	Accommodation for 10 team members and drivers	459	
	Meal expenses for 10 team members	764	
	Incentives for 54 interview participants	103	
	Honorarium for local staff	267	
Manpower for background survey and intervention (2014 trip)	Air-tickets and road transportation costs for 24 team members		19,200
	Accommodation for 24 team members and drivers		1100
	Meal expenses for 24 team members		2000
	Incentives for 100 interview participants		200
	Honorarium for local staff		300
Intervention materials	Printing 5 posters and 100 flyers		130
	ORS souvenirs: 100 plastic teaspoons and cups		25
	100 disaster kits		380
	Polaroid films		100

Expenses were solicited from various sources, including CUHK's ICARE programme and CCOUC development fund. Although the cost of intervention per participant was relatively high due to travel expenses, the project also served other purposes: training and education of students, academic exchange, research and raising public awareness.

3.4.2. Training People and Building Sustainable Programmes

Our programme provides villagers with education and equipment for disaster preparedness. Since most villagers live in poor rural areas, giving them disaster kits, ORS recipes and utensils reduces problems related to affordability and access. The equipment can be re-used, and they can demonstrate their acquired knowledge to family and friends back home. In this way, the programme trains villagers to pass on their knowledge and use their new skills in times of need.

As well as training villagers, the programme trains students and staff. CCOUC has ongoing health promotion programmes in a wide range of disaster-prone rural villages in China. This trip was part of CCOUC's Ethnic Health Minority Project, ongoing since 2009. Due to the mix of team member experience in CCOUC trips, students and staff learn from each other. Experienced team members will take up additional responsibility in future trips. This includes leading teams and dealing with logistics.

Lessons learnt from each trip inform the next trip. Graduate students could obtain academic credit for participating or as part of a global health elective "field action lab". Some used the collected data to write their master's thesis. Medical students were also recruited from CUHK's Global-Physician Leadership Stream and Medical Outreachers, which aims to train holistic future physicians. Thus, this trip is a building block in multiple programmes.

3.4.3. Raising Public and Political Awareness

After the flood in August 2012, WZQ and CCOUC contacted the chief of Hongyan village and visited the village on an exploration mission. The village chief agreed there was a need for health needs assessment and programme development. CCOUC staff discussed future trip logistics with him and confirmed his support, serving as the access point to Hongyan village. Public awareness of the intervention was crucial for sufficient participation. The chief helped spread the details to the villagers. Households previously approached for surveys were also informed. When the intervention was about to start, the loudspeaker microphone reminded villagers to attend.

4. Discussion

Lack of disaster preparedness is a problem found in many disaster-prone areas globally. Therefore, international information about disaster kits and treatment of gastroenteritis is available. However, although rural ethnic minority groups comprise a significant proportion of those living in disaster-prone areas in China, there is a lack of research focusing on these communities [30]. Literature review alerted us of the need to avoid generalizing other research findings, as there is a difference between ethnic and non-ethnic minorities: The higher illiteracy rate, different language and occupations among the Yi minority [31] meant that different strategies were needed to overcome communication barriers. Our study revealed that a worrying proportion described deteriorating general health over the years. Villagers had a poor health baseline, even in normal times outside the disaster period. Since the average age was only 42.2 and the predominant occupation was agriculture, this deterioration might affect not only their quality of life but also livelihood. Further data shed light on possible reasons for the predominantly gastrointestinal problems in the village: A similarly high proportion of respondents to those reporting diarrhoea in the last three months did not have a regular handwashing habit, despite having stable access to water sources [31]. In addition, more than half of the respondents drank water without treatment [15]. The lack of healthcare access is typical of low-income rural villages in remote areas [32,33]. Together with our findings in the determinants of lack of disaster preparedness section indicating a lack of knowledge regarding the consequences and treatment of diarrhoea, we conclude that there is a great health need in this aspect; empowering villagers through education on the severity of diarrhoea and how to make ORS could vastly improve lives by preventing dehydration, despite the lack of healthcare access.

The low number of fatalities were likely due to the slow-onset nature of the disaster, which allowed time for evacuation. Most villagers had no preparation before the flooding and less than half felt empowered. Nevertheless, it is encouraging that the community was close-knit enough to communicate and look out for each other as a village. This could have implications for health-EDRM, as knowledge gained by the 100 villagers from the intervention could potentially be passed onto other villagers through informal conversation and advice. Most villagers were forced to move after the flood, and thus any health-EDRM items must be essentials that are easy to prepare and carry. Despite a willingness to prepare disaster kits, there was a lack of knowledge regarding preparation, thereby leading to lack of possession of disaster kits. Research shows that disaster kits may be the most cost-effective means of reducing mortality in these settings [34]. Incorporation of ORS and disaster kit preparation in a health-EDRM programme would therefore address health needs for this community.

Apart from the Health Belief Model, another model that has been used in health-EDRM programmes is the Precaution Adoption Process Model (PAPM). One study explored the correlation between the HBM and the PAPM and found that perceived benefits and perceived barriers in the HBM predicted adoption stage in PAPM [35]. Given the emphasis on perceived barriers, future health-EDRM programmes could explore whether there are significant barriers apart from knowledge and poverty. The importance of community involvement was echoed by the World Health Organization, which listed it as a strategy for achieving the Sendai Framework priorities [36].

Although the project managed to gather information specific to local villagers, there are a few limitations. Our surveys had high response rates (ranging from 93–100%), but the quality of responses was hampered by language barriers. Translators were needed for surveys as most villagers could not speak Putonghua. In addition, convenience sampling was used, as households were far apart. Without random sampling, selection bias is likely. Our focus groups gathered more in-depth information regarding villagers' opinions. However, focus groups are limited by small sample size, and villagers might concur with each other as a result of peer pressure. Our semi-structured interview with the village chief informed us of the village disaster plan and response system. However, this only represented one person's opinion, and it was difficult to ascertain whether participant recall bias, such as inaccurate recall of events, existed.

Although community involvement was crucial, gaining access was not easy. Securing political support from the village chief was crucial, with trust built up slowly through a previous trip and ongoing communication. The village chief was helpful in providing an overview of the village situation, local input, and village access. Planning the health promotion programme required much logistical support, using limited time and resources. Due to these pressures, team members found themselves under stress in a new environment. Pairing team members with different levels of experience and capabilities eased the adjustment of new team members. In addition, incorporating evaluation during the planning stage ensured that the programme could be thoroughly and efficiently evaluated by comparing changes before and after the program.

Health promotion during the post-disaster period was a good opportunity as villagers would be more aware of the impact of a disaster and eager to learn about disaster preparedness. However, communication was important to manage expectations. As disaster was fresh in their minds, they desired infrastructure reconstruction, which could not be delivered through this program. Nevertheless, the health promotion programme on Disaster Preparedness for Yi-minority community in Sichuan Province in China was successfully delivered in March 2014.

5. Conclusions

Based on this experience of using Nutbeam's planning model to develop a tailored health-EDRM programme, future programmes could be planned and expanded to different disaster-prone areas. To be successful, it is essential that health-EDRM programmes address local health needs and priorities. Using a planning model ensures a systematic approach to planning and is useful for defining the scope of an intervention, particularly where scant pre-existing information is available regarding the local situation. The planning model can serve as a framework for organizing and combining multiple sources of information, thereby translating evidence-based planning into a health promotion programme applicable to the local context.

Author Contributions: Conceptualization, G.T. and E.Y.Y.C.; Data curation, G.T.; Formal analysis, G.T.; Funding acquisition, E.Y.Y.C.; Investigation, G.T., E.Y.Y.C. and S.L.; Methodology, G.T.; Project administration, E.Y.Y.C.; Resources, E.Y.Y.C. and S.L.; Supervision, E.Y.Y.C.; Writing—original draft, G.T.; Writing—review & editing, G.T.

Acknowledgments: This work was supported by the CCOUC field research fund, the Chow Tai Fook Charitable Foundation, the I-CARE Programme (The Chinese University of Hong Kong), and the Wu Zhi Qiao Charitable Foundation.

Conflicts of Interest: The authors declare no conflict of interest. The founding sponsors had no role in the design of the study; in the collection, analyses, or interpretation of data; in the writing of the manuscript, and in the decision to publish the results.

References

1. Institute of Development Studies. Rural Disaster Risk-Poverty Interface. 2008. Available online: http://www.ids.ac.uk/publication/rural-disaster-risk-poverty-interface (accessed on 1 March 2016).
2. Prevention Web. Poverty and Inequality. Available online: http://www.preventionweb.net/risk/poverty-inequality (accessed on 1 March 2016).
3. Chan, E.Y.Y.; Kim, J.H.; Lin, C.; Cheung, E.Y.L.; Lee, P.P.Y. Is Previous Disaster Experience a Good Predictor for Disaster Preparedness in Extreme Poverty Households in Remote Muslim Minority Based Community in China? *J. Immigr. Minority Health* **2014**, *16*, 466–472. [CrossRef] [PubMed]
4. Woersching, J.; Snyder, A. Earthquakes in El Salvador: A descriptive study of health concerns in a rural community and the clinical implications, part I. *Disaster Manag. Response* **2003**, *1*, 105–109. [CrossRef]
5. Woersching, J.; Snyder, A. Earthquakes in El Salvador: A descriptive study of health concerns in a rural community and the clinical implications, part II. *Disaster Manag. Response* **2004**, *2*, 10–13. [CrossRef] [PubMed]
6. United Nations Office for Disaster Risk Reduction. Sendai Framework for Disaster Risk Reduction. Available online: https://www.unisdr.org/we/coordinate/sendai-framework (accessed on 1 April 2016).
7. United Nations Office for Disaster Risk Reduction. Hyogo Framework for Action. Available online: https://www.unisdr.org/we/coordinate/hfa (accessed on 1 April 2016).
8. United Nations Office for Disaster Risk Reduction. Terminology. Available online: https://www.unisdr.org/we/inform/terminology (accessed on 1 April 2016).
9. United Nations. Building Disaster Resilient Communities. 2007. Available online: http://www.unisdr.org/files/596_10307.pdf (accessed on 1 April 2016).
10. International Federation of Red Cross and Red Crescent Societies. China and Cambodia: Integrated Programming and Cooperation with Local Authorities Boost Communities' Disaster Preparedness. Available online: http://www.ifrc.org/Global/Case%20studies/Disasters/cs-dm-china-cambodia-en.pdf (accessed on 1 April 2016).
11. Charitable Foundation Cartier. Preparing for Natural Disasters in Western China. Available online: http://www.cartiercharitablefoundation.org/en/commitment/programs/planning-and-preparing-for-natural-disasters-in-western-china (accessed on 1 April 2016).
12. Centre for Research on the Epidemiology of Disasters. Annual Disaster Statistical Review 2013: The Numbers and Trends. Available online: http://reliefweb.int/report/world/annual-disaster-statistical-review-2013-numbers-and-trends (accessed on 1 April 2016).
13. Emily, Y.Y.; Chan, Y.J.; Zhu, P.; Lee, S.D.; Liu, C. Impact of disaster preparedness intervention in Yi-minority community in Sichuan Province, China. In Proceedings of the 12th Asia Pacific Congress on Disaster Medicine, Tokyo, Japan, 17–19 September 2014.
14. Emily, Y.Y.; Chan, Y.J.; Zhu, P.; Lee, S.D.; Liu, C. The Evaluation on Disaster Preparedness Interventions in Post-flooding Yi Minority Community in Sichuan Province, China. In Proceedings of the 19th World Congress on Disaster & Emergency Medicine, Cape Town, South Africa, 21–24 April 2015.
15. Chan, E.Y.Y.; Guo, C.; Lee, P.; Liu, S.; Mark, C.K.M. Health Emergency and Disaster Risk Management (Health-EDRM) in Remote Ethnic Minority Areas of Rural China: The Case of a Flood-Prone Village in Sichuan. *Int. J. Disaster Risk Sci.* **2017**, *8*, 1–8. [CrossRef]
16. Yoder, P.S.; Hornik, R.C. Perceptions of severity of diarrhoea and treatment choice: A comparative study of HealthCom sites. *J. Trop. Med. Hyg.* **1994**, *97*, 1–12. [PubMed]
17. Thomas, T.N.; Leander-Griffith, M.; Harp, V.; Cioffi, J.P. Influences of Preparedness. Knowledge and Beliefs on Household Disaster Preparedness. *Morb. Mortal. Wkly. Rep.* **2015**, *64*, 965–971. [CrossRef] [PubMed]
18. Ejeta, L.T.; Ardalan, A.; Paton, D. Application of Behavioral Theories to Disaster and Emergency Health Preparedness: A Systematic Review. *PLoS Curr. Disasters* **2015**, *1*, 1. [CrossRef] [PubMed]
19. Lewis, G.; Sheringham, J.; Kalim, K.; Crayford, T. *Mastering Public Health: A Postgraduate Guide to Examinations and Revalidation*; Royal Society of Medicine: London, UK, 2008.
20. Teitler-Regev, S.; Shahrabani, S.; Benzion, U. Factors Affecting Intention among Students to Be Vaccinated against A/H1N1 Influenza: A Health Belief Model Approach. *Adv. Prev. Med.* **2011**, *1*, 353207. [CrossRef] [PubMed]

21. Taylor, P.; Yang, Z.J. Predicting Young Adults' Intentions to Get the H1N1 Vaccine: An Integrated Model. *J. Health Commun.* **2014**, *20*, 1–11.
22. Nexøe, J.; Kragstrup, J.; Søgaard, J. Decision on influenza vaccination among the elderly. A questionnaire study based on the Health Belief Model and the Multidimensional Locus of Control Theory. *Scand. J. Prim. Health Care* **1999**, *17*, 105–110. [CrossRef] [PubMed]
23. Semenza, J.C.; Ploubidis, G.B.; George, L.A. Climate change and climate variability: Personal motivation for adaptation and mitigation. *Environ. Health* **2011**, *10*, 46. [CrossRef] [PubMed]
24. Bradley, D.T.; McFarland, M.; Clarke, M. The Effectiveness of Disaster Risk Communication: A Systematic Review of Intervention Studies. *PLoS Curr. Disasters* **2014**, *22*, 1. [CrossRef] [PubMed]
25. Ardalan, A.; Naieni, K.H.; Mahmoodi, M.; Zanganeh, A.M.; Keshtkar, A.A.; Honarvar, M.R.; Kabir, M.J. Flash flood preparedness in Golestan province of Iran: A community intervention trial. *Am. J. Disaster Med.* **2010**, *5*, 197–214. [CrossRef] [PubMed]
26. Eisenman, D.P.; Glik, D.; Gonzalez, L.; Maranon, R.; Zhou, Q.; Tseng, C.H.; Asch, S.M. Improving Latino disaster preparedness using social networks. *Am. J. Prev. Med.* **2009**, *37*, 512–517. [CrossRef] [PubMed]
27. Clerveaux, V.; Spence, B. The Communication of Disaster Information and Knowledge to Children Using Game Technique: The Disaster Awareness Game (DAG). *Int. J. Environ. Res.* **2009**, *3*, 209–222.
28. Tanes, Z. Earthquake Risk Communication with Video Games: Examining the Role of Player-Game Interaction in Influencing the Gaming Experience and Outcomes. Ph.D. Thesis, Purdue University, West Lafayette, IN, USA, 2011.
29. Tanes, Z.; Cho, H. Goal setting outcomes: Examining the role of goal interaction in influencing the experience and learning outcomes of video game play for earthquake preparedness. *Comput. Hum. Behav.* **2013**, *29*, 858–869. [CrossRef]
30. Chan, E.Y.Y. *Building Bottom-Up Health and Disaster Risk Reduction Programmes*; Oxford University Press: Oxford, UK, 2018.
31. CCOUC (Collaborating Centre for Oxford University and CUHK for Disaster and Medical Humanitarian Response). *The Ethnic Minority Health Project: Trip Report for Hongyan, Sichuan*; CCOUC: Hong Kong, China, 2014.
32. Chan, E.Y.Y. Bottom-up disaster resilience. *Nat. Geosci.* **2013**, *6*, 327–328. [CrossRef]
33. Du, F.; Kobayashi, H.; Okazaki, K.; Ochiai, C. Research on the disaster coping capability of a historical village in a mountainous area of China: Case study in Shangli, Sichuan. *Procedia Soc. Behav. Sci.* **2016**, *218*, 118–130. [CrossRef]
34. Kelman, I. *Disaster Mitigation is Cost Effective*; World Bank: Washington, DC, USA, 2013.
35. Jassempour, K.; Shirazi, K.K.; Fararooei, M.; Shams, M.; Shirazi, A.R. The impact of educational intervention for providing disaster survival kit: Applying precaution adoption process model. *Int. J. Disaster Risk Reduct.* **2014**, *10*, 374–380. [CrossRef]
36. WHO (World Health Organization). Health Emergency and Disaster Management Fact Sheets 2017. Available online: https://www.who.int/hac/techguidance/preparedness/risk-management-overview-december2017.pdf (acessed on 1 January 2019).

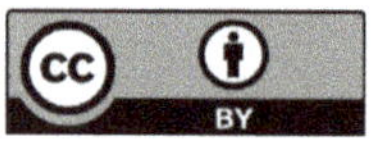

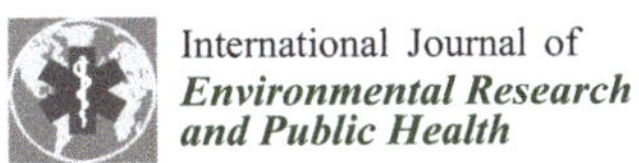
International Journal of
Environmental Research and Public Health

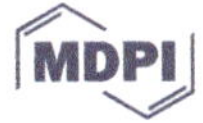

Commentary

WHO Thematic Platform for Health Emergency and Disaster Risk Management Research Network (TPRN): Report of the Kobe Expert Meeting

Ryoma Kayano [1,*], Emily YY Chan [2], Virginia Murray [3], Jonathan Abrahams [4] and Sarah Louise Barber [1]

1 World Health Organization Centre for Health Development, Kobe 651-0073, Japan; barbers@who.int
2 Collaborating Centre for Oxford University and Chinese University of Hong Kong for Disaster and Medical Humanitarian Response (CCOUC), School of Public Health and Primary Care, The Chinese University of Hong Kong, HongKong, China; Emily.chan@cuhk.edu.hk
3 Public Health England, London SE1 8UG, UK; Virginia.Murray@phe.gov.uk
4 Country Health Emergency Preparedness and International Regulations Department, WHO Health Emergencies Programme, World Health Organization, CH-1211 Geneva, Switzerland; abrahamsj@who.int
* Correspondence: kayanor@who.int; Tel.: +81-78-230-3100

Received: 31 January 2019; Accepted: 30 March 2019; Published: 6 April 2019

Abstract: The WHO Thematic Platform for Health Emergency and Disaster Risk Management Research Network (TPRN) was established in 2016 in response to the Sendai Framework for Disaster Risk Reduction 2015–2030. The TPRN facilitates global collaborative action for improving the scientific evidence base in health emergency and disaster risk management (Health EDRM). In 2018, the WHO convened a meeting to identify key research questions, bringing together leading experts from WHO, TPRN, World Association for Disaster and Emergency Medicine (WADEM), and the Japan International Cooperation Agency, and delegates to the Asia Pacific Conference on Disaster Medicine (APCDM). The meeting identified research questions in five major areas for Health EDRM: health data management, psychosocial management, community risk management, health workforce development, and research methods and ethics. Funding these key research questions is essential to accelerate evidence-based actions during emergencies and disasters.

Keywords: health emergency and disaster risk management (Health EDRM); Sendai Framework for Disaster Risk Reduction 2015–2030; WHO Thematic Platform for Health EDRM; health data; psychosocial; risk communication; capacity building; research methods; ethics

---

1. Introduction

Over the past few decades, the frequency of disasters has increased as a result of a number of risk drivers including unplanned urbanization and unmitigated climate change. The impact of many of these disasters on human health has also become more severe, due in part to increasing numbers of vulnerable populations, including older persons. The 2015 Third UN World Conference on Disaster Risk Reduction (WCDRR) established the Sendai Framework on Disaster Risk Reduction 2015–2030 (SFDRR), which introduced a framework for action across the disaster risk management (DRM) continuum (prevention, preparedness, response, and recovery) and sought to enhance the resilience of communities and health and social systems. With more than 30 references to health issues specifically, the framework includes health in its goal as "the substantial reduction of disaster risk and losses in lives, livelihoods and health ... ." [1]. It also emphasizes the importance of improving the scientific evidence base to advance health emergency and disaster risk management (Health EDRM).

In response, World Health Organization (WHO) established the WHO Thematic Platform for Health EDRM Research Network (TPRN) to promote global collaboration among academia [2,3], government officials and other stakeholders to generate better scientific evidence to inform policy and practice for managing health risks associated with emergencies and disaster. In 2017, leaders of this research network published a review paper on the Sendai Framework implementation and recommendations on Health EDRM research [4,5]. The paper highlighted the critical importance of research before, during and after disasters (not only the acute phase) and gave consideration to the following: a holistic approach, including physical, mental and psychosocial health and well-being; identifying populations at risk with specific health needs; standardization of needs assessments, standardization of evaluation methodologies and reporting systems for countries, communities and individual cases; multidisciplinary and multi-sectoral approaches; and a review of research for informing better policy development and implementation.

To accelerate research in Health EDRM, the WHO organized a meeting to identify key research gaps and questions by convening the leading experts from WHO, World Association for Disaster and Emergency Medicine (WADEM), and Japan International Cooperation Agency (JICA), and delegates to the Asia Pacific Conference on Disaster Medicine (APCDM). The WHO Kobe Center (WKC) organized the meeting as one of the programs during APCDM 2018 on 17 October 2018, in Kobe, Japan [6].

2. Materials and Methods

The purpose of the meeting was to identify concrete research questions based on the established overarching priorities in line with the published reviews of research needs conducted by the coordinators of the WHO Thematic Platform for Health EDRM Research Network (TPRN) [4,5]. The selection of the research themes, meeting participants and research questions were conducted as below.

As a first step, an open-ended consultation was conducted with the ten TPRN coordinators. Background information from the above-mentioned references [4,5] was shared for the consultation. Through this process, the first draft of the expert meeting agenda with potential discussion themes and background information was developed. Based on the potential discussion themes, 25 participants from 10 countries for the expert meeting were selected based on their global expertise in responding to health emergencies and natural disasters in consultation with the TPRN coordinators and APCDM organizers. They included the WHO Health-EDRM responsible officers in headquarters and regional offices in the Asia Pacific Region (Western Pacific Region and Southeast Asia Region), the TPRN co-chairs and representatives from international, regional or national organizations and societies involved in Health-EDRM (Public Health England, the Chinese University of Hong Kong, WADEM, Association of South-East Asian Nations (ASEAN) Secretariat, JICA, Government of Thailand, Japan Disaster Medical Assistance Team Secretariat; and leading researchers selected based on their previous academic works and Health-EDRM related activities.

As a second step, another consultation to finalize the major research themes was conducted with all of the potential 25 participants to obtain their feedback, and five major discussion themes were selected (Table 1). Based on the final confirmed meeting themes, participants were then selected to cover all the five research themes through consultation with stakeholders. Through this process, 32 experts from 12 countries (Australia, Canada, Hong Kong, India, Indonesia, Japan, Myanmar, New Zealand, Philippines, Thailand, UK, USA) were selected for the expert meeting. The meeting agenda with the five major discussion themes and their background information was shared with all the participants.

As a third step, the expert meeting was conducted as a session of APCDM. Two rounds of group discussions were conducted. The discussion on each theme was facilitated by a lead discussant selected based on their expertise and previous research under each area in Health-EDRM (Table 1). After the group discussions, a plenary discussion was conducted to integrate the results of the group discussions and reach consensus among the participants.

3. Key Research Gaps and Questions in Five Key Research Areas

The process resulted in a series of questions listed in Table 1.

Table 1. Key research questions in five major areas.

Area	Research Questions
Area 1 Health data management before, during and after emergencies and disasters Lead discussant: Tatsuhiko Kubo, University of Occupational and Environmental Health, Japan	(a) What are the national and regional challenges inhibiting implementation of the WHO standardized medical data collection systems after emergencies and disasters? (b) What is the broader health-related data needed to inform effective Health emergency and disaster risk management (EDRM), i.e., community vulnerabilities, hospital functional status, infrastructure, lifelines and health workforce?
Area 2 Psychosocial management before, during and after emergencies and disasters, and other medium and long-term effects on the public health and health system Lead discussant: Yoshiharu Kim, National Center for Neurology and Psychiatry, Japan	(a) How can mental health and psychosocial risk be classified using longitudinal and multi-centric studies? (b) How can methods for screening, diagnosis and treatment for affected people be standardized across different settings? (c) How can assets associated with greater community resilience be identified before, during, and after disaster?
Area 3 Community emergency and disaster risk management, including risk literacy and addressing needs of sub-populations Lead discussant: Emily Y.Y. Chan, The Chinese University of Hong Kong	(a) What architecture is needed to support research in Health EDRM including consensus among disciplines and ethics? (b) How can research be better translated to policy and practice across different backgrounds and contexts? (c) What kind of technology for information and data management and communication is needed for risk communication, emergency response and research design?
Area 4 Health workforce development for health emergency and disaster risk management Lead discussant: Jonathan Abrahams, World Health Organization	(a) How can different countries strengthen Health EDRM through disaster risk management training programs, and what strategies will support retention, motivation and deployment of trained people? (b) What are the best practices for sustaining the development of the local health workforce for Health EDRM, fostering positive interactions between external support workers and the local workforce, and enabling the transition to recovery and post-event Health EDRM? (c) What is the common knowledge or competencies required for Health EDRM?
Area 5 Research methods and ethics Lead discussant: Virginia Murray, Public Health England	(a) What are the definitions of research methods and technical terms for Health EDRM? (b) How can impact evaluation methods for intervention and qualitative–quantitative mixed methods be standardized? (c) How can the publication process for Health EDRM research become more systematic and effective? (d) What are the challenges and best practices in addressing national health system, cultural and religious issues before, during and after interventions?

The first research area was health data management before, during and after emergencies and disasters. Experts highlighted the significant progress made through the development of the WHO Emergency Medical Team (EMT) Minimum Data Set (MDS) in 2017 [7], enabling standardized data collection and reporting by EMTs dispatched to emergency areas. However, it was noted that implementation was not optimal. Further research is needed on reducing the implementation barriers in national and regional contexts, and the supplementary data required for broader public health action.

The second area was psychosocial management. Experts identified research priorities in the classification of mental health and psychosocial risk, standardization of methods for screening, diagnosis and treatment, and the identification of characteristics of risk and resilience among affected individuals and communities.

The third research area was community risk management and risk literacy. Experts identified the need to strengthen the components of research architecture to support research for Health EDRM, the means to translate research to policy and practice, and research to advance the technology of information and data management and communication for risk communication for Health EDRM, with the focus on an effective and localized risk communication approach to meet the requirements of the local community.

The fourth area was health workforce development. Experts identified knowledge gaps in a common understanding of relevant knowledge and competencies required for the Health EDRM workforce as well as the contents for in-house training/professional development and their interaction with stakeholders, and in understanding how to sustain the development of the local health workforce for Health EDRM, foster positive interactions between external support workers and the local workforce and the effective transition to recovery, integrating measures to reduce risks of future events and build stronger systems. More understanding is needed about how countries can strengthen Health EDRM through disaster risk management training programs, and how they are able to retain, motivate and utilize trained personnel, including for deployment.

The fifth area was research methods and ethics. To move beyond case studies, key research priorities including the basic definitions of research methods and technical terms in the field of Health EDRM setting, standardizing impact evaluation methodologies, and promoting publication of result in a systematic way. Lastly, the group identified the need for best practices in addressing national health systems, and cultural and religious issues. A research methods resource and book were thought to be important additions to the TPRN tools.

4. Follow-Up Actions

The expert meeting focused on identifying the key research needs in five major areas through formulating research questions. Specific approaches in responding to each research question should be discussed and implemented with additional studies and literature reviews conducted in a systematic way. These include: (a) conducting more implementation research using currently available health data collection tools (Area 1); (b) standardization of monitoring of long-term psychological consequences, and validation of individual-level and community-level interventions for better psychological consequences (Area 2); (c) identifying the existing challenges for better translation of research findings to policy and programs (Area 3); (d) conducting an inventory of the existing workforce development programs and identifying essential components of training programs (Area 4); and (e) integrating existing knowledge about research methods for Health-EDRM by developing guidance by global experts (Area 5). These follow-up actions are addressed in greater detail in the later theme-based articles.

Given this background, the meeting concluded with the commitment to organize an annual TPRN meeting and utilize other forums in collaboration with partner organizations to promote and update knowledge and experience in Health EDRM research. The meetings will update progress in the key research areas, and further expert consultations will be held to identify further research gaps and possible sources of funding. In 2019, the WKC will function as the secretariat of TPRN in collaboration with WHO HQ. The WHO will establish an information sharing platform to facilitate interactions among TPRN participants about Health EDRM research and science, as well as opportunities for funding, conferences and collaborative research.

5. Conclusions

The expert meeting contributed to setting forth some key research gaps to be addressed for the advancement of Health EDRM research. Successful implementation will require further research collaborations through the TPRN initiative, partnerships and resource mobilization.

The expert meeting did not reach consensus through blind rating, voting or a structured questionnaire-based approach, which are recommended by Delphi Method. This limitation will be addressed during the next follow-up expert meeting.

Author Contributions: Conceptualization, R.K. and E.Y.Y.C.; Writing-Original Draft Preparation, R.K.; Writing-Review & Editing, E.Y.Y.C., V.M., S.L.B. and J.A.; Project Administration, R.K., J.A.

Funding: This research received no external funding.

Acknowledgments: The opinions contained in the paper are those of its authors and, except where specifically stated, are not intended to represent the official policies or positions of the WHO. The expert meeting was organized under the collaboration among WHO, APCDM 2018, and JICA. The authors express their gratitude to the following individuals who contributed substantially to meeting organization: Shinichi Nakayama (APCDM) and Masako Tani (Project for Strengthening the ASEAN Regional Capacity on Disaster Health Management (ARCH Project), JICA). The authors thank all the meeting participants who contributed to achieving the results (in alphabetical order of their last name): Myo Nyein Aung (Chiang Mai Rajabhat University, Thailand), Nilesh Buddh (WHO Regional Office for South East Asia), Cheuk Pong Chiu (The Chinese University of Hong Kong, China), Shinichi Egawa (Tohoku University, Japan), Paul Farrell (WADEM), Ferdinal Moreno Fernando (ASEAN Secretariat), Sayaka Gomei (Dokkyo Medical University, Japan), Mélissa Généreux (University of Sherbrooke, Canada), Teodoro Herbosa (University of the Philippines, Philippines), Shuichi Ikeda (ARCH Project, JICA), Tatruro Kai (Saiseikai Senri Hospital, Japan), Hiroshi Kato (Hyogo Institute for Traumatic Stress), Yoshiharu Kim (National Center for Neurology and Psychiatry, Japan), Yuichi Koido (Japan Disaster Medical Assistance Team (DMAT) Secretariat, Ministry of Health, Labor and Welfare, Japan), Tomoko Komagata (Tokyo Medical and Dental University, Japan), Tatsuhiko Kubo (University of Occupational and Environmental Health, Japan), Sonoe Mashino (University of Hyogo, Japan), Yasushi Nakajima (ARCH Project, JICA), Toshiyuki Ojima (Hamamatsu University School of Medicine, Japan), Yasuhiro Otomo (Tokyo Medical and Dental University, Japan), Heather Papowitz (WHO Regional Office for the Western Pacific), Philip Schluter (University of Canterbury, New Zealand), Phumin Silapunt (Chulabhorn Hospital, Thailand), Yosuke Takada (Okayama University, Japan), Sho Takahashi (University of Tsukuba, Japan), Nobuyo Tsuboyama-Kasaoka (National Institute of Health and Nutrition, Japan), Shiori Usami (Kumamoto University, Japan).

Conflicts of Interest: The authors declare no conflicts of interest.

References

1. Sendai Framework for Disaster Risk Reduction 2015–2030. Available online: https://www.unisdr.org/we/inform/publications/43291 (accessed on 02 April 2019).
2. WHO Thematic Platform for Health Emergency and Disaster Risk Management. Available online: http://www.who.int/hac/techguidance/preparedness/WHO-Thematic-Platform-Health-EDRM-Terms-Reference-2018.pdf?ua=1 (accessed on 02 April 2019).
3. WHO Thematic Platform for Health Emergency and Disaster Risk Management Research Network. Available online: http://www.who.int/hac/techguidance/preparedness/WHO-Thematic-Platform-Health-EDRM-Research-Network-2018.pdf?ua=1 (accessed on 02 April 2019).
4. Chan, E.Y.Y.; Murray, V. What are the health research needs for the Sendai Framework. *Lancet* **2017**, *390*, e35–e36. [CrossRef]
5. Lo, S.T.T.; Chan, E.Y.Y.; Chan, G.K.W.; Murray, V.; Abrahams, J.; Ardalan, A.; Kayano, R.; Yau, J.C.W. Health Emergency and Disaster Risk Management (Health-EDRM): Developing the Research Field within the Sendai Framework Paradigm. *Int. J. Disaster Risk Sci.* **2017**, *8*, 145–149. [CrossRef]

6. Asian Pacific Conference for Disaster Medicine. 2018. Available online: http://www.apcdm2018.org/index.html (accessed on 02 April 2019).
7. Benin-Goren, O.; Kubo, T.; Norton, I. Emergency Medical Team Working Group for Minimum Data Set. *Prehosp. Disaster Med.* **2017**, *32* (Suppl. S1), S96. [CrossRef]

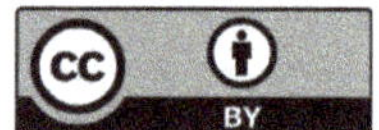

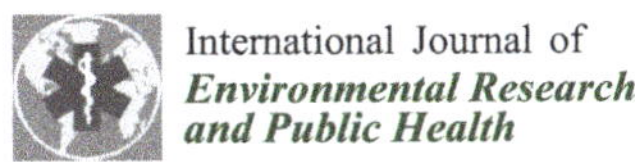
International Journal of
Environmental Research and Public Health

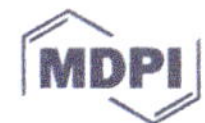

Communication

Is "Perceived Water Insecurity" Associated with Disaster Risk Perception, Preparedness Attitudes, and Coping Ability in Rural China? (A Health-EDRM Pilot Study)

Janice Ying-en Ho [1], Emily Ying Yang Chan [1,2,*], Holly Ching Yu Lam [2], May Pui Shan Yeung [1], Carol Ka Po Wong [2] and Tony Ka Chun Yung [2]

1 Division of Global Health and Humanitarian Medicine, Jockey Club School of Public Health and Primary Care, The Chinese University of Hong Kong, Hong Kong; janice.ho@link.cuhk.edu.hk (J.Y.H.); may.yeung@cuhk.edu.hk (M.P.S.Y.)

2 Collaborating Centre for Oxford University and CUHK for Disaster and Medical Humanitarian Response, The Chinese University of Hong Kong, Hong Kong; hollylam@cuhk.edu.hk (H.C.Y.L.); wongcarol@cuhk.edu.hk (C.K.P.W.); yungtony@cuhk.edu.hk (T.K.C.Y.)

* Correspondence: emily.chan@cuhk.edu.hk; Tel.: +852-2252-8411

Received: 27 February 2019; Accepted: 7 April 2019; Published: 8 April 2019

Abstract: Water security is essential for maintaining health and well-being, and for reducing a population's vulnerability in a disaster. Among resource-poor villagers in China, water-related disasters and climate change may increasingly affect people's water security. The purpose of this study was to explore the relationship between perceived water security and disaster risk perception in a rural ethnic minority community. A cross-sectional household survey was conducted in 2015 in Xingguang village, Chongqing, China, examining the association between villagers' perceptions of household water security, disaster risk, and sociodemographic variables. Among 52 household representatives, 84.6% relied on rainwater as their main water source and 63.5% reported having insufficient water on a regular basis. Only 32.7% perceived themselves to be living in a high-risk area, of which climate-related disasters such as storms (44.4%) and droughts (38.9%) were the most frequently reported disasters in their area. Insufficient water quantity, previous disaster experience, and household members on chronic disease medication were found to be associated with higher disaster risk perception. Perceived water security indicators were not found to be predictors of preparedness attitudes and coping ability. Addressing water sufficiency in both disaster risk reduction strategies and long-term water management will be necessary to improve the health and livelihood of rural villagers in the coming decades.

Keywords: water security; disaster risk; risk perception; rural; China; Health-EDRM

---

1. Introduction

Water is a basic necessity of life and health, with communities requiring the provision of accessible safe drinking water at an affordable cost to meet their basic needs [1]. Lack of access to clean adequate water supplies is an indirect contributing risk factor of disaster through poorer hygiene and water-related diseases that diminish health and increase a population's vulnerability. On the contrary, adequate water supplies enable households to not only have enough for personal consumption and hygiene but also to build livelihoods, invest in opportune projects, and facilitate community development and poverty eradication [2] (pp. 5, 22). This capacity "to safeguard sustainable access to adequate quantities of acceptable quality water for sustaining livelihoods, human well-being and socio-economic development" is also known as water security [1]. Maintaining water security in communities not only protects health and sustains development but can also help reduce a population's vulnerability and increase the resilience of households when disaster inevitably strikes. Water-related disasters comprise 90% of the world's natural disasters [3]. Disasters such as floods, droughts, and storms can greatly affect communities in their development, livelihoods, and health. At the intersection of health and disaster risk reduction is the emerging field of Health Emergency Disaster Risk Management (Health-EDRM), which emphasizes the need to understand the direct and indirect health risks of hazards and to use multisectoral approaches to strengthen evidence-based guidelines and build community health resilience [4]. Health risks in emergencies and disasters should be minimized through a systematic analysis and management of risks across the entire disaster cycle, which should include considerations of the following aspects: "(1) hazard and vulnerability reduction to prevent and mitigate risks, (2) preparedness, (3), response, and (4) recovery measures" [5]. In terms of water, if a community already experiences water insecurity prior to a disaster, this problem will be magnified when sudden or slow-onset disastrous events occur, thus affecting the vulnerability status, preparedness, response, and recovery in a disaster. Inadequate water security and unreliable water systems could compound disaster risk [6–8] and have a direct effect on disaster response if water systems fail when they are most needed for survival after a disaster [8] and for emergency healthcare and infrastructural services [9]. A community's water security is also vulnerable to disaster impacts, as water systems or sources may be damaged by the disasters [6]. Especially with climate change, which will disrupt the hydrological cycle and heighten the frequency and intensity of hydro-meteorological hazards [10], the water security of many communities will be left increasingly at risk unless they take adaptation measures.

Disaster risk perception is an intuitive judgement made by lay persons and may be divergent from objective scientific assessments of disaster risk [11]. In terms of water-related disaster risks such as floods, risk perception research is still in its infancy and many studies take on a non-theoretical approach to risk perception, although measures such as risk characteristics, coping abilities, and preparedness attitudes are often assessed [12]. Research has found risk perception to be affected by prior disaster experience and trust in authorities, with less consistent associations with socio-demographic characteristics, cultural factors, and the influence of media [12,13]. However, environmental conditions and external physical factors have rarely been assessed in relation to a person's risk perception, and water security has not been suggested amongst such contextual factors.

As securing water at the household level is a cornerstone and foundation to water security [2], there is a need to understand the water insecurity and disaster risk perception at the household and community level. This is particularly true in the context of a rural village, where water systems may be decentralized, thus leaving room for variability amongst different households. Increased reliability and provision of water service can increase the adaptive capacity of a household in the face of disaster impacts and improve household resilience [2]. By understanding the linkage between communities' water security and disaster risk perception, this can empower the development of water resources management with a consideration towards disaster risk reduction and climate adaptation, contributing to the emergency resilience of the communities [2,14].

As water insecurity problems in a community could be magnified in the occurrence of disasters, this paper seeks to explore the current state of perceived household water security and disaster risk among an ethnic minority village community in Chongqing, China. Perceived water security is measured in this study through self-reported responses adapted from WHO 2011 Guidelines for drinking water quality, 4th Ed. Vol 1 [15]. The aim of this study is to assess the associations of disaster risk perception with perceived water security indicators and socio-demographic characteristics. The study hypothesized that in a rural water-scarce area, perceived water insecurity would be associated with greater disaster risk perception, preparedness attitudes, and coping ability.

Our study was conducted during a health needs assessment trip to Xingguang village in Lutang Township, Pengshui Miao and Tujia Autonomous County, Chongqing Direct-Controlled Municipality, China. In a recent climate change impact assessment, Chongqing was identified as highly vulnerable to future climate change impacts, especially in terms of its water resources [16]. Located in a disaster-prone region, the local community has had frequent exposure to hydro-meteorological risks such as drought, landslides, floods, and storms. The rural village has a largely decentralized water system, and individual households often rely on rooftop collection of rainwater. The village is administratively divided into nine sub-villages and has a total population of approximately 2000 villagers, with average incomes around the international poverty line ($1.90 USD per day per person). It is also ethnically diverse, with minorities such as the Miao (苗族) and Tujia (土家族) ethnicities, as well as the majority ethnicity of Han Chinese.

2. Materials and Methods

A pilot cross-sectional stratified sample household survey was conducted in the Xingguang village community in Lutang Township, Chongqing China in February 2015. Households were stratified according to their sub-village and surveys were completed in all nine sub-villages. Within each cluster, we aimed to reach a 10% representation of each sub-village population by simple random sampling. This sampling format is similar to other studies conducted elsewhere [17,18] and enables a representative understanding of different locations throughout the village, limiting the over-accumulation of household surveys from one or two sub-villages. However, this method only takes characteristics of the individual village into account, thus limiting generalizability to other villages. Trained interviewers conducted the face-to-face surveys with each household representative, with the language support of local translators. Each interview took approximately 20–30 minutes. Verbal consent was obtained from all participants. Ethics approval was obtained from the Survey and Behavioural Research Ethics Committee of the Chinese University of Hong Kong. All data were double entered and cleaned by trained staff.

The survey questionnaire of the health needs assessment consisted of 10 sections, with this analysis focusing on the data provided from three sections, namely, (1) respondent background and household characteristics, (2) water and sanitation, and (3) disaster risk perception. The respondent background and household characteristics section included sociodemographic measures such as ethnicity, gender, position as household head, age, education level, occupation, main source of income, annual household income, migrant workers in family, household members with chronic disease, and household members on chronic disease medication. Annual income per capita was calculated by dividing the annual household income by the total number of household members. The water and sanitation section was comprised of general indicators (main source of drinking water, storage of water) and self-reported water security indicators adapted from WHO 2011 Guidelines for drinking-water quality [15]: quality (measured as protection of water source, and boiling of drinking water), quantity (sufficiency of water), accessibility (time needed to fetch water), affordability (money spent on water), and reliability of water (stability of water supply). The outcomes assessed in the disaster risk perception section included the following measures: risk perception (perception of living in a high-risk disaster area), preparedness attitudes (measured as importance of keeping extra medication for a disaster [19], and the necessity of a disaster bag [20]), and coping ability (perceived ability to protect their family's health and safety in the case of a disaster). The measure of previous personal disaster experience, which was also from this section, was included in the analyses as an exposure.

Descriptive analyses were conducted on the perceptions of water security, disaster risk, and sociodemographic variables. Variables were simplified into binary categorical variables for the univariate analysis. Univariate analyses were conducted using Chi-squared test on the disaster risk perception variables, as associated with subjective water security indicators and sociodemographic variables. A backward stepwise multivariable logistic regression was conducted for each of the disaster risk perception outcomes, which included sociodemographic variables of age, gender, education, and annual per capita income, and variables with $p < 0.2$ in the univariate analyses. After the significant variables were identified in the backward models, the models were re-run while controlling for age and gender. These final models, inclusive of significant variables from the backward logistic regressions and controlled for age and gender, are reported in this paper. Significance level for the multivariable analyses was set at $p \leq 0.05$. All statistical analyses used SPSS version 20.0 (SPSS Inc., Chicago, IL, USA).

3. Results

3.1. Descriptive Analyses

Around the time of the survey, Xingguang village was reported to include 540 households and approximately 2300 residents [21]. Our final study sample was comprised of 52 household representatives from the village community. The sociodemographic characteristics of the surveyed households are shown in Table 1. The median household size was five members, and the median annual household income was 20,000 RMB (equivalent to ~$2940 USD). After calculations, the median annual income per capita was 3571 RMB (equivalent to ~$525 USD).

Table 1. Sociodemographic characteristics of participants and their households in Xingguang village, Chongqing, China ($N = 52$).

Participants	n	%	Households	n	%
Gender			**Main source of household income**		
Male	36	69.2	Farming	25	48.1
Female	16	30.8	Working	25	48.1
Age			Others	2	3.8
16–24	6	11.5	**Annual income per capita ($N = 43$)**		
25–44	16	30.8	≤2500 RMB (≤$1 USD/day)	18	41.9
45–64	23	44.2	2501–5000 RMB (≤$2 USD/day)	10	23.3
≥65	7	13.5	5001–7500 RMB (≤$3 USD/day)	7	16.3
Ethnicity			>7500 RMB (>$3 USD/day)	8	18.6
Miao	11	21.2			
Tujia	4	7.7	**Household members who are …**		
Han	37	71.2	**Migrant workers**		
Household Head			None	5	9.6
Yes	32	61.5	1	25	48.1
No	20	38.5	2	13	25.0
Education			3–5	9	17.3
No Schooling	7	13.5	**With chronic disease**		
Primary School	21	40.4	Yes	35	67.3
Middle School	16	30.8	No	17	32.7
High School	5	9.6	**On chronic disease medication ($N = 47$)**		
College or Higher	3	5.8	Yes	22	46.8
Occupation [1]			No	25	53.2
Farmer	21	40.4			
Employee	15	28.8			
Others	16	30.7			

[1] Other occupations included the following: business person, teacher, student, household work, unemployed, and retired.

Indicators of perceived water security among the surveyed households are shown in Figure 1. Most of the participants used rainwater as their main source of drinking water (84.6%) and reported having an unreliable (37.3% often no water or 54.9% occasionally no water) and insufficient (63.5%) quantity of water. Only 5.8% of respondents had a protected water source and, although half of the households stored their water, less than half of those that stored their water kept the water container covered (38.4%, $N = 10/26$). However, over 70% of the households did not need to use money to buy water (76.9%), had access within 5 minutes (76.9%, $N = 48$), and boiled their water (73.1%).

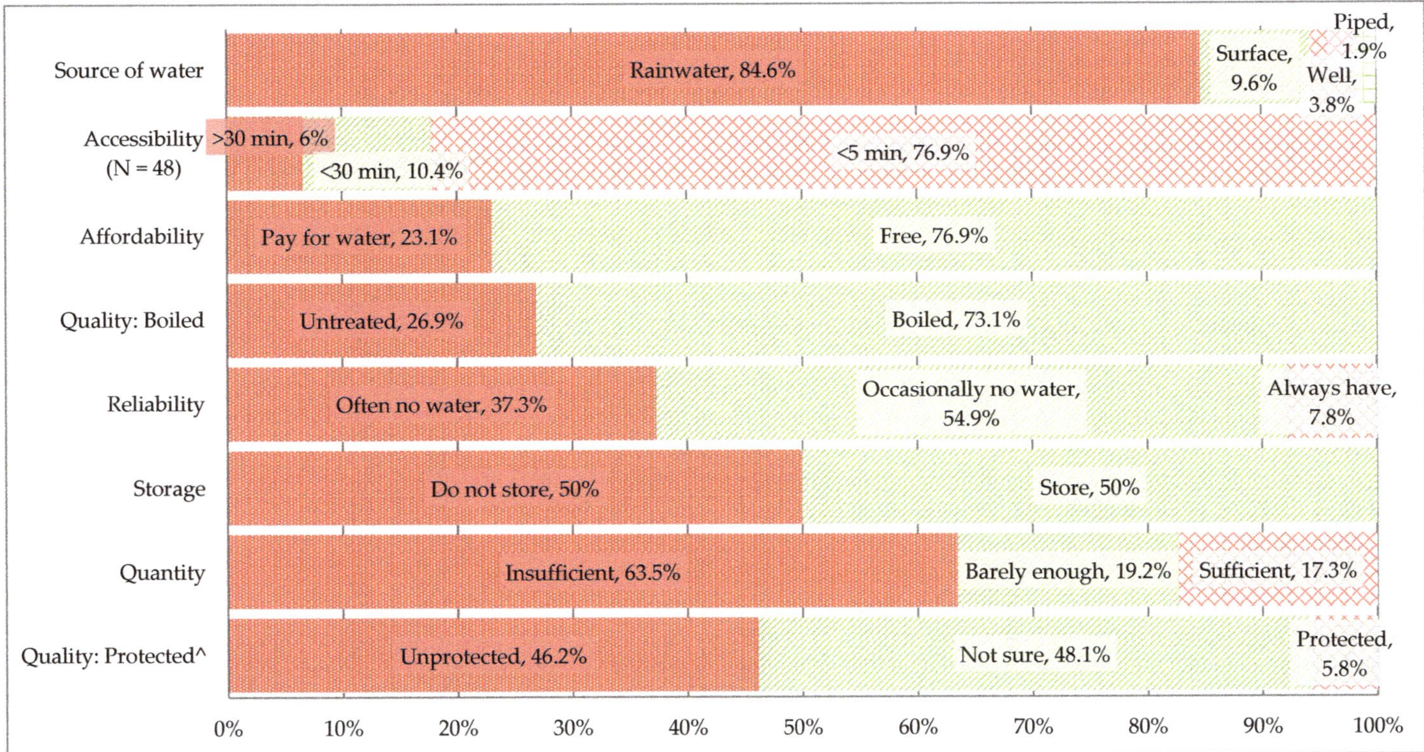

Figure 1. Descriptive statistics of water security indicators adapted from WHO guidelines [15] among households in the Xingguang village community, Chongqing, China ($N = 52$). ^ Protection indicates that the water source quality was protected from runoff water, bird droppings, and animals with a well-lining or casting, and a cover.

In terms of disaster risk perception indicators, over half of the respondents (60.8%) reported to have personally experienced a disaster during their lifetime, namely, floods (25.8%), storms (25.8%), snowstorms (22.6%), or droughts (12.9%), among others. However, only 32.7% of respondents believed they were living in a high-risk disaster area, of which storms (44.4%), droughts (38.9%), floods (22.2%), and snowstorms (11.1%) were the most frequently reported disasters in their area. In terms of disaster preparedness attitudes, 47.7% out of 44 respondents agreed to the importance of keeping extra medications for a disaster. Only 34.6% reported the necessity of a disaster bag, although most reported having the following emergency items at home: a flashlight (98.1%), lighter (100%), and emergency blanket (86.5%), with the exception of a whistle (3.8%). Finally, only 34.6% believed they had the ability to protect their family's health and safety in the case of a disaster.

3.2. Multivariable Analyses

Results from the multivariable analyses are shown in Table 2. Perception of living in a high-risk disaster area was found to be associated with insufficient quantity of water (Adjusted Odds Ratio, AOR = 30.48, 95% CI: 1.79–520.47), previous personal disaster experience (AOR = 37.17, 95% CI: 1.44–957.29), and household members on chronic disease medication (AOR = 23.68, 95% CI: 1.49–377.65), after adjusting for gender, age, and annual per capita income. Perceived importance of keeping extra medication for a disaster, as an indicator of disaster preparedness attitudes, was found to be associated with household members with chronic disease (AOR = 4.66, 95% CI: 1.08–20.04), after adjusting for gender, age, and annual per capita income. However, the preparedness attitude of disaster bag necessity was not found to be significantly associated with any predictors. Coping ability, as demonstrated through the perceived ability to protect their family's health and safety in the case of a disaster, also was not observed to have any significant associations in the backward logistic regression model.

Other perceived water security indicators were not found to be associated with the disaster risk outcomes. Although some perceived water security indicators (such as drinking water source, water storage, and water affordability) were associated with disaster risk outcomes in our univariable analyses, they were no longer associated with disaster risk outcomes in the multivariable analyses.

Table 2. Multivariable analyses of disaster risk outcomes in Xingguang village, Chongqing, China.

Outcome	Variable	Adjusted Odds Ratio (95% CI)	p-Value
Risk perception: Living in a high-risk disaster area (N = 46) [1]			
	Female	0.51 (0.05, 5.76)	0.584
	45 or older	2.39 (0.24, 24.32)	0.462
	Insufficient quantity water	30.48 (1.79, 520.47)	0.018 *
	Personal disaster experience	37.17 (1.44, 957.29)	0.029 *
	Household member on chronic disease medication	23.68 (1.49, 377.65)	0.025 *
	Per capita income (Ref: >5000 RMB)		
	≤5000 RMB	16.03 (0.92, 278.92)	0.057
	Refuse to answer	1578.1 (6.65, 374,389.16)	0.008 *
Preparedness attitude: Importance of keeping extra medication for a disaster (N = 44) [2]			
	Female	0.96 (0.21, 4.34)	0.954
	45 or older	0.48 (0.12, 1.88)	0.289
	Household member with chronic disease	4.66 (1.08, 20.04)	0.039 *
	Per capita income (Ref: >5000 RMB)		
	≤5000 RMB	0.81 (0.17, 3.81)	0.79
	Refuse to answer	0.07 (0.01, 0.98)	0.048 *
Preparedness attitude: Necessity of disaster bag (N = 50) [3]			
	Nil		
Coping ability: Perceived ability to protect in disaster (N = 52) [4]			
	Nil		

The following variables had $p < 0.2$ in the univariate analyses and were included in the backward stepwise logistic regression models: [1] main source of drinking water, water quantity, previous personal disaster experience, and household members on chronic disease medication (or, alternately, household members with chronic disease); [2] water storage, ethnicity, occupation, and household members with chronic disease; [3] education, previous personal disaster experience, and household members on chronic disease medication; [4] water affordability. Each backward logistic regression analysis included age, gender, education, and annual per capita income. * Statistically significant at $p < 0.05$.

4. Discussion

Overall, our study found that Xingguang village in Chongqing, China, faced vulnerabilities in their perceived water security. The Xingguang village has been obligated to rely on the collection of rainwater as their main source of drinking water despite the low quantity, relatively low reliability, and potential risks of poor quality reported among the majority of the respondents in the village. This indicates a water-scarce context where there is no better alternative source of water resources available. Our findings support the premise that some aspects of perceived water insecurity could further exacerbate the village's disaster risk perception. Although only one-third of respondents perceived themselves to be in a high-risk disaster area, our findings showed that perceived insufficient water quantity was positively associated with higher disaster risk perception. This demonstrates that within a community that regularly experiences insufficient water quantities, the awareness of their disaster risk is influenced by this external circumstance.

Consistent with previous research, prior disaster experience was found to be associated with a higher perceived disaster risk [12,13,22], while sociodemographic variables, such as age and gender, were not found to be associated [12,13]. Moreover, those on chronic disease medications were more likely to feel at risk of disasters than those who do not take medications, although the preparedness attitude for supplying extra medications was associated with chronic disease persons in general. These results indicate that those who have had relevant experiences related to their vulnerabilities (such as previous disasters or chronic diseases) seem to have greater risk awareness and express more willingness to protect themselves. By enabling more community members to identify their health-related disaster risks and corresponding preparedness actions, this would help lower the vulnerability of the community.

Preparedness attitude (perceived necessity of a disaster bag) and coping ability (perceived ability to protect one's family in a disaster) were relatively low, with only one-third of respondents in agreement. However, we could not identify any water security or sociodemographic predictors for these two outcomes among a rural population. This indicates that the ability to prepare or cope with disasters is not impaired or impacted by the community's frequent issues of water insecurity. These two outcomes were also not associated with age or gender, although education might potentially have some effect on coping ability, as it was found to be marginally significant ($p = 0.088$) but did not remain in the final model. Higher risk perception, prior disaster experience, and resources-related variables, such as income, were not found to be associated with preparedness attitudes of a disaster bag, or respondents' coping ability. As this household survey was conducted during the needs assessment phase of our project, our results indicate the disaster preparedness attitudes and coping ability prior to any disaster education interventions in the community. Thus, increased awareness through a disaster education intervention may be applicable to community members and could be beneficial towards developing an appropriate attitude in regard to disaster preparedness. Additionally, respondents did report possessing common household items that would be useful in the case of a disaster. This indicates that they possess the necessary resources to respond to potential disasters but could be further guided in their awareness and educated on the applicability of their resources.

Our findings on the association between insufficient water and high-risk perception is aligned with the premise that if a community regularly experiences water insecurity then this problem may be objectively exacerbated when sudden or slow-onset disastrous events occur. As such, more should be done to develop the water supply of households in the village, to decrease their vulnerability, and increase their resilience to respond to forthcoming water-related disasters. Literature has shown that those with higher levels of perceived risk are more likely to engage in risk reduction behaviors [23,24]. Households could be guided to better harness the use of rainfall collection, such that they could collect greater quantities of water. Community development should be conducted with the awareness of the risks natural disasters pose to the water supply. Disaster risk reduction activities could be carried out to address this association [25], such as spatial hazard mapping of water insecure households. This may contribute to identifying a vulnerable group in the village that may be more exposed to water insecurity or disaster hazards. Risk assessments can be further conducted to prevent or mitigate the effect of disasters on their water supply. Early warning systems can be put into place for different types of water-related disasters (such as droughts, floods, etc.), such that the villages can ensure a timely response and collect or prepare their water resources sufficiently in the case of emergencies.

Other water security indicators were not found to be associated with disaster risk perception, which supports the argument that adequate water quantity is of greater importance than water quality in water-scare conditions [26]. However, despite the non-significant associations, care should be taken to ensure that the increase of water quantity does not come at the cost of other water security indicators that would further increase the vulnerability of the villagers. Appropriate storage containers could be identified that can maintain the quality of water and protect it from potentially hazardous elements. These actions would in turn not only reduce the disaster risk of the community, but also further enhance the community's water security.

Our study faced limitations in terms of its cross-sectional study design, small sample size, and missing data. We were unable to include objective assessments of water security indicators, such as water quantity measures or measures of chemical or microbiological contaminants. Additionally, we had no information on respondents' actual disaster preparedness or coping ability and were only able to assess their attitudes towards it. Our findings cannot be attributed as causation. Excessive amounts of predictor variables would have reduced the power of the analysis, nevertheless we tried to standardize our findings by adjusting for gender and age in the final models. As this was only a pilot study with limited sample size, future research could help tease out possible relationships between water security and disaster risk perception or further identify any associations.

5. Conclusions

As far as we know, our study is the first to examine the relationship between water security and disaster risk perception and responses, and our results identified a relationship between insufficient water quantity and disaster risk perception. These findings support the hypothesis that external physical factors, namely inadequate water quantity, can be a contextual factor which affects disaster risk perception. If a community already experiences water insecurity prior to a disaster, its vulnerability will be magnified when affected by sudden or slow-onset disastrous events. With rapid socioeconomic development in China, water security will be challenged and exacerbated. Our study identifies that in a water insecure rural village, perceived insufficient water quantity is associated with higher disaster risk perception, but not preparedness attitudes and coping ability. Water security, particularly sufficiency of water quantity, is an important consideration not only in objective disaster risk assessments but also among disaster risk perceptions and disaster risk management. Particularly in a rural decentralized context, it is essential to consider and develop long-term water management in the lens of disaster risk reduction, as well as disaster risk reduction strategies with an awareness of water sufficiency levels. Such a two-pronged Health-EDRM approach would be valuable to combat future water security challenges and improve the health and livelihoods of disaster-prone rural villages.

Author Contributions: Conceptualization: E.Y.Y.C. and J.Y.H.; Methodology: E.Y.Y.C., J.Y.H., and M.P.S.Y.; Formal Analysis: J.Y.H.; Investigation: M.P.S.Y. and T.K.C.Y.; Resources: E.Y.Y.C.; Data Curation: H.C.Y.L.; Writing—Original Draft Preparation: J.Y.H.; Writing—Review and Editing: J.Y.H., E.Y.Y.C., H.C.Y.L., M.P.S.Y., C.K.P.W., and T.K.C.Y.; Visualization: J.Y.H.; Supervision: E.Y.Y.C.; Project Administration: H.C.Y.L. and C.K.P.W.; Funding Acquisition: E.Y.Y.C.

Funding: This research was supported by the Chow Tai Fook Charity Foundation and the Jockey Club School of Public Health and Primary Care (SPHPC) Medical Humanitarian Response and Disaster Development Fund.

Acknowledgments: The authors would like to acknowledge the EMHP-CCOUC team members who participated in the 2015 Xingguang field trip and collected the data to make this study possible: Kelvin WK Ling, Carman KM Mark, Chun Wai Yee, Chung Po Lam, Lucille C But, Chaoqin Chen, Pui Yee Tina Cheng, On Wa Ng, and Wing Yi To.

Conflicts of Interest: The authors declare no conflict of interest.

References

1. United Nations University Institute for Water Environment & Health. *Water Security & the Global Water Agenda: A UN-Water Analytical Brief*; United Nations University: Hamilton, ON, Canada, 2013.
2. Asian Development Bank; Asia-Pacific Water Forum. *Asian Water Development Outlook 2013: Measuring Water Security in Asia and the Pacific*; Asian Development Bank: Mandaluyong, Philippines, 2013.
3. World Water Assessment Programme (WWAP). *Managing Water under Uncertainty and Risk*; United Nations Educational, Scientific and Cultural Organization (UNSECO): Paris, France, 2012.
4. Lo, S.T.T.; Chan, E.Y.Y.; Chan, G.K.W.; Murray, V.; Abrahams, J.; Ardalan, A.; Kayano, R.; Yau, J.C.W. Health Emergency and Disaster Risk Management (Health-EDRM): Developing the Research Field within the Sendai Framework Paradigm. *Int. J. Disaster Risk Sci.* **2017**, *8*, 145–149. [CrossRef]
5. World Health Organization; Public Health England; United Nations Office of Disaster Risk Reduction (UNISDR). *Emergency Risk Management for Health: Overview*; World Health Organization: Geneva, Switzerland; Public Health England: London, UK; United Nations Office of Disaster Risk Reduction (UNISDR): Geneva, Switzerland, 2013.
6. Schipper, L.; Pelling, M. Disaster risk, climate change and international development: Scope for, and challenges to, integration. *Disasters* **2006**, *30*, 19–38. [CrossRef] [PubMed]
7. Shi, W.; Xia, J.; Gippel, C.J.; Chen, J.; Hong, S. Influence of disaster risk, exposure and water quality on vulnerability of surface water resources under a changing climate in the Haihe River basin. *Water Int.* **2017**, *42*, 462–485. [CrossRef]
8. Phan, H.L.; Winkler, I.T. Water Security. In *Research Handbook on Disasters and International Law*; Breau, S.C., Samuel, K.L.H., Eds.; Edward Elgar Publishing: Cheltenham, UK, 2016.
9. Centers for Disease Control and Prevention (CDC). Water, Sanitation, & Hygiene (WASH)-Related Emergencies & Outbreaks. Available online: https://www.cdc.gov/healthywater/emergency/index.html (accessed on 5 November 2018).
10. Asian Development Bank. *Disaster Risk Assesment For Project Preparation: A Practical Guide*; Asian Development Bank: Mandaluyong, Philippines, 2017.
11. Ho, M.C.; Shaw, D.; Lin, S.; Chiu, Y.C. How do disaster characteristics influence risk perception? *Risk Anal.* **2008**, *28*, 635–643. [CrossRef] [PubMed]
12. Kellens, W.; Terpstra, T.; De Maeyer, P. Perception and communication of flood risks: A systematic review of empirical research. *Risk Anal.* **2013**, *33*, 24–49. [CrossRef] [PubMed]
13. Wachinger, G.; Renn, O.; Begg, C.; Kuhlicke, C. The risk perception paradox—Implications for governance and communication of natural hazards. *Risk Anal.* **2013**, *33*, 1049–1065. [PubMed]
14. Asian Development Bank. *Water-Related Disasters and Disaster Risk Management in the People's Republic of China*; Asian Development Bank: Mandaluyong, Philippines, 2015.
15. World Health Organization. *Guidelines for Drinking-Water Quality*, 4th ed.; World Health Organization: Geneva, Switzerland, 2011.
16. Asian Development Bank. 24: Climate Change Impact Assessment. In *Chongqing Urban-Rural Infrastructure Development Demonstration II Project (RRP PRC 45509): Linked Documents*; Asian Development Bank: Mandaluyong, Philippines, 2013.
17. Chan, E.Y.Y.; Lam, H.C.Y.; Chung, P.P.W.; Huang, Z.; Yung, T.K.C.; Ling, K.W.K.; Chan, G.K.W.; Chiu, C.P. Risk Perception and Knowledge in Fire Risk Reduction in a Dong Minority Rural Village in China: A Health-EDRM Education Intervention Study. *Int. J. Disaster Risk Sci.* **2018**, *9*, 306–318. [CrossRef]
18. Thorogood, M.; Connor, M.D.; Hundt, G.L.; Tollman, S.M. Understanding and managing hypertension in an African sub-district: A multidisciplinary approach. *Scand. J. Public Health Suppl.* **2007**, *69*, 52–59. [PubMed]
19. Chan, E.Y.; Sondorp, E. Medical Interventions following Natural Disasters: Missing out on Chronic Medical Needs. *Asia-Pac. J. Public Health* **2007**, *19*, 45–51. [CrossRef] [PubMed]
20. Pickering, C.J.; O'Sullivan, T.L.; Morris, A.; Mark, C.; McQuirk, D.; Chan, E.Y.; Guy, E.; Chan, G.K.; Reddin, K.; Throp, R.; et al. The Promotion of 'Grab Bags' as a Disaster Risk Reduction Strategy. *PLoS Curr. Disasters* **2018**. [CrossRef]

21. Wu Zhi Qiao (Bridge to China) Charitable Foundation. *Investigation Report on the Village of Xingguang Village, Lutang Township, Pengshui County, Chongqing (Chinese)*; Wu Zhi Qiao (Bridge to China) Charitable Foundation: Hong Kong, China, 2014.
22. Chan, E.Y.; Kim, J.H.; Lin, C.; Cheung, E.Y.; Lee, P.P. Is previous disaster experience a good predictor for disaster preparedness in extreme poverty households in remote Muslim minority based community in China? *J. Immigr. Minor. Health* **2014**, *16*, 466–472. [CrossRef] [PubMed]
23. Lepesteur, M.; Wegner, A.; Moore, S.A.; McComb, A. Importance of public information and perception for managing recreational activities in the Peel-Harvey estuary, Western Australia. *J. Environ. Manag.* **2008**, *87*, 389–395. [CrossRef] [PubMed]
24. Martin, W.E.; Martin, I.M.; Kent, B. The role of risk perceptions in the risk mitigation process: The case of wildfire in high risk communities. *J. Environ. Manag.* **2009**, *91*, 489–498. [CrossRef] [PubMed]
25. Baas, S.; Ramasamy, S.; de Pryck, J.D.; Battista, F. *Disaster Risk Management Systems Analysis: A Guide Book*; 1684 8241; Food and Agriculture Organization of the United Nations: Rome, Italy, 2008.
26. Bostoen, K.; Kolsky, P.; Hunt, C. Improving Urban Water and Sanitation Services: Health, Access and Boundaries. In *Scaling Urban Environmental Challenges: From Local to Global and Back*; Marcotullio, P.J., McGranahan, G., Eds.; Earthscan: London, UK, 2007; pp. 106–131.

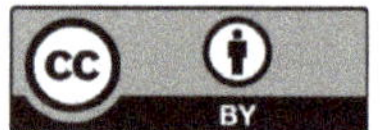

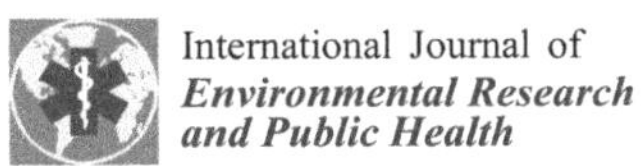
International Journal of *Environmental Research and Public Health*

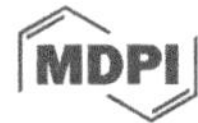

Communication

Psychosocial Management Before, During, and After Emergencies and Disasters—Results from the Kobe Expert Meeting

Mélissa Généreux [1,2,*], Philip J. Schluter [3,4], Sho Takahashi [5,6], Shiori Usami [7], Sonoe Mashino [8], Ryoma Kayano [9] and Yoshiharu Kim [10]

1 Sherbrooke Hospital University Centre, Eastern Townships Integrated University Centre in Health and Social Services, Sherbrooke, QC J1J 3H5, Canada
2 Department of Community Health Sciences, Faculty of Medicine and Health Sciences, Université de Sherbrooke, Sherbrooke, QC J1G 1B1, Canada
3 School of Health Sciences, University of Canterbury—Te Whare Wānanga o Waitaha, Christchurch 8140, New Zealand; philip.schluter@canterbury.ac.nz
4 Primary Care Clinical Unit, School of Clinical Medicine, The University of Queensland, Brisbane QLD 4006, Australia
5 Department of Disaster Psychiatry, University of Tsukuba, Tsukuba 305-8575, Japan; takahashi.sho.fn@u.tsukuba.ac.jp
6 Ibaraki Prefectural Medical Center of Psychiatry, Kasama 309-1717, Japan
7 Department of Mental Health and Psychiatric Nursing, Faculty of Life Sciences, Kumamoto University, Kumamoto 860-8555, Japan; susami@kumamoto-u.ac.jp
8 Research Institute of Nursing Care for People and Community, University of Hyōgo, Akashi 673-8588, Japan; sonoe_mashino@cnas.u-hyogo.ac.jp
9 World Health Organization Centre for Health Development, Kobe 651-0073, Japan; kayanor@who.int
10 National Institute of Mental Health, National Center for Neurology and Psychiatry, Kodaira 187-0031, Japan; kim@ncnp.go.jp
* Correspondence: melissa.genereux@usherbrooke.ca; Tel.: +1-819-829-3400 (ext. 42453)

Received: 31 January 2019; Accepted: 1 April 2019; Published: 12 April 2019

Abstract: Emergencies and disasters typically affect entire communities, cause substantial losses and disruption, and result in a significant and persistent mental health burden. There is currently a paucity of evidence on safe and effective individual- and community-level strategies for improving mental health before, during, and after such events. In October 2018, the World Health Organization (WHO) Centre for Health Development (WHO Kobe Centre) convened a meeting bringing together leading Asia Pacific and international disaster research experts. The expert meeting identified key research needs in five major areas, one being "Psychosocial management before, during, and after emergencies and disasters". Experts for this research area identified critical gaps in observational research (i.e., the monitoring of long-term psychological consequences) and interventional research (i.e., the development and evaluation of individual- and community-level interventions). Three key research issues were identified. First, experts underscored the need for a standardized and psychometrically robust instrument that classified the mental health/psychosocial risk of people within both a clinical and community setting. Then, the need for a standardization of methods for prevention, screening, diagnosis, and treatment for affected people was highlighted. Finally, experts called for a better identification of before, during, and after emergency or disaster assets associated with greater community resilience.

Keywords: health emergency and disaster risk management (Health-EDRM); Sendai Framework for Disaster Risk Reduction; WHO Thematic Platform for Health-EDRM Research Network; post-traumatic stress disorder; mental health impacts; psychosocial management; community resilience

1. Introduction

Large-scale emergency and disaster events, resulting from natural, technological, or human causes, often affect entire communities. They invariably yield significant human and capital injuries and losses coupled with prolonged social and infrastructure disruption. Moreover, emergencies and disasters typically place a significant and persistent mental health burden on those directly and indirectly affected, together with those who respond and their associated services. As a result, public health organizations are charged with intervening and helping citizens and communities cope in the aftermath of emergencies and disasters. The public health response during and after emergencies and disasters has historically focused on protecting populations from immediate threats [1]. However, the role of public health and health systems in providing sustained psychosocial support for directly and indirectly affected victims, the long-term monitoring of psychological profiles, and delivering ongoing strategies for enhancing resilience may be just as important [2].

In October 2018, the World Health Organization (WHO) Centre for Health Development (WHO Kobe Centre) convened a meeting in order to identify key emergency and disaster research needs. A panel of invited experts from the WHO, WHO Thematic Platform for Health Emergency and Disaster Risk Management (Health-EDRM) Research Network (TPRN), World Association for Disaster and Emergency Medicine, and the Japan International Cooperation Agency, along with delegates to the Asia Pacific Conference for Disaster Medicine 2018, was convened [3]. The panel was informed by multiple sources, including the progress and implementation of the Sendai Framework on Disaster Risk Reduction 2015–2030 [4], documentation from the 3rd UN World Conference on Disaster Risk Reduction (including the establishment of TPRN), and literature on the recommended Health-EDRM research activities [5–8]. After a review of these documents, together with appraising existing projects and activities, five major areas of research need were identified. These were clustered and named under the following banners: (i) Health data management before, during, and after emergencies and disasters; (ii) Psychosocial management before, during, and after emergencies and disasters, and other medium- and long-term effects on the public health and health systems, the topic of this paper; (iii) Community emergency and disaster risk management, including risk literacy and addressing needs of sub-populations; (iv) Health workforce development for health emergency and disaster risk management; and, (v) Research methods and ethics.

2. Material and Methods

The content of this discussion paper arises from the WHO Kobe Centre convened panel's deliberations, based on available evidence and their expertise in psychosocial management before, during, and after emergencies and disasters. The lead discussant (Yoshiharu Kim), the rapporteur (Mélissa Généreux), and the other experts who participated to the discussion ($n = 7$) primarily sought to (i) identify critical gaps in scientific evidence in this major area of research, as well as (ii) discuss concrete research questions and issues, with the aim of potentially resolving these gaps through collaboration among Asian Pacific regional and global researchers and related stakeholders. Additionally, the panel aimed to assess knowledge-to-practice gaps in order to better integrate current expertise and research in this area for each disaster management phase.

3. Results

A consensus emerged among the expert panel that there is currently a paucity of evidence on safe and effective individual- and community-level strategies for monitoring and improving psychosocial health and building resilience before, during, and after emergencies and disasters.

3.1. Critical Research Gap Identification

The discussion on critical gaps in scientific evidence led to the identification of three priorities in research, namely the monitoring of long-term psychological consequences; the need for individual-level interventions; and the need for community-level interventions. Each of these identified gaps are now described in turn.

3.1.1. Monitoring of the Long-Term Psychological Consequences

In order to strengthen current psychosocial strategies to promote health and wellbeing before, during, and after emergencies and disasters, the monitoring of people's psychological profile needs to be harmonized or standardized. Such standardized monitoring enables population patterns to be followed over time, across the phases of the emergency or disaster, and provides an empirical characterization of recovery for the whole population and various important subgroups. Moreover, it would enable national and international comparisons to be drawn and facilitate a better understanding of community-level psychosocial wellbeing. Ideally, any standardized instrument would be derived from routinely collected information, thereby reducing participant burden and also being available before, during, and after emergencies and disasters. Many studies have reported both persistent adverse outcomes (notably post-traumatic stress disorders (PTSD) or symptoms (PTSS), anxiety, and depression) and positive outcomes (e.g., post-traumatic growth, and closer sense of community) for years following exposure to natural or anthropogenic disasters. Moreover, these positive and negative effects have been observed among those directly affected by the emergency or disaster, and also among those peripherally affected, such as workers and caregivers, and the wider population. However, community-level profiles are often left unmeasured prior to emergencies or disasters, making longitudinal recovery patterns difficult to fully ascertain. This is further compounded by the fact that specific sub-groups are often disproportionally impacted, may have differential recovery periods, and that the impact may vary greatly according to exposure type and intensity [9–15]. Children and youth, the elderly, those socioeconomically deprived, and disabled people frequently carry this disproportionate burden. Although standardization of exposure and outcome measures is desirable and central, this should not preclude the additional use and reporting of other culturally or geographically specific measures. Various indigenous and other groups of people around the globe define health and wellbeing in different but equally valid ways, and this should be acknowledged and respected in any form of reporting or monitoring.

3.1.2. Individual-Level Interventions

To better understand the psychosocial risks, vulnerabilities, and capacities following an emergency or disaster, a wide range of individual-level interventions need to be developed and evaluated, both in clinical and community-based settings. Such interventions should include, but are not limited to, self-care programs, humanitarian support, psychological first aid, prevention, screening and diagnosis tools for both health and non-health workers, and medication required for various types of sequelae mental health problems [16,17]. Preventive interventions are thought to be especially important to reduce the risk of PTSD and depression among workers who are acutely exposed [18], including first responders (e.g., fire, police, emergency medical staff). It is also critical to ensure that validated clinical interventions and tools can be shared and used more widely, through training, guidelines, repositories, and communication and dissemination strategies. Guidelines for the appropriate use of the interventions and tools must be clearly articulated, and their misuse must be avoided.

3.1.3. Community-Level Interventions

In a similar vein to the above, there is a need to further develop and evaluate community-level strategies, such as psychosocial education (before emergency or disaster), addressing the unmet psychosocial needs through self-help groups and dynamic group psychotherapy (after emergency or disaster), cultivating community resilience, empowering the citizens, and mobilizing the community (before, during, and after emergency or disaster) [19–22]. An evidence base of interventions that have empirically demonstrated successful implementation and efficacy needs to be developed and established. As for individual-level interventions, there is an added need for enhanced knowledge translation strategies so that lessons learned from community-level interventions can be pooled, shared, and used on a broader basis.

3.2. Proposed Research Questions and Issues

Concrete research questions were proposed to meet each of the identified knowledge gaps. The first question pertained to the classification of people exposed to a disaster according to their level of psychosocial need. Currently, multiple and often inconsistent definitions are employed. It was advocated that an epidemiological tool (i.e., a standardized and psychometrically robust instrument) should be developed and validated for the classification of risk (e.g., high-risk, mid-risk, and low-risk) for people exposed to an emergency or disaster. Drawing on the social determinants of health framework, a wide range of risks and assets previously documented in the scientific literature should underpin the construction of this tool [23–25]. Broadly, it is likely to include the following:

- Before emergency or disaster: pre-existing risk and protective factors;
- During emergency or disaster: exposure to primary stressors, human and material losses;
- After emergency or disaster: exposure to secondary stressors, and access and use of local resources.

As the emergency or disaster impacts invariably extend beyond the clinical setting, the tool should be suitable for patients within that setting but also for persons within the wider community (e.g., conducting a community health survey). As such, it is likely the tool will have robust screening rather than definitive clinical exposure diagnostic properties. The validation of this tool should be performed using longitudinal and multi-centric studies, and should focus on its ability to predict various outcomes, like PTSD, other psychological symptoms (including psychological distress, anxiety, and depressive symptoms), maladaptive behaviors (including alcohol and drug abuse), self-care, quality of life, and positive outcomes (including post-traumatic growth).

The need to standardize interventions delivered to people exposed to a disaster using evidence-based best practices was also stressed. Panel members suggested the development and validation of methods to screen, diagnose, and treat people exposed to a disaster in clinical and community-based settings. Such clinical tools should frame emerging practices, such as risk screening by community members, by ensuring that they are both effective and safe, and by underlining the conditions for success of such methods.

Finally, panel members called for a better identification of what makes a community resilient, through an assessment of before, during, and after emergency or disaster assets (i.e., characteristics, strengths, and resources) that are associated with greater community resilience. Local knowledge should be considered in the same manner as scientific knowledge. Having been through a unique and informative experience, the local health workforce involved in psychosocial management must draw and share lessons in the aftermath of a disaster (in close collaboration with researchers and community members) through case studies. Guidelines for their reporting of these studies should include the following.

- What were the needs and assets in the local community?
- How and by whom were these needs and assets addressed?
- What were the barriers and the success factors for sustaining resilience and recovery?

Standards (or format) to report case studies should facilitate the pooling and the sharing of such local evidence. Moreover, respective roles of health and non-health sectors need to be clarified, as community resilience absolutely requires a cross-sectoral approach. In time, these case studies could be subjected to meta-analyses in order to distill common features that transcend each unique emergency or disaster-ravaged community.

4. Discussion

The current research gaps and priorities in psychosocial management after emergencies and disasters identified by the expert panel are, perhaps unsurprisingly, mirrored within the literature. The lack of long-term observational and interventional research [8,26–28], challenges in systematically collating and delivering lessons learned from events, and difficulties in creating and sustaining effective community engagement [29–31] have all been described before. However, this paper is among the first that attempts to draw the various threads of these research needs together.

Although the before, during, and after phases of emergency and disaster management are all important, the panel asserted that local efforts in psychosocial management are mostly oriented toward the short-term after the event. Once the emergency or disaster is over, medical, psychosocial, and public health teams are often required to revert to and resume their regular tasks as quickly as possible. Long-term psychosocial recovery is perhaps the most challenging task because of the burden on professionals (e.g., accumulating workload) and organizational factors (e.g., weakening political commitment). As a result of this fatigue, monitoring of long-term psychological health consequences is not usually done (with a few exceptions) [25,32], much less in a standardized manner.

Another critical area that is typically overlooked in the post-event landscape is the evaluation of psychosocial interventions provided during the recovery phase of an emergency or disaster, which are typically not routinely carried out. Such evaluations would provide the necessary evidence for establishing standards and best practices [26]. Due to the often unpredictable nature of emergencies or disasters, it is often impossible to conduct randomized or prospective cohort studies that capture the before, during, and after phases of the event. Instead, within this emergency or disaster setting, interventional research should exploit apposite tailored natural experiment designs. These will often be shaped by pragmatic considerations, such as resources, expertise, and data availability, but are likely to include pre–post, interpreted time series, and change point study designs. Together with the standard cross-sectional or repeated measure studies often initiated following an event, a richer empirical evidence base will emerge. With the increasing availability of routinely collected data and greater ability for matching and tracking individuals over time, these data sources are likely to have increased utility in emergency and disaster research. With data sufficiency, the psychosocial profiles within affected communities could be monitored by measuring changes before, during, and after the emergency or disaster and comparing these patterns to unaffected control communities [33]. Finally, learning from past events should be systematized, notably through case studies, as they are likely to inform the identification and sharing of common international problems and solutions.

The importance of identifying and leveraging existing assets at the community level was also raised. Working from existing capacities was strongly valued among the panel. However, communities typically remain poorly engaged in disaster management. Indeed, often after an emergency or disaster, various sectors within the community, particularly those disproportionately affected, experience heightened barriers which contribute to further physical and social exclusion, and pursuant disengagement. Evidence-based efficacious strategies to mobilize local knowledge and expertise before, during, and after a disaster are yet to be developed [34].

Finally, the discussion of our expert panel on solutions to fill psychosocial management knowledge and knowledge-to-practice gaps before, during, and after emergencies and disasters aligned with the priorities set by the 2015–2030 Sendai Framework for Disaster Risk Reduction [35]. Indeed, the Sendai Framework emphasizes the requirement for *"improving the knowledge of government representatives at all levels through the sharing of experiences, lessons learned and good practices"* (Paragraph 24g) and *"ensuring that local knowledge and practices complete, as appropriate, scientific knowledge of disaster risk assessment"* (Paragraph 24i) [4].

5. Conclusions

It is hoped that this delineation and discussion on key research issues in psychosocial management will contribute to the identification and implementation of concrete solutions that foster the creation and the use of knowledge for psychosocial support and resilience building before, during, and after emergencies and disasters. As for other major Health-EDRM research areas, psychosocial management requires collaboration between experts, decision makers, practitioners, and communities in order to facilitate coordinated responses when and where they are most needed. It is critical that psychosocial strategies developed to support victims and communities affected by emergencies and disasters are validated and that knowledge gained from these experiences is shared and used as much as possible.

Author Contributions: Conceptualization: M.G., Y.K.; Methodology: M.G., Y.K.; Original Draft Preparation: M.G.; Writing—Review and Editing: Y.K., P.J.S., S.T., S.U., S.M., R.K.; Project Administration: R.K.

Funding: This research received no external funding.

Acknowledgments: The opinions contained in the paper are those of its authors and, except where specifically stated, are not intended to represent the official policies or positions of the WHO.

Conflicts of Interest: The authors declare no conflict of interest.

References

1. Généreux, M.; Petit, G.; Maltais, D.; Roy, M.; Simard, R.; Boivin, S.; Shultz, L.M.; Pinsonneault, L. The public health response during and after the Lac-Mégantic train derailment tragedy: A case study. *Disaster Health* **2015**, *2*, 1–8.
2. Spittlehouse, J.K.; Joyce, P.R.; Vierck, E.; Schluter, P.J.; Pearson, J.F. Ongoing adverse mental health impact of the earthquake sequence in Christchurch, New Zealand. *Aust. N. Z. J. Psychiatry* **2014**, *48*, 756–763. [CrossRef] [PubMed]
3. Asian Pacific Conference for Disaster Medicine 2018. Available online: http://www.apcdm2018.org/index.html (accessed on 31 January 2019).
4. Sendai Framework for Disaster Risk Reduction 2015–2030. Available online: https://www.unisdr.org/we/inform/publications/43291 (accessed on 31 January 2019).
5. WHO Thematic Platform for Health Emergency and Disaster Risk Management. Available online: http://www.who.int/hac/techguidance/preparedness/WHO-Thematic-Platform-Health-EDRM-Terms-Reference-2018.pdf?ua=1 (accessed on 31 January 2019).
6. WHO Thematic Platform for Health Emergency and Disaster Risk Management Research Network. Available online: http://www.who.int/hac/techguidance/preparedness/WHO-Thematic-Platform-Health-EDRM-Research-Network-2018.pdf?ua=1 (accessed on 31 January 2019).
7. Chan, E.Y.Y.; Murray, V. What are the health research needs for the Sendai Framework. *Lancet* **2017**, *390*, E35–E36. [CrossRef]
8. Lo, C.T.T.; Chan, E.Y.Y.; Chan, G.K.W.; Murray, V.; Abrahams, J.; Ardalan, A.; Kayano, R.; Chung, J.; Yau, W. Health Emergency and Disaster Risk Management (Health-EDRM): Developing the Research Field within the Sendai Framework Paradigm. *Int. J. Disaster Risk Sci.* **2017**, *8*, 145–149. [CrossRef]
9. Galea, S. The long-term health consequences of disasters and mass traumas. *CMAJ* **2007**, *176*, 1293–1294. [CrossRef]
10. Galea, S.; Nandi, A.; Vlahov, D. The epidemiology of post-traumatic stress disorder after disasters. *Epidemiol. Rev.* **2005**, *27*, 78–91. [CrossRef]
11. Goldmann, E.; Galea, S. Mental health consequences of disasters. *Ann. Rev. Public Health* **2014**, *35*, 169–183. [CrossRef]
12. Neria, Y.; Nandi, A.; Galea, S. Post-traumatic stress disorder following disasters: A systematic review. *Psychol. Med.* **2008**, *38*, 467–480. [CrossRef]
13. Hull, A.M.; Alexander, D.A.; Klein, S. Survivors of the Piper Alpha oil platform disaster: Long-term follow-up study. *Br. J. Psychiatry* **2002**, *181*, 433–438. [CrossRef] [PubMed]
14. Bromet, E.J.; Havenaar, J.M.; Guey, L.T. A 25 year retrospective review of the psychological consequences of the Chernobyl accident. *Clin. Oncol.* **2011**, *23*, 297–305. [CrossRef] [PubMed]
15. Généreux, M.; Maltais, D. Three years after the tragedy: How the Le Granit community is coping. *Bull. Vis. Santé Publique* **2017**, *34*, 1–8.

16. Usami, U.; Takahashi, N.; Kayano, R. Development of specific care strategies to maintain and recover survivors' health after disasters-intervention program to prevent PTSD and depression after Kumamoto earthquake: Case report. In Proceedings of the International Conference on Nursing, Pharmacy, Traditional Medicine and Health Cciences, TKP Conference, Osaka, Japan, 28–30 September 2018.
17. Kim, Y. Great East Japan earthquake and early mental-health-care response. *Psychiatry Clin. Neurosci.* **2011**, *65*, 539–548. [CrossRef] [PubMed]
18. Suzuki, Y.; Fukasawa, M.; Obara, A.; Kim, Y. Mental health distress and related factors among prefectural public servants seven months after the great East Japan earthquake. *J. Epidemiol.* **2014**, *24*, 287–294. [CrossRef] [PubMed]
19. Usami, S. Kumamoto earthquake, certified nurse specialist in mental health and psychiatric nursing to prevent PTSD. *J. Jpn. Assoc. Group Psychother.* **2017**, *33*, 18–22.
20. O'Sullivan, T.L.; Kuziemsky, C.E.; Corneil, W.; Lemyre, L.; Franco, Z. The EnRiCH community resilience framework for high-risk populations. *PLoS Curr.* **2014**. [CrossRef]
21. Généreux, M.; Petit, G.; Roy, M.; Maltais, D.; O'Sullivan, T. The "Lac-Mégantic tragedy" seen through the lens of the EnRiCH community resilience framework for high-risk populations. *Can. J. Public Health* **2018**, *109*, 261–267. [CrossRef]
22. Leadbeater, A. Community leadership in disaster recovery: A case study. *Aust. J. Emerg. Manag.* **2013**, *28*, 41–47.
23. Norris, F.H.; Friedman, M.J.; Watson, P.J.; Byrne, C.M.; Diaz, E.; Kaniasty, K. 60,000 disaster victims speak: Part I. An empirical review of the empirical literature, 1981–2001. *Psychiatry* **2002**, *65*, 207–239. [CrossRef]
24. Warsini, S.; West, C.; Dip, E.G.; Mills, J.; Usher, K. The psychosocial impact of natural disasters among adult survivors: An integrative review. *Issues Ment. Health Nurs.* **2014**, *35*, 420–436. [CrossRef]
25. Morgan, J.; Begg, A.; Beaven, S.; Schluter, P.; Jamieson, K.; Johal, S.; Johnston, D.; Sparrow, M. Monitoring wellbeing during recovery from the 2010–2011 Canterbury earthquakes: The CERA Wellbeing Survey. *Int. J. Disaster Risk Reduct.* **2015**, *14*, 96–103. [CrossRef]
26. Birnbaum, M.L.; Daily, E.K.; O'Rourke, A.P.; Kushner, J. Research and evaluations of the health aspects of disasters, part VI: Interventional research and the disaster logic model. *Prehosp. Disaster Med.* **2016**, *31*, 181–194. [CrossRef]
27. Tsutsumi, A.; Takashi, I.; Ito, A.; Thronicroft, G.; Patel, V.; Minas, H. Mental health mainstreamed in new UN disaster framework. *Lancet Psychiatry* **2015**, *2*, 679–680. [CrossRef]
28. Suzuki, Y.; Fukasawa, M.; Nakajima, S.; Narisawa, T.; Keiko, A.; Kim, Y. Developing a Consensus-Based Definition of "Kokoro-no Care" or Mental Health Services and Psychosocial Support: Drawing from Experiences of Mental Health Professionals Who Responded to the Great East Japan Earthquake. *PLoS Curr.* **2015**. [CrossRef]
29. Gamboa-Maldonado, T.; Marshak, H.H.; Sinclair, R.; Montgomery, S.; Dyjack, D.T. Building capacity for community disaster preparedness: A call for collaboration between public environmental health and emergency preparedness and response programs. *J. Environ. Health* **2012**, *75*, 24–29.
30. Jong, S.V.Z. Let's Talk Oil Spill Risk. Lessons Learned from Coastal Communities in British Columbia, Canada. Chapter 8. In *Responses to Disasters and Climate Change. Understanding Vulnerabilities and Fostering Resilience*; Taylor and Francis Group: Florida, FL, USA, 2016; pp. 83–92.
31. Svendsen, E.R.; Whittle, N.C.; Sanders, L.; McKeown, R.E.; Sprayberry, K.; Heim, M.; Caldwell, R.; Gibson, J.J.; Vena, J.E. GRACE: Public health recovery methods following an environmental disaster. *Arch. Environ. Occup. Health* **2010**, *65*, 77–85. [CrossRef]
32. Généreux, M.; Maltais, D.; Petit, G.; Roy, M. Monitoring adverse psychosocial outcomes one and two years after the Lac-Mégantic train derailment tragedy (Eastern Townships, Quebec, Canada). *Prehosp. Disaster Med.* **2019**. In press.
33. Schluter, P.J.; Hamilton, G.J.; Deely, J.M.; Ardagh, M.W. The impact of integrated health system changes, accelerated due to an earthquake, on emergency department attendances and acute admissions: A Bayesian change-point analysis. *BMJ Open* **2016**, *6*, e010709. [CrossRef]

34. Lichtveld, M.; Kennedy, S.; Krouse, R.Z.; Grimsley, F.; El-Dahr, J.; Bordelon, K.; Sterling, Y.; White, L.; Baelow, N.; DeGruy, S.; et al. From design to dissemination: Implementing community-based participatory research in postdisaster communities. *Am. J. Public Health* **2016**, *106*, 1235–1242. [CrossRef]
35. Aitsi-Selmi, A.; Murray, V. The Sendai framework: Disaster risk reduction through a health lens. *Bull. World Health Organ.* **2015**, *93*. [CrossRef]

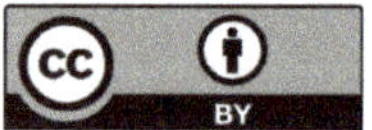

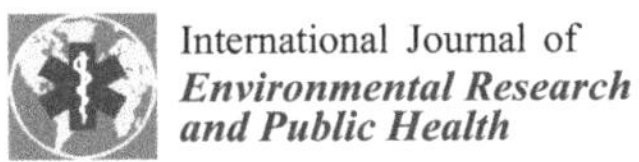
International Journal of
Environmental Research and Public Health

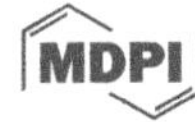

Article

Factors Influencing the Response to Infectious Diseases: Focusing on the Case of SARS and MERS in South Korea

Kyu-Myoung Lee [1] and Kyujin Jung [2,*]

1 Department of Public Administration, Korea University, Seoul 02841, Korea; joanna528@korea.ac.kr
2 Department of Public Administration and the Graduate School of Governance, Sungkyunkwan University, Seoul 02841, Korea
* Correspondence: kjung1@skku.edu; Tel.: +82-2-760-0253

Received: 31 January 2019; Accepted: 9 April 2019; Published: 22 April 2019

Abstract: Following the 2003 the severe acute respiratory syndrome (SARS) and the 2015 Middle East Respiratory Syndrome (MERS) outbreak in South Korea, this research aims to explore and examine the factors influencing the response to infectious diseases, which encompasses both communicable and non-communicable diseases. Through a qualitative research method, this research categorizes the factors as inputs, processes and outputs and applies them into the 2003 SARS and MERS outbreak in South Korea. As the results conducted meta-analyses to comprehensively analyze the correlations of factors influencing disaster response from a Korean context, the findings show that the legislative factor had direct and indirect influence on the overall process of infectious disease response and that Leadership of the central government, establishment of an intergovernmental response system, the need for communication, information sharing and disclosure and onsite response were identified as key factors influencing effective infectious disease response.

Keywords: infectious diseases; meta-analyses; severe acute respiratory syndrome (SARS); Middle East Respiratory Syndrome (MERS); South Korea

---

1. Introduction

Recently, a wide array of disasters, including earthquakes, forest fires, various infectious disease outbreaks and marine accidents have occurred in Korea. Accordingly, the importance of disaster response has drawn more attention than it ever has in Korea, which was once considered a safe zone from various disasters. However, following the recent and sudden increase in the frequency of disasters, sufficient learning and legislature, as well as policy-making processes in Korea have exposed limitations in the disaster management system, relative to other countries and regions where disasters have occurred more frequently. The recent efforts to change the disaster response system after certain disasters has exposed many limitations. Under such circumstances, it is difficult to respond appropriately to disasters and there are limitations to avoiding or reducing social and economic losses caused by disasters.

After the sinking of MV Sewol, also called the Sewol ferry disaster, in 16 April 2014, the Korea Coast Guard was dissolved and the Ministry of Public Safety and Security (MPSS) took on the role of a control tower. Every episode of failed disaster response was always blamed on the lack of a control tower. Therefore, the introduction of MPSS was expected to be a panacea for effective disaster response. However, the initial response still failed during subsequent disasters, including in the Middle East respiratory syndrome (MERS) outbreak, the Geyongju earthquake and various marine accidents, which confirmed that the disaster response was still not being effectively executed. When President Moon took office, the new government underwent reorganization and in July 2017, MPSS was integrated into and absorbed by the Ministry of Interior and Safety. In 2018, the Department of Disaster and Safety Management within the Ministry of Interior and Safety took over the responsibilities that used to belong to MPSS.

Despite the persisting limitations in disaster response and management, studies related to disaster response continued to discuss the need to achieve the common goal of effective disaster management within a network with participation from regional government, central government, private organizations, citizen's groups and military units based on independence and autonomy [1–11]. Moreover, other studies outlined factors influencing disaster management and response from a macroscopic perspective and analyzed disaster management and response through awareness surveys [8,12–14]. Discussions on disaster resilience have been increasing in recent years. The term "resilience" refers to a concept that demonstrates the attributes of the ecosystem as a system, which has become a social science concept [15] and is being applied in disaster management. After a disaster, our society requires resilience to return to normalcy following the disaster's physical and social impact. This can be regarded as part of the recovery phase of disaster management. Resilience includes not only a physical system but also disaster resilience at the organizational level, which is the ability to cooperate in coordinating key resources by going above and beyond for the community and minimizing operational confusion [16]. Despite the various disaster-related studies in Korea and abroad mentioned above, studies about disasters within the context of Korea, where discussions on disasters have only recently begun, have been qualitatively and quantitatively insufficient. Therefore, in addition to the existing studies, diverse and comprehensive discussions consisting of identification and securement of resources for disaster management; information sharing; timely and accurate communication and coordination with relevant agencies; networking processes that organically link disaster prevention and preparedness during non-disaster times; response during a disaster; recovery after a disaster; and learning from the experience of the disaster; are needed for effective disaster response. However, as the present study focused on disaster response, its discussion section did not cover recovery that includes resilience.

Moreover, the present study focused on infectious diseases. Despite not being the first infectious disease outbreak in Korea, responses to the severe acute respiratory syndrome (SARS) outbreak in 2003 and the Middle East respiratory syndrome (MERS) outbreak in 2015 had completely different outcomes. In 2003, upon identification of the outbreak of an emerging infection known as SARS in China, immediate nationwide preventive measures and an organic cooperation system involving the central government, health centers and quarantine stations nationwide were implemented. In the end, approximately over 8000 people worldwide, including in China, were infected and approximately 770 people died. However, Korea had only three confirmed SARS patients and no deaths; as a result, Korea was assessed as a model nation for SARS prevention by the World Health Organization (WHO). By 2015, however, more than 10 years later, Korea's reputation regarding infectious disease response had been tarnished by systematic problems and the absence of disaster management and communication capacity. After the MERS outbreak, everyone felt the need for an in-depth examination of issues concerning how the infectious disease response system in Korea had changed over the past 10 years; the role of the central government, experts and the onsite command system and organizations at regional level; and how to solve some of those problems.

Despite the growing interest in and the need for further research, there are only few studies on the factors that determine the success and failure of infectious disease response and the responses to administrative and policy aspects. Therefore, the present study aimed to conduct a systematic investigation into the factors that influence disaster response, focusing specifically on infectious diseases by examining cases of outbreaks of infectious diseases that have occurred in Korea. The study aimed to analyze the correlations of the factors that influence infectious diseases by conducting a review of articles, precedent studies and other publications.

2. Theoretical and Institutional Background

2.1. Infectious Diseases

The present study conducted an in-depth review of the concept of infectious disease and infectious disease response, which are the subjects of its theoretical review. In the past, the terms "contagious" or "communicable disease" were generally used. However, because the term "communicable diseases" implied diseases that were transmitted from one person to another, which further implied difficulties in controlling them, the term was changed to "infectious diseases," which encompasses both communicable and non-communicable diseases. For effective prevention and management of infectious diseases, the existing "Parasitic Disease Prevention Act" and "Communicable Disease Prevention Act" were merged. According to the "Infectious Disease Control and Prevention Act," infectious diseases include Class 1–5 of infectious diseases, designated infectious diseases, WHO-monitored infectious diseases, bioterror infectious diseases, sexually transmitted diseases, zoonotic infectious diseases and healthcare-associated infections.

Korea has experienced outbreaks of diseases that were traditionally regarded as "diseases that occur in developing countries," such as hepatitis A, tuberculosis, chicken pox and malaria, while cholera patients were identified for the first time in 15 years in 2016. Moreover, despite continued outbreaks of emerging infectious diseases since the SARS outbreak, there have been no noticeable changes in prevention and response measures. With the subsequent occurrence of the MERS and Zika virus in Korea and the re-emergence of cholera, an infectious disease that had not been experienced for a while, public anxiety about health safety is growing. According to the Infectious Diseases Surveillance Yearbook published by the Korea Center for Disease Control and Prevention (KCDC), the level of imported infectious diseases has been increasing every year, with 300–400 newly reported cases every year since 2010.

Experts have warned that this is only the beginning of the war against infectious diseases, due to the following reasons. With the changing global environment and increased human migration, prevention of emergence or re-emergence of infectious diseases is fundamentally impossible. Moreover, infectious diseases tend to evolve along with advances in medical technology and emerging infectious diseases are difficult to handle since they spread quickly and have no readily available treatment. In particular, knowledge about the characteristics, route of infection and control measures of emerging infectious diseases are lacking or uncertain and it is difficult to predict when, where and how these diseases may emerge. Moreover, globalization has brought with it an increased level of international trade and travel. Therefore, Korea, which has a high foreign trade dependency, is constantly exposed to the risk of imported infectious diseases.

Despite the growing anxiety and concerns about infectious diseases, studies on infectious disease response and control are lacking. After the MERS outbreak, numerous studies on the response to this outbreak were conducted [17–37]. However, most of the studies focused mostly on medicine and communication, with relatively fewer studies focusing on administrative fields [38–46]. Studies in the medical field must precede the response to infectious diseases, so that information and knowledge about the infectious disease can be applied in response measures. However, if the national infectious disease response system is not ready when an actual infectious disease outbreak occurs, then medical determination and response, as well as crisis management and communication cannot be executed properly. This is because medical response, crisis management and communication are sub-elements in such a national-scale system. Therefore, it is important to conduct studies on infectious diseases and responses in every specialty. However, there is also need for comprehensive discussions that include the establishment of laws; regulations; resources; information on infectious disease response from administrative and policy perspectives; information sharing system; and the establishment of an international cooperation system and national response system involving the central government, the regional government, private organizations and the public for effective response when an actual infectious disease outbreak occurs.

In addition to infectious diseases being difficult to handle, the MERS outbreak in 2015 also revealed that even if prevention and response measures are in place, a failed initial response can lead to an unanticipated increase in the rate and scope of infection transmission. Moreover, disaster responses do not always pan out as planned and uncertainties and complexities that emerge after the disaster must be handled. Therefore, it is necessary to identify government-level responses and make effort to improve the response system. However, previous studies on responses to infectious diseases are still lacking despite the importance of this issue. Accordingly, the present study was conducted with the consciousness of the need to analyze response systems based on past response experiences in order to effectively respond to future infectious diseases, which are a threat. The present study analyzed two cases of infectious disease outbreaks based on the factors that influence response to disaster, as identified through existing studies and theories and aimed to derive factors that have a strong influence on the effectiveness of actual disaster response.

In the following section, the factors that influence disaster response will be categorized from a system theory perspective to form a categorization framework.

2.2. Factors That Influence Disaster Response

Factors that influence disaster response have been identified through numerous studies over several years. Most of the studies on disaster response analyzed actual cases by applying analytical tools based on major variables presented in existing studies and theories [14,47–54] or they analyzed the factors that influence disaster response by administering questionnaire surveys to members of agencies associated with disaster response [12,55,56]. Therefore, instead of comprehensively examining the factors influencing disaster response, these studies handled the subject at a macroscopic level, focusing on the major variables. The present study aimed to organize factors and variables that influence the entire process of disaster response from a comprehensive and systematic perspective and categorize these factors and variables based on a system theory perspective in order to present an analytical framework. This concept and context are similar to those of Perry [57], who claimed that influencing factors of disaster response that are derived without classifying according to disaster types do not need different analytical frameworks since they can be described and analyzed according to the factors presented and they only differ in intensity according to the type of disaster.

The present study reviewed existing studies, focusing on those with "disaster response" and "effective disaster response" as the outcome variables. The factors that influence disaster response can be broadly categorized into financial resources, human resources, physical resources, information, education and training, leadership, intergovernmental relationships, onsite response, information sharing, environmental context, characteristics of disaster and the legal/institutional environment.

Resources that influence disaster response can be categorized into financial, human and physical resources.

Financial resources include the government's budget for disaster response, funding to support processes involved in disaster response and support from the government or community [50–53]. Therefore, financial resources can be regarded as the disaster-related budget, the disaster management fund and financial support measures for processes entailed in Korea's disaster response system.

Human resources included disaster response-related organizations and agencies, education and training of relevant organizations and the general public and utilization of specialists. Existing studies have pointed out that the establishment of disaster response-related organizations or crisis management centers and the securement of specialists have a very significant influence on disaster response [49,51,52,55,58,59]. This is because identification of disaster response-related organizations and agencies must come first to allow effective communication about disaster response and secure accountability in disaster response [55]. Moreover, education and training for disaster response organizations and their members has been mentioned as an element that allows effective disaster response [49,51]. Lastly, physical resources refer to securement of disaster management-related resources and establishment of disaster management facilities. As indicated in the study by Lindell et al. [51], securement of disaster response and management resources within the organization allows timely and accurate disaster response, which was expressed as disaster response equipment in the study by Jung [56]. Such physical resources can be viewed as disaster management resources and facilities and whether the expansion of negative-pressure units and emergency isolation units have occurred also influences the response to infectious diseases.

Other influencing factors besides resource-related factors include education and training. Knowledge can be explained as a collection of disaster-related information and information sharing in advance, where information about different types of disasters must be collected before the occurrence of a disaster. Factors associated with disaster information have a positive effect on disaster response, as indicated in the study by Kim [60], which reported that when a disaster information system is established the recognition of the importance of information quality and higher information quality had a positive effect on achieving disaster management duties.

Next, leadership, intergovernmental relationships and communication, onsite response and information sharing have been identified as factors that influence disaster response. First, leadership in the context of this paper refers to leadership in the central government, which can be divided into leadership from the President and leadership from central organizations and agencies. The President's level of interest in disaster management and response and the governance style in running an organization, were analyzed as factors that have significant influence on disaster response [61]. Moreover, onsite leadership by the heads of organizations and agencies must be demonstrated in a timely manner, especially in initial disaster response, in order to prevent the disaster from spreading [50,53,56,59,62]. Second, intergovernmental relationships and communication are also factors that influence effective disaster response [50,52,53,63,64]. In addition, network was also pointed out as a factor that influences disaster response. Existing studies tended to use the concepts of network and inter-organizational cooperation without clearly differentiating them but both network and inter-organizational cooperation were analyzed as factors that positively influence disaster response [54,63,64]. One of the reasons inter-organizational communication and coordination, network and cooperation have been identified as important influencing factors is that appropriate allocation and utilization of disaster response-related resources are essential for effective disaster response. Accordingly, the present study analyzed intergovernmental relationships in order to comprehensively examine intergovernmental and inter-organizational relationships, communication and cooperation.

Information sharing has also been identified as an important factor in disaster response. Information sharing between organizations and with the general public after a disaster was found to have a positive influence on actual disaster response. In particular, a study by Hyun [6] found that information disclosure-related legislation, the organization's budget, personal awareness and attitude and information quality influenced the effectiveness of disaster management. Among various factors influencing disaster management and response, factors associated with disaster-related information disclosure and sharing were tested for their influence on the effectiveness of disaster management. The results showed that greater information quality in information disclosure and sharing and greater personal awareness and attitude positively influenced the effectiveness of disaster management. Effective disaster response may comprise sub-variables from its outcome aspect. In a study by Denise [65], the effectiveness of disaster response was determined by measuring life loss, property damage, satisfaction of stakeholders, society's resilience, operational efficiency and budget maximization. Moreover, a study by Byun (2014) examined fire service organizations and thus effectiveness was determined by evaluating fire containment and rescue, while efficiency was represented by reduction in damage and cost-effectiveness.

Other factors influencing disaster response include environmental factors [55,56,58,59], disaster characteristics [51,55,59] and legislative factors [3,51,55,66].

2.3. Introduction of Cases

2.3.1. SARS

SARS stands for Severe Acute Respiratory Syndrome. It has a latency period of 10 days, after which the victim experiences high fever (≥38 °C), coughing and respiratory distress. It is transmitted by respiratory routes to medical staff and family members who come in close contact with the patient. Complete cure is possible if treatment is administered early, where approximately 90% of infected patients recover easily within one week. However, SARS may rapidly become severe for elderly or frail patients or for patients with chronic illness, yielding a mortality rate of approximately 3.5%.

SARS became known worldwide on 11 February 2003, when the Chinese health authority announced that 305 patients with SARS had been identified in China between November 16, 2002 and 9 February 2003, five of whom had died. WHO, which had strengthened its surveillance activities in the Asian region after identifying the likelihood of the emergence of influenza, issued a worldwide warning on 12 March 2003. According to the official statistics released by WHO in November 2003, between November 2002 and July 2003, a total of 8098 suspected SARS cases from a total of 28 countries were identified and a total of 774 SARS related deaths were reported. Consequently, SARS emerged as the first new disease in the 21st century that was highly contagious and severe and its transmission through international air travel received special attention.

Since February 2003, when SARS became known for the first time, Korea continued to monitor SARS outbreak trends through WHO data and recognized the need for national quarantine measures. Accordingly, guidelines for strengthening nationwide SARS quarantine measures were passed down on 12 February 2003 and on March 16 the Korean government issued a SARS alert, in keeping with the announcement of the global SARS alert by WHO and established a quarantine system. With NIH playing a central role, all healthcare institutions, including 12 national quarantine stations and 242 health centers, maintained a 24-hour emergency operation-ready status as part of the emergency SARS quarantine measures. Moreover, a quarantine system was established by designating 41 hospitals as isolation treatment hospitals according to regions. In addition, the policy of measuring people's body temperature as they entered the country through airports and sea ports was implemented in order to detect SARS inflow from overseas and to prevent the disease from spreading. Furthermore, follow-up investigations were conducted on people who entered Korea from SARS-risk regions and a system through which patients suspected of being infected could be transported immediately for isolation and treatment was put in place. Moreover, additional isolation measures were implemented for people who came in contact with infected patients to prevent the disease from spreading further, in addition to preventing the import of SARS. Recommendations were made to refrain from traveling to high-risk regions to further prevent the import of SARS into Korea and to encourage precautions during travel.

During the response process to the outbreak, a meeting for city and provincial quarantine officials and experts was held on 3 April 2003. On 23 April 2003, a discussion was held on measures of blocking the importation of SARS and preventing its spread. The decision to implement government-wide response measures by setting up a central SARS measures headquarter, led by the Minister of Health and Welfare and satellite stations at city and province levels was made. Subsequently on 28 April 2003, a government-wide comprehensive SARS situation room was introduced and Prime Minister Kun Goh released a general public statement, urging active cooperation from the general public regarding the response measures taken by the government. Eventually, WHO declared on 17 June 2003 that Korea had won the war against SARS, effectively subduing SARS in less than 100 days after the global SARS alert was issued [67].

2.3.2. MERS

MERS stands for Middle East respiratory syndrome. The outbreak of MERS coronavirus started on 24 April 2015 following its introduction into Korea by a 68-year-old male, who worked in floriculture and was returning home to Korea after a visit to the Middle East. The patient was treated at a clinic for a fever he developed seven days after arriving in Korea but his condition did not improve. After his visit to the clinic, he received inpatient treatment for three days at Pyeongtaek St. Mary's Hospital and was subsequently discharged. Because of continued symptoms of high fever and respiratory distress, he visited another clinic and was eventually admitted to a single-bed unit at the Samsung Medical Center in Seoul on 18 May 2015. The staff at Samsung Medical Center had learned that the patient had visited the Middle East and based on a suspicion of MERS, the doctor in charge requested KCDC to perform further testing on the patient the following day (19 May 2015). The diagnostic test performed by NIH detected Middle East Respiratory Syndrome CoronaVirus: (MERS-CoV) genes in the patient. Following the announcement of these findings on 20 May 2015, identification of the first MERS patient in Korea was officially reported [68].

As shown in Figure 1, the first MERS patient in Korea visited multiple clinics and large hospitals for treatment over a 10-day period since the symptoms first appeared, during which time he came in contact with family members, other patients and medical staff, resulting in many cases of secondary infection.

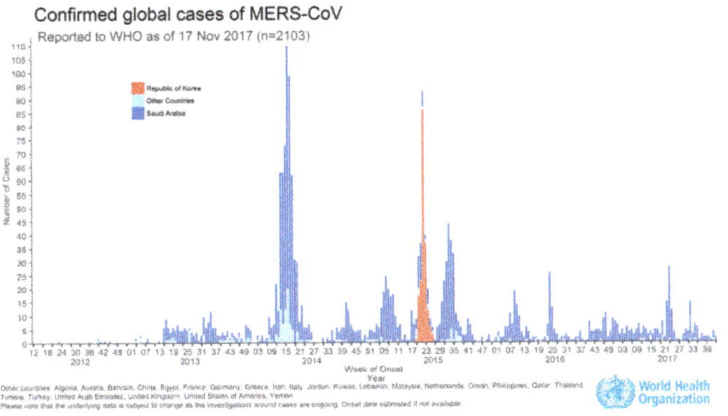

Figure 1. Confirmed global cases of MERS-CoV (source: https://www.who.int/emergencies/mers-cov/en/).

As shown in the graph above, the highest number of confirmed MERS cases outside of the Middle East region was found in Korea.

The response to MERS completely exposed contradictions in the national quarantine system, as well the healthcare system. KCDC and local government entities all proved inadequate in their ability to respond to the public health crisis caused by this infectious disease. There was confusion due to lack of clarity in the delegation of roles between the central and regional governments and the cooperation system between health authorities and medical institutions did not operate smoothly either. Most medical institutions, including general hospitals, small-to-medium-sized hospitals and clinics, were not prepared to deal with healthcare-associated infections and as a result the infection continued to spread among patients and medical staff. In addition, problems in the transport and referral system for confirmed or suspected patients were discovered, while compensation for medical institutions and research and development of emerging infectious diseases became points of contention. Moreover, medical staff who participated in the isolation and treatment of MERS patients complained about job-related burden and stress.

The MERS outbreak exposed fundamental problems in the public healthcare system and vulnerabilities in the national quarantine system but the solutions to these problems have not been clearly identified to date. The MERS outbreak caused restrictions in Korean citizens' day to day lives and significantly impacted the national economy. The socioeconomic impact of MERS has still not been accurately assessed. What is clear at this point is that the entire Korean society has become more interested in infectious diseases and that infectious diseases have become an agenda directly linked to public safety.

Moreover, people recognized that in order to respond to emerging infectious diseases it is necessary to continually assess and monitor infectious diseases that occur worldwide and establish manuals based on up-to-date knowledge through research, specialists and timely crisis analysis during the response process. In addition, the need to establish an infectious disease response network and partnerships between medical institutions and local government, as well as a central government, was also presented.

3. Study Design

3.1. Factor Categorization

The objective of this study was to inductively explore the factors that influence response based on studies related to disaster and infectious disease response. For this, a meta-analysis method called successive approximation was used [69]. Prior to inductive exploration of the factors that influence disaster response, sample articles were used to categorize these factors. The study also aimed to perform successive meta-analyses to present a model based on detailed explanation and revision of the previously established factors influencing disaster response. Accordingly, the present study used a rough model based on the categorization of the factors influencing disaster response presented in existing studies to perform meta-analyses on SARS and MERS cases.

In summary, after establishing the initial model, several rounds of meta-analyses were performed to refine the model. Accordingly, the incomplete preliminary theoretical framework, which can be viewed as the initial model, represented simplification and categorization of major factors through existing disaster response-related studies. The study aimed to conduct successive analyses based on the incomplete framework to present a refined model by revising the factors and the relationships between them. Accordingly, precedent studies previously examined in Chapter 2 were used to derive the factors influencing disaster response from a system perspective. On a review of numerous studies, it was discovered that the duties assigned to various organizations and agencies and the factors that actually influence disaster response show regularity [47,70,71]. Therefore, based on such regularity, the study aimed to categorize these factors according to timelines from a system theory perspective.

First, the studies that presented communication, coordination, cooperation and network from the process level as the mediating variables for effective disaster response included those by [3,50,55,71]. Other studies selected the process level variable as one variable among many independent variables in analyzing the influence on effective disaster response. It was commonly pointed out that resources related to disaster response influenced the outcome of disaster response through the interactions and coordination between organizations and agencies in the response process.

Kapucu [71] analyzed the influence of the system, organizational environment, tools for organizational capability and cooperation and the decision-making process of actors in the entire process on effective disaster response. The system was a variable that included organizational structure, culture and goals, while the environment included time pressure, uncertainty and complexity of the situation. Capability was a factor that involved decision-making support, communication tools, previous cooperation experience, flexibility in responding to disaster and immediate response capability, while actors included the number of stakeholders, experts, interdependence and trust. The study examined whether these independent variables influenced effective disaster response through cooperative decision-making processes, meaning open and honest exchange of opinions, shared model construction, negotiation and utilization of relevant knowledge and information. The proposed research model was used to conduct social network analysis through content analysis, in addition to in-depth case analysis on countries that were victims of terrorist attacks, including the US, Indonesia, Turkey, Spain and the UK. Moreover, a study by Lindell et al. [51] also revealed that various resources influenced disaster planning and such process had a significant influence on the efficiency of disaster response. On the basis of these studies, a framework consisting of independent variables having an influence on the effectiveness of disaster response through the disaster response processes was constructed. Even in studies that do not present process variables as mediating factors, the majority of process variables were selected as independent variables for analysis and thus it is necessary to reorganize and categorize the variables that were presented in previous studies.

As shown in Figure 2 the present study selected the factors influencing disaster response presented in existing studies and categorized them largely into environment, inputs and process based on system theory. This model was presented because disasters act as a single system that includes the aforementioned factors, regardless of their type (natural or social disaster) [54,72–74]. The strength of the influencing factors may vary depending on the type of disaster but because they were described and analyzed by the factors that are presented below, analyzing or describing social and natural disasters using different frameworks is unnecessary [57]. Based on the categorization of the influencing factors shown in the figure below, the study aimed to conduct future meta-analyses to explore detailed factors and identify the relationships between these factors.

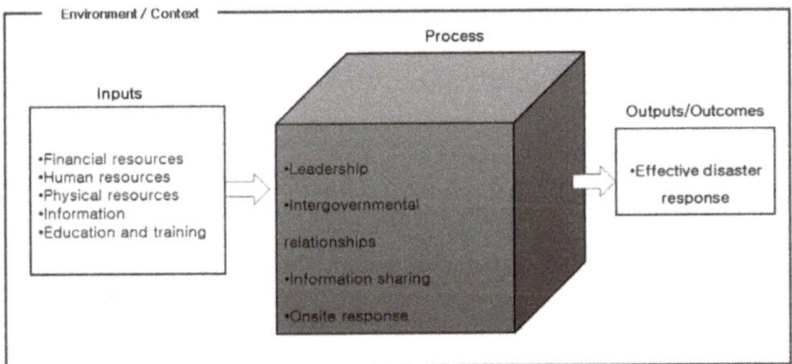

Figure 2. Categorization of the factors influencing disaster response.

3.2. Scope and Method of Analysis

For inductive exploration of the factors influencing infectious disease response, meta-analyses were performed based on the aforementioned factor categorization framework and in-depth interviews were conducted for testing and supplementation.

The present study used previous studies on disaster response to compile a list of the factors influencing disaster response and presented a theoretical framework. Moreover, the factors influencing disaster response were explored through case review, while qualitative meta-analysis was performed to identify the correlations between the factors. Qualitative meta-analysis was conducted to allow a comprehensive analysis of qualitative studies [60]. This method of analysis is different from meta-analysis which integrates results from existing empirical studies using a quantitative method [75,76]. The approach in qualitative meta-analysis involves interpretive analysis, which strives to include major concepts that appeared in individual qualitative studies but at the same time, generate a higher-level concept that can connect these concepts to a higher dimensional theoretical structure to allow for comprehensive understanding of the phenomenon and possibility of new interpretation and theoretical creation [77].

Therefore, the major goal of qualitative meta-analysis is to contribute to knowledge. From this perspective, Schreier et al. [78] listed theory building, theory explication and theory development as the three overlapping goals of qualitative meta-analysis. In the present study, the factors influencing disaster response were reviewed from existing studies in the theory building process and organized from a system theory level. Subsequently, meta-analysis was performed to explore factors through Korean studies and articles and interviews. The protocol was constructed through data collection and analysis and effort was made to ensure reliability and validity of the study [79].

Using this approach, the study was conducted systematically, from the data collection stage to the final analysis. After comprehensively collecting data, including domestic research articles, media reports and audit reports from the Board of Audit and Inspection (BAI) of Korea related to SARS and MERS cases, data to be analyzed were selected on the basis of the inclusion and exclusion criteria. The data collection method will be discussed in more detail in the data collection section.

The collected data were codified and categorized on the basis of the meta-analysis framework consisting of the factors influencing disaster response extracted from existing studies and theories. As shown in Figure 3, for the influencing factors identified from the data, the factor and source were recorded, and evidence of the correlation was identified. The evidence included statistical data, media reports, interviews with experts and claims made by authors. With this coding process, consistency of the results when the same analysis is performed by different researchers can be maintained and this can be used to ensure reliability.

ID	Coder	Govern ance ty pe	Data name	Category (content/source)	Environmental factors	Input factors	Gov. process factors	Outcome
					1. Disaster characteristics 2. Administrative and politic al factors (political party, nat ional assembly, media, etc.) 3. Legislation 4. Sociocultural environmen t 5. Economic environment 6. Others	1. Financial resources 2. Human resources 3. Physical resources/infrastructure 4. Information 5. Education and training 6. Others	Factors corresponding to the gover nance process This varies according to the type of governance 1. Leadership 2. Intergovernmental relationships and response system (including inte r-organizational communication) 3. Information sharing 4. Onsite response 5. Others	Effective disaster response 1. Life and property damage 2. Stakeholder satisfaction 3. Resilience

Evidence (content)	Evidence (validity/reliability)	Remarks
Reliable worker interviews, official govern ment data, media reports, researcher case a nalyses, statistical analysis, and others	Use a 10-point scale (1 – very low, 5 – average, 10 – very high)	Details

Figure 3. Coding framework.

Data for meta-analysis were collected from various sources, including listed academic journals, articles from daily and weekly periodicals and audit reports from BAI. Duplicate items were eliminated based on search results and data that met the objective of the present study were selected through in-depth reviews and discussions with fellow researchers.

Academic articles were limited to those published in journals listed in the National Research Foundation of Korea, while duplicate articles and articles with low correlation to the research question were excluded. The period of data of academic articles was from 2003 (SARS outbreak) to 2017 (at the time of the research). All searched articles were tallied and data were selected through validity testing and unanimity with fellow researchers.

Media reports were collected from daily and weekly periodicals to provide information that was not covered in academic articles. The search process used the Naver news site and the official home pages of each newspaper. The search keywords were disaster case names: SARS, MERS and different variations of these terms in Korean. Additionally, data that mentioned a disaster name along with the term "response" were reviewed. To eliminate political bias, Chosun Ilbo, Donga Ilbo, Kyunghyang Shinmun and Hankyoreh were selected from daily periodicals, while Weekly Chosun, Weekly Donga, Weekly Kyunghyang and Hankyoreh 21 were selected from weekly periodicals. The period included in data collection was set to one year to include the infection outbreak and response period between January and December 2003 for SARS and between January and December 2015 for MERS. Lastly, the homepage of BAI was searched for BAI audit reports on SARS and MERS but since audit reports for SARS did not exist only MERS cases were analyzed. Among the 59 cases that appeared as search results for MERS, the results that were unrelated to the selected cases were excluded. As a result, a total of 38 cases of audit reports for various organizations were selected for the analysis (Table 1).

Table 1. Analysis of targets.

Category		SARS	MERS
Academic articles	Total search results	110 cases	229 cases
	Selected for analysis	0 cases	4 cases
Media reports	Total search results	120 cases	2416 cases
	Selected for analysis	5 cases	28 cases
BAI audit reports	Total search results	0 cases	59 cases
	Selected for analysis	0 cases	38 cases

4. Analysis of Results

The results of factors coded and explored based on aforementioned media reports, BAI audit reports, academic articles and in-depth interviews are provided here. To effectively demonstrate the results of exploring the factors influencing disaster response, analysis was performed by identifying how each factor, as an independent factor, influenced other factors; and by gathering evidence of the relationship between time, cause and outcomes.

The present study underwent the process of identifying and testing correlations through a meta-analysis of the factors influencing infectious disease response. The analysis results on the factors influencing infectious disease response were as follows.

Legislation, sociocultural factors and disaster characteristics were identified as the environmental factors influencing disaster response. With respect to SARS, although there was no legislative system for disaster response and management, some respiratory transmission diseases, including SARS, were temporarily designated as "infectious diseases subject to quarantine and surveillance" for onsite response. Enactment and amendment of laws have procedural and time requirements and thus quarantine or isolation was made possible by presenting them as subjects of quarantine and surveillance following the decree of the Minister of Health and Welfare, which actually had a positive influence on onsite response. Moreover, while legislation for MERS was in place, it was incomplete and not detailed enough. This caused confusion in the response process because of the possibility of arbitrary decisions and because it contained inaccurate information about infectious diseases, it had a negative influence on onsite response. Consequently, MERS spread to other patients, leading to a failed initial response. Moreover, unlike the SARS outbreak, when international public health crisis was declared, there was no announcement of an international public health crisis with MERS, which caused a lack of awareness on the importance of prevention and response.

Financial resources, human resources, physical resources, information and education and training were identified as the input factors influencing disaster response. Human resources also acted as a mediating factor in the relationship between legislation and the effectiveness of response to infectious diseases. In the processes of responding to SARS and MERS, problems related to human resources, especially epidemiologists, were identified. This was also very apparent in the correlations. Although epidemiological investigation in infectious disease response is very important for preventing the spread of infectious diseases and for timely response, an insufficient number of epidemiologists made it impossible to keep up with the rate at which the disease was spreading and since public health physicians were mostly responsible for epidemiological investigation, a lack of specialization was also a serious problem. Moreover, budget, the proportion of public healthcare and infection control infrastructure, such as negative-pressure units, were also found to be insufficient during both SARS and MERS outbreaks. One of the factors that was identified as being important in the correlation analysis was education and training. Since everyone may experience an actual disaster, simulated training according to given scenarios and education for response personnel are very important.

Leadership, intergovernmental relationships, information sharing and onsite response were identified as the process factors influencing response to infectious disease outbreak, while information sharing was found to influence stakeholder satisfaction. With respect to leadership, as mentioned earlier, the role of the prime minister and the president was an important factor in the implementation of timely and effective disaster response. During the SARS outbreak, Prime Minister Kun Goh was at the forefront, urging the public and departments to cooperate. On the other hand, during the process of responding to MERS, the control tower changed at least twice and the president made it clear through the spokesperson that the Blue House was not the control tower. During this process, the intergovernmental relationship was not smooth either. Moreover, poor information sharing and communication between departments and between the central and local government caused confusion and increased the level of distrust among the general public. Among the process factors, intergovernmental relationships, information sharing and onsite response were independent variables that influenced the outcome and acted as mediating factors between legislation and outcome.

Lastly, although not presented in existing analytical frameworks, the factors identified through meta-analysis and interviews were interest and cooperation from the private sector (volunteerism). With respect to interest, an analysis of SARS cases showed that the interest of local citizens, meaning regional self-centeredness, caused the designation of SARS quarantine hospitals to be nullified, acting as a factor that interfered with infectious disease response. These factors were confirmed in the interview results. The interest of the agency in charge of the control tower emerged as a factor that interfered with the infectious disease response, albeit at a different level than the interest of local citizens. The agency in charge of determining the disclosure of information was the MOHW and because the same agency was responsible for both promoting actual related projects and managing disaster, conflict of interest did not allow immediate response measures to be implemented.

Cooperation from the private sector (volunteerism) was a factor that did not appear in the meta-analysis but was identified in interviews with workers. Its correlations were not analyzed in the meta-analysis data of the present study and existing studies did not discuss the role of volunteers in infectious disease response either. However, resource support for self-quarantine patients in actual infectious disease response was lacking but active participation by volunteers played a major role in helping to slow the spread of MERS and to successfully implement self-quarantine.

Moreover, the hidden context of correlations identified through interviews, which was not identified in existing articles, was education and training. Education and training was analyzed as a factor influencing infectious disease response, while the interview results revealed that education and training not only had a direct influence on response but also had an impact on the relationship between the people in charge of disaster response. Timely response was made possible by relationships built between people in charge of disaster response through continued training, which may be attributed to the uniqueness of Korean culture.

As shown earlier, the factors influencing infectious disease response in Korea were very diverse and they became more refined and detailed when compared to categorization of factors presented in the introduction of this paper. These were factors identified through meta-analyses and in-depth interviews and should be considered in the improvement of the infectious disease response system in Korea. A comprehensive model that summarizes the aforementioned exploration of the influencing factors is shown in Figure 4.

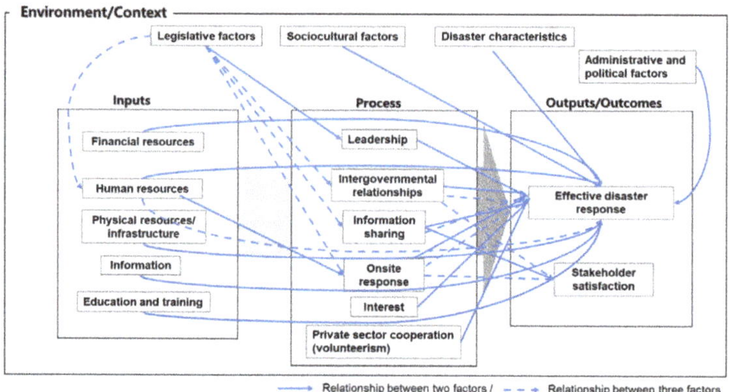

Figure 4. Model of factors influencing infectious disease response in Korea.

5. Conclusions

The present study conducted meta-analyses to comprehensively analyze the correlations of factors influencing disaster response from a Korean context. For inductive exploration of the factors influencing infectious disease response in Korea, the present study collected and selected reliable data from academic research on infectious disease response conducted in Korea, newspaper articles and audit reports from BAI. The reason for limiting the studies to those conducted within Korea was based on the determination that it was necessary to review how well domestic studies and articles explained domestic cases. The objective was to use the findings to point out the limitations of infectious disease-related studies in Korea and to present factors influencing infectious disease response within a Korean context.

The analysis results confirmed that, overall, the studies Korea focused on factors from the process aspect when analyzing the factors influencing infectious disease response. A summary of other major findings are as follows:

First, among environmental factors, the legislative factor had direct and indirect influence on the overall process of infectious disease response. Other environmental factors were regarded as factors influencing disaster response based on their correlations but the legislative factor was considered especially important. Disaster-related legislation enacted in various forms including basic laws, manuals and code of conduct should be systematic and exhibit high integrity to allow timely and accurate response in crisis situations. However, owing to insufficiencies in many aspects, it had a negative influence throughout the entire response process.

The legislative factor indirectly influenced disaster response, making it an important factor that influences the overall disaster response process. In other words, human resource was identified as the mediating factor in the relationship between the legislative factor, human resources and onsite response. On the other hand, intergovernmental relationships, information sharing and onsite response were identified as the mediating factors in the relationships between the legislative factor, intergovernmental relationships and the effectiveness of disaster response; the relationship between the legislative factor, information sharing and the effectiveness of disaster response and the relationship between the legislative factor, onsite response and the effectiveness of disaster response, respectively. Along with the determination of mediating factors, the study also found that the establishment of legislation had an overall impact on infectious disease response.

Second, the results showed that most input factors, including physical resources, human resources and information were insufficient. Within a Korean context, it is believed that this problem stemmed from the lack of a disaster response system or many studies related to disaster response, as indicated by the fact that basic laws about disaster management were implemented in Korea from 2004. Considering that the systematization of disaster response following the passing of basic related laws was relatively recent, more detailed issues, such as securement of resources, did not draw attention until a disaster actually occurred, leading to gradual improvement. Therefore, factors related to these resources showed insufficiencies no matter which case was reviewed. However, considering the differences in the timeframes of the cases raises concern on whether the experience gained from the disaster response system is actually being used as an asset to improve the disaster response system in Korea.

Third, major findings regarding process factors were as follows. Leadership of the central government, establishment of an intergovernmental response system, the need for communication, information sharing and disclosure and onsite response were identified as key factors influencing effective infectious disease response. Existing studies have found that information sharing occurred top-down, from the central government to local government [80]. Even so, information sharing was correlated with process factors. Nondisclosure of hospital names by the government had an impact on the spread of infectious diseases and on failed initial response. Further, the general public voluntarily shared information and made the effort to share accurate information, such as creating a MERS map and sharing information on websites. In addition, the interests of local citizens and departments also acted as a factor that interfered with effective infectious disease response.

By analyzing the factors influencing infectious disease response within a Korean context, the present study presents the following theoretical and policy implications. Theoretically, the study established a model of factors influencing infectious disease response by performing inductive exploration on the factors influencing infectious disease response in Korea, which was utilized for comprehensive analysis. Policy-wise, the study aimed to emphasize the need for improvement of infectious disease response-related legislation, strengthening the authority of KCDC, which currently serves as the control tower, qualitative and quantitative supplementation of disaster response-related human resources, legal grounds for the authority of response personnel and preparation of protective measures. Lastly, since the importance of information collection and sharing and cooperation between agencies was demonstrated, it is necessary to establish a system for information sharing and disclosure, as well as a cooperation system involving the central government, the local government, health centers and medical institutions.

Author Contributions: K.M. designed study and collected data; K.J. gave an important advice on analyzing data; and K.M. and K.J. wrote the paper.

Funding: This work was supported by the Ministry of Education of the Republic of Korea and the National Research Foundation of Korea (NRF-2016S1A3A2924832) as well as the National Research Foundation of Korea (NRF-2016S1A3A2924956).

Acknowledgments: This study summarizes the doctoral dissertation of Kyu-Myung Lee (2018).

Conflicts of Interest: The authors declare no conflict of interest.

References

1. Kapucu, N. Interorganizational Coordination in Dynamic Context- Networks in Emergency Response Management. *Connections* **2005**, *26*, 33–48.
2. Kapucu, N. Interorganizational Coordination in Complex Environments of Disasters—The Evolution of Intergovernmental Disaster Response Systems. *JHSEM* **2009**, *6*. [CrossRef]
3. Schneider, S.K. Government Response to Disaster: The Conflict between Bureaucratic Procedures and Emergent Norms. *Public Adm. Rev.* **1992**, *52*, 135–145. [CrossRef]
4. Moynihan, D.P. *The Dynamics of Performance Management: Constructing Information and Reform*; Georgetown University Press: Washington, DC, USA, 2008.
5. Robinson, S.E.; Eller, W.S.; Gall, M.; Gerber, B.J. The core and periphery of emergency management networks. *Public Manag. Rev.* **2013**, *15*, 344–362. [CrossRef]
6. Hyun, S.H.; Lee, B.K.; Kim, K.W.; Chu, B.J. A Comparative Study on Emergency System of Local Government: Focus on the Marine Environmental Damage by Oil Pollution in South Korea and Japan. *Korean Public Adm. Rev.* **2009**, *43*, 273–306.
7. Boo, H.W.; Dudley, L.S. Management of Emergent Networks during Disasters—A Meta synthesis. *Korean J. Policy Stud.* **2012**, *27*, 23–42.
8. Cho, J.M.; Ryu, S.I. Relationship between Effectiveness of Disaster Management and Cooperative Factors of Agencies in Disaster Management. *J. Korean Assoc. Crisis Emerg. Manag.* **2010**, *2*, 1–13.
9. Lee, E.H. MERS Isolation Patient—A Public Enemy? *Issue Diagn.* **2015**, *212*, 1–24.
10. Yoo, S.D.; Jeon, S.H. A Study on the Implementation Factors and Collaborative Governance of Disaster Management Policy: Focusing on the Recognition of Local Governments Officials. *Korean Gov. Rev.* **2016**, *23*, 87–115.
11. Cho, N.H.; Chai, W.H. Building the Governance System for the Effective Disaster Management of Local Government: Focusing on Buchon City. *Korean Assoc. Policy Sci.* **2008**, *12*, 227–254.
12. Hyun, M.J. An Empirical Study on the Factors of Effective Disaster Management: Focused on the Disclosure and Sharing of Information of the Local Government. Ph.D. Thesis, University of Seoul, Seoul, Korea, 2016.
13. Chae, J.; Woo, S.C. The Study on the Factors Affecting the Effectiveness of Disaster Management in Governance—Focused Recognition of Fire Officials. *Fire Sci. Eng.* **2009**, *234*, 79–90.
14. Jo, S.J. Improvement of administrative response system of infectious diseases: An information-process perspective. *J. Gov. Stud.* **2016**, *11*, 77–109.
15. Palmboom, G.; Willems, D. Dealing with Vulnerability: Balancing Prevention with Resilience as a Mehod of Governance. In *Vulnerability in Technological Cultures: New Directions in Research and Governance*; Hommels, A., Mesman, J., Bijker, W.E., Eds.; The MIT Press: Cambridge, MA, USA, 2014; pp. 267–284.
16. Jung, K.D.; Yoon, Y.K.; Seo, J.S.; Im, P.J.; Sin, S.W. A study on urban railway passenger's safety strategy for emergency: A focus on the MERS case. In Proceedings of the 2015 Korean Society for Railway General Meeting and Fall Conference, Yeosu, Korea, 22 October 2015; pp. 1357–1362.
17. Kim, K.H. Uncertainties of International Standards in the MERS CoV Outbreak in Korea: Multiplicity of Uncertainties. *Korean J. Environ. Sociol.* **2016**, *20*, 317–351.
18. Kim, M.C. A Reflection on Korean MERS Crisis in 2015: Socio-Medical Approach. *Korean J. Sci. Technol. Stud.* **2016**, *16*, 5–22.
19. Kim, M.K.; Lee, E.J. The Study on Behavior Intention of Health Protection Affected by News Media and News Usage, News Reliability on MERS Outbreak. *Media Perform. Arts Res.* **2016**, *11*, 119–144.
20. Kim, W.J. A Study on the Impact of the Epidemic Disease on the Number of Books Checked Out of the Public Libraries: Based on the Middle East Respiratory Syndrome Coronavirus. *J. Korean Soc. Inf. Manag.* **2015**, *32*, 273–287.
21. Kim, E.S. A Social Analysis of the Limitation of Governmental MERS Risk Communication. *Crisisonomy* **2015**, *11*, 91–109. [CrossRef]
22. Kim, J.H. A Study on the Use of Twitter by Local Government for Coping with Disaster. *Korean Assoc. Public Soc.* **2016**, *6*, 5–30. [CrossRef]
23. Nam, J.H. MERS: 70 Days of Records. *Kwanhun J.* **2015**, *136*, 16–22.
24. Park, H.G.; Kim, S.H.; Yang, J.A. The Effects of Exposure to MERS Information and Issue Involvement on Perceived Information Influence, Disease Prevention and Information Sharing. *J. Media Econ. Cult.* **2016**, *14*, 7–48. [CrossRef]
25. Seo, M.H. Effects of Risk Information Seeking and Processing on MERS Preventive Behaviors and Moderating Roles of SNS Use during 2015 MERS Outbreak in Korea. *Korean J. Commun. Inf.* **2016**, *78*, 116–140.

26. Sung, H.G. Impacts of the Outbreak and Proliferation of the Middle East Respiratory Syndrome on Rail Transit Ridership in the Seoul Metropolitan City. *J. Korea Plan. Assoc.* **2016**, *51*, 163–179. [CrossRef]
27. Ahn, J.C. The age of infectious diseases, where is the reporting standing. *Broadcast Rep.* **2016**, *25*, 28–29.
28. Oh, H.Y.; Cho, A.R.; Park, J.A.; Gil, E.H. Contents and Quality of Online News Articles on Preventive Food for MERS during MERS Outbreak in South Korea. *Crisisonomy* **2015**, *11*, 167–184. [CrossRef]
29. Yoo, W.H.; Jung, Y.G. The Roles of Interpersonal Communication between Exposure to Mass Media and MERS-Preventive Behavioral Intentions: The Moderating and Mediating Effects of Face-to-Face and Online Communication. *Korean J. Broadcast. Telecommun. Stud.* **2016**, *30*, 121–151.
30. Yoon, J.T. The Study of Effectiveness of MERS on the Law and Remaining Task. *Korean Soc. Law Med.* **2015**, *16*, 263–291.
31. Lee, M.A.; Hong, J.H. Semantic Network Analysis of Government's Crisis Communication Messages during the MERS Outbreak. *J. Korea Contents Assoc.* **2016**, *16*, 124–136. [CrossRef]
32. Lee, I.W. Policy PR and Crisis Management Communication: The Case of Seoul Metropolitan Government on MERS. *J. Soc. Sci.* **2016**, *42*, 67–104.
33. Jang, K.E.; Baek, Y.M. How did MERS Outbreak Become a Political Matter?: How Political Ideology Moderates the Effect of Multidimensional Health Locus of Control Beliefs on Citizens' Attribution Process of MERS Outbreak. *Korean J. Commun Stud.* **2016**, *6*, 36–65. [CrossRef]
34. Jang, S.J.; Hah, S.T. News Frames about Political Leaders of Different Genders in National Crises: A Comparative Analysis of A(H1N1) in 2009 and MERS in 2015. *J. Political Commun.* **2016**, *41*, 109–147.
35. Jeon, H.J. An Analysis of Risk Communication—A Case Study of MERS—CoV in Korea. *Crisisonomy* **2016**, *12*, 143–155. [CrossRef]
36. Jung, H.J.; Choi, A.L.; Lee, G.J.; Kim, J.Y.; Jeong, S.Y. Turnover intention of nurses that were cohort quarantined during the Middle East Respiratory Syndrome (MERS) outbreak. *J. Korea Acad.-Ind. Coop. Soc.* **2017**, *18*, 175–184.
37. Cho, G.Y.; Yoo, J.S. Estimating economic loss from MERS-CoV. *KERI Insight* **2017**, *20*, 1–16.
38. Choi, B.D. Geography of MERS outbreak and politics of bio-power. *Space Environ.* **2015**, *53*, 173–192.
39. Kim, B.C.; Kim, J.I. Risk Society and Bureaucratic Responsibility: A Comparative Analysis between Sewol Ferry Disaster and MERS-CoV. *Korean Soc. Public Adm.* **2016**, *26*, 379–407.
40. Park, D.K.; Jang, C.Y. Directions for Crisis Management: Lessons from MERS in South Korea. In Proceedings of the Korean Association for Public Administration Winter Conference, Chungcheongbuk-do, Korea, 23–25 June 2016; pp. 245–259.
41. Park, C.S.; Baek, D.S. An Analysis of Blame Avoidance Behaviors from the Failure of Initial Governmental Responses to MERS. *Korean J. Public Adm.* **2017**, *55*, 41–76.
42. Seo, K.H.; Lee, J.C.; Kim, K.H.; Lee, E. A Review on the Korea's National Public Health Crisis System. *Public Policy Rev.* **2015**, *29*, 219–242.
43. Seo, J.H. Future issues and the direction of healthcare system reform in Korea brought on by MERS crisis. *Korea Public Adm. Forum* **2015**, *150*, 30–37.
44. Ahn, Y.H. Status and task of infection prevention by regional local government as viewed through the MERS outbreak. *Korea Local Adm. Rev.* **2015**, *64*, 20–23.
45. Lee, P.S. Four problems and improvement measures of public-private cooperation system for infection prevention viewed from MERS outbreak. *Korea Local Adm. Rev.* **2015**, *64*, 26–29.
46. Chun, J.S.; Lee, S.Y. The Study on Medical Privatization Policy Change through ACF and Policy Network Model. *Korean Soc. Public Adm.* **2015**, *26*, 385–414.
47. Drabek, T.E. Managing the Emergency Response. *Public Adm. Rev.* **1985**, *45*, 85–92. [CrossRef]
48. Rijpma, J.A. Complexity, Tight-coupling and Reliability: Connecting Normal Accidents Theory and High Reliability Theory. *J. Conting. Crisis Manag.* **1997**, *5*, 15–23. [CrossRef]
49. Cohen, S.; Eimicke, W.; Horan, J. Catastrophe and the Public Service: A Case Study of the Government Response to the Destruction of the World Trade Center. *Public Adm. Rev.* **2002**, *62*, 24–32. [CrossRef]
50. Kapucu, N. Interagency Communication Networks during Emergencies: Boundary Spanners in Multiagency Coordination. *Am. Rev. Public Adm.* **2006**, *36*, 207–225. [CrossRef]
51. Lindell, M.K.; Prater, C.S.; Perry, R.W. *Fundamentals of Emergency Management*; FEMA: Washington, DC, USA, 2006.
52. Céline, T.; Resodihardjo, S.L. All the best laid plans conditions impeding proper emergency response. *Int. J. Prod. Econ.* **2010**, *126*, 7–21.
53. Lee, Y.C. Causes and Management Strategies of Natural Disasters: Three Cases and AHP Analysis. Ph.D. Thesis, Incheon National University, Incheon, Korea, 2007.

54. Ryu, S.I. Comparative Study on Disaster Response Systems of Local Government with Reference to Network Approach. *Korean Public Adm. Rev.* **2007**, *41*, 287–313.
55. Lee, J.E. A Study of Crisis Management Policy in Korea: An Analysis of Multi-Organizational Relationships in the Implementation Structure. Ph.D. Thesis, Yonsei University, Yonsei, Korea, 2000.
56. Byun, S.H. Uniformed Rank System and Its Effects on Organizational Performance: Effectiveness and Efficiency for Disaster Response of the Fire Service Organizations in Korea. Ph.D. Thesis, Hanyang University, Seoul, Korea, 2014.
57. Perry, R. *Comprehensive Emergency Management: Evacuating Threatened Populations*; JAI Press: Greenwich, CT, USA, 1985.
58. Jung, S.H. Analysis on Determinants of Efficiency in Disaster Management System in Regional Governments. Ph.D. Thesis, Kyungnam University, Changwon, Korea, 2010.
59. Park, G.W. A Study on Factors Affecting Efficiency of Disaster Management System. Master's Thesis, Incheon National University, Incheon, Korea, 2008.
60. Kim, H.Y. A Study on the Effects of the Quality of Information on Disaster Response Performance. Master's Thesis, Dongguk University, Seoul, Korea, 2006.
61. Sa Kong, J.J. The Effect of Presidential Leadership on Crisis Management Performance: Focused on The Cases of National Crisis over The Infectious Respiratory Disease. Master's Thesis, University of Seoul, Seoul, Japan, 2016.
62. Lee, J.Y.; Park, K.G.; Jo, K.H.; Kim, O.I. A Study on Establishing National Crisis Management system—AHP Approach. *Korean J. Policy Anal. Eval.* **2004**, *15*, 347–367.
63. Hwang, E.H. An Impact of Interorganizational Relationship Characteristics on the Cooperation and Performance in Disaster Management. Ph.D. Thesis, Dongguk University, Seoul, Korea, 2011.
64. Moon, B.H. A Study on Disaster Management Governance System. Ph.D. Thesis, Honam University, Eodeung-daero, Korea, 2015.
65. Thompson, D.D. Building Effectiveness in Multi-State Disaster Management Systems: The Case of the Caribbean Disaster and Emergency Response Agency. Ph.D. Thesis, The Pennsylvania State University, University Park, PA, USA, 2010.
66. Jeong, S.H.; Song, B.J.; Kwon, G.H. The Analysis about the Potential Effects of Local Overnment's Disaster Control Type on the Efficiency of Its Disaster Control System. *Korean Soc. Public Adm.* **2010**, *21*, 85–406.
67. Choi, W.K. The end of SARS. *Kyunghyang Shinmun*, 19 June 2003.
68. Park, S.J. Collaborative Networks for the Infrequent Emergency Management: A Comparative Analysis on the Case of Controlling MERS. Master's Thesis, Hanyang University, Seoul, Korea, 2017.
69. Ansell, C.; Gash, A. Collaborative Governance in Theory and Practice. *J. Public Adm. Res. Theory* **2008**, *18*, 543–571. [CrossRef]
70. Dynes, R.R. *Organized Behavior in Disaster*; Heath Lexington Books: Lexington, MA, USA, 1970.
71. Perry, R.W.; Lindell, M.K.; Tierney, K.J. *Facing the Unexpected: Disaster Preparedness and Response in the United States*; Joseph Henry Press: Washington, DC, USA, 2001.
72. Kapucu, N. *The Network Governance in Response to Acts of Terrorism: Comparative Analyses*; Routledge: Abingdon-on-Thames, UK, 2012.
73. Kim, Y.S. A Study on the Establishment of Integrated Disaster Management System by Local Governments. *Korean Assoc. Local Gov. Stud.* **1998**, *2*, 59–78.
74. Kwon, H.C. A Study of Semantic Network Analysis of Newspaper Articles on MERS Situation: Comparing Conservative and Progressive News Media. *J. Korean Acad. Commun. Healthc.* **2016**, *11*, 63–80.
75. Na, J.H. Qualitative Meta-Synthesis on Training and Workplace Experiences of Individuals with Disabilities: Focusing on Practical Issues of Applying Qualitative Meta-Synthesis. *Disabil. Employ.* **2008**, *18*, 135–158.
76. Glass, G.V. Primary, Secondary and Meta-Analysis of Research. *Educ. Res.* **1976**, *5*, 3–8. [CrossRef]
77. Glass, G.V.; McGaw, B.; Smith, M.L. *Meta-Analysis in Social Research*; Sage Publications: Beverly Hills, CA, USA, 1981.
78. Sandelowski, M.; Docherty, S.; Emden, C. Focus on Qualitative Methods Qualitative Metasynthesis: Issues and Techniques. *Res. Nurs. Health* **1997**, *20*, 365–371. [CrossRef]

79. Yin, R.K. *Case Study Research Design and Methods: Applied Social Research and Methods Series*, 2nd ed.; Sage Publications Inc.: Thousand Oaks, CA, USA, 1994.
80. Kim, K.; Andrew, S.A.; Jung, K. Public Health Network Structure and Collaboration Effectiveness during the 2015 MERS Outbreak in South Korea: An Institutional Collective Action Framework. *Int. J. Environ. Res. Public Health* **2017**, *14*, 1064. [CrossRef]

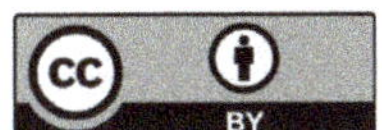

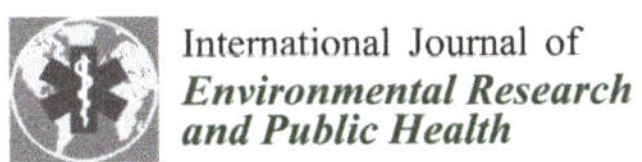
International Journal of
Environmental Research and Public Health

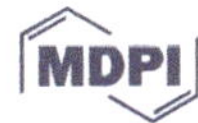

Article

Food-Related Health Emergency-Disaster Risk Reduction in Rural Ethnic Minority Communities: A Pilot Study of Knowledge, Awareness and Practice of Food Labelling and Salt-intake Reduction in a Kunge Community in China

Emily Ying Yang Chan [1,2,3,*], Holly Ching Yu Lam [1], Eugene Siu Kai Lo [1], Sophine Nok Sze Tsang [1], Tony Ka Chun Yung [1] and Carol Ka Po Wong [1]

1 Collaborating Centre for Oxford University and CUHK for Disaster and Medical Humanitarian Response (CCOUC), JC (Jockey Club) School of Public Health and Primary Care, Faculty of Medicine, Chinese University of Hong Kong, Hong Kong, China; hollylam@cuhk.edu.hk (H.C.Y.L.); euglsk@cuhk.edu.hk (E.S.K.L.); sophinetsang@cuhk.edu.hk (S.N.S.T.); yungtony@cuhk.edu.hk (T.K.C.Y.); wongcarol@cuhk.edu.hk (C.K.P.W.)

2 Nuffield Department of Medicine, University of Oxford, Oxford OX3 7BN, UK

3 François-Xavier Bagnoud Center for Health & Human Rights, Harvard University, Boston, MA 02138, USA

* Correspondence: emily.chan@cuhk.edu.hk

Received: 21 March 2019; Accepted: 24 April 2019; Published: 26 April 2019

Abstract: Food safety and unhealthy dietary pattern are important global health problems. Understanding food-related health needs and providing corresponding support are important to health risk reduction. A needs assessment, education intervention for food labelling, and another intervention for salt-intake reduction were conducted in a rural Kunge community in Yunnan, China in 2014, 2015 and 2016, respectively. Not checking the expiry date of packaged food (37.1%) and a high salt diet (53.9%) were the most common problems in the community. Both topics were selected for education intervention. Pre- and post-intervention questionnaires were used to evaluate the effectiveness. Education interventions were found effective in improving food-health-related knowledge, changing attitudes toward behaviors such as willingness to read food labels before buying and consuming packaged food. However, no significant improvements were found for the attitudes toward not consuming expired food, controlling salt-intake, and decreasing the consumption of cured food. Health education was shown to be effective in promoting food-health-related knowledge but was limited in changing relevant behaviors in a rural ethnic minority community.

Keywords: food-related health; risk reduction; rural; ethnic minority; food label; salt; food safety; education intervention; Health-EDRM

---

1. Introduction

Globally, food safety and unhealthy dietary have always been major health concerns for societies. According to World Health Organization (WHO) [1], food safety is the "assurance that food will not cause harm to the consumer when it is prepared and/or eaten according to its intended use". It has been a persistent problem in China and has caused different foodborne illnesses and food poisoning incidents over-time [2]. In addition, inappropriate dietary behavior is also prevalent in China, leading to significant rates of non-communicable diseases. For example, high salt consumption is associated with hypertension, cardiovascular disease and strokes [3]. This study focuses on two food-related health topics: food labelling and salt consumption in rural China population with education intervention.

Food safety issues are often multifaced. For example, suboptimal food safety system (for example regulation violations during transportation or storage) could lead to large scale food-borne disease outbreaks in a community. On the individual level, insufficient food safety knowledge could lead to incorrect food-process or consumption and to food-borne illness eventually [4,5]. Relevant food-related knowledge, awareness, and practices vary from place to place and were shown to be different between urban and rural [6]. A study from Nigeria [6] found that the practices of checking food labels and expiry date were significantly different between rural and urban population. More rural respondents thought that checking food labels and expiry dates did not have a significant impact on health than urban respondents. The lower awareness of food safety among rural population might contribute to their vulnerability, especially among ethnic minorities. In China, selling expired and rotten food has been reported to be prevalent in rural villages [7–9]. In the Food Safety Situation Investigation Report of China 2008 [10], expired food, no food labelling and hygiene of packaged food were the top food safety concerns listed by the rural villagers.

In terms of unhealthy food consumption, high salt intake has been recognized as a critical problem due to its association with hypertension [3]. Hypertension is a major public health problem and the leading disease among populations aged 40 or above in China [11–13]. According to the China Statistical Yearbooks Database data [14], the 2013 prevalence of hypertension in China's rural regions was 12.31%, which was about three-fold greater than the prevalence data previously collected in 2008 (3.85%). Furthermore, it was found that Yunnan was one of the regions with the highest prevalence of hypertension in China [15]. Hence, salt intake reduction is considered as one of the preventive measures against the increase in non-communicable diseases in China [16]. Moreover, a study [17] that investigated the salt consumption habits among 21 countries found China has the highest rate of salt consumption; 80 percent of the population in China had a mean sodium intake higher than 5 g/day (the recommended maximum salt intake for adults by the WHO [3]). In particular, hypertension prevalence in rural regions was found higher than those in urban regions [18,19]. This might be due to the suboptimal medication [20] and inadequate knowledge [21] in rural regions. Therefore, salt intake-related health issues need to be emphasized, especially health interventions to reduce salt consumption and the risk of hypertension. During disasters, a high proportion of chronic diseases such as hypertension would further increase the health vulnerability of the community [22]. Furthermore, food safety would be an important health determinant for resilience. Therefore, ensuring food safety and enhancing dietary knowledge and practices are non-negligible for health-related emergency and disaster risk management (Health-EDRM) in the household level [23].

To tackle health risk-associated food safety and high salt intake problems among China's rural villagers, understanding villagers' practices and promoting relevant knowledge are essential. The authors and the team have developed a 1.5-year project to: 1) understand the current practices regarding food safety and salt intake of China rural villagers, 2) to promote food safety and salt intake knowledge through delivering education interventions to China rural villagers and 3) to evaluate the effectiveness of the education interventions. The target population of this project was a subgroup of an ethnic minority group in rural Yunnan, China—the Kunge. Yunnan is an earthquake-prone province in China. Keeping reserves of packaged food is a common practice in disaster-prone communities [24,25]. This project not only aimed to enhance the food-related health status of the community, but also to increase their capacity for Health-EDRM in rural community. This case study presents the background, methods, and findings of the project.

Project Background and Study Context: Kunge People in Xishuangbanna Dai Autonomous Prefecture in Yunnan

In 2009 the Ethnic Minority Health Project (EMHP) was established in China by the authors and the team, with a core mission to develop and evaluate effective interventions of bottom-up Health-EDRM for vulnerable populations in remote areas of the country. One of the 14 project sites, Xishuangbanna Dai Autonomous Prefecture in Yunnan, was chosen to be one of the study areas on the basis of studying the risk of disaster and health situation which affected the ethnic minority group. The Yunnan ethnic minority health project was initiated in 2014.

The Kunge people reside in Kunge Mountain, Mengyang township, Jinghong city, Xishuangbanna Dai Autonomous Prefecture in Yunnan. It is one of the Xishuangbanna's ethnic groups, officially classified as a branch of the Bulang ethnic group by the People's Republic of China (PRC), and accounts for no more than 2500 residents in China [26]. There are total six Kunge groups in a Mengyang township with a total population of around 1600 [27]. To the authors' knowledge, there were only a few articles exploring the Kunge population and those all were related to the language [26,27]. Bulang people have their own dialogue and religious beliefs. Males and females made up a similar proportion of the village population. Most of the population were farmers, mainly growing rice, sweet corns, tea, and rubber. The average annual household income was approximately RMB 3000–4000 (approximately USD 1.34–1.79 per day, which is lower than the official poverty line of USD 1.90 per day, defined by the World Bank 2015 [28]). Their income mainly comes from exporting agricultural products to other areas in the region. The villagers generally had a regular pattern of life and spent most of their daytime working on farms. In the estimation from our team field visit, there were 140 households with 608 residents living in ManBangTang Village in 2016.

A total of three visits were made in 2014, 2015 and 2016, respectively. A needs assessment was performed in 2014. Although agricultural activity provides the main food source for the Kunge people, as per our interviews in the 2014 visit, all villagers reported the practice of purchasing packaged food, supplied from the local food companies and markets in Mengyang township. Besides packaged food, consumption of salt-cured food, pickled vegetables, and salted meat were also reported. During the needs assessments in ManBangTang, villagers were found to use a generous amount of salt during cooking.

Based on the findings in the literature review and needs assessment conducted in November 2014, two interventions, targeting food labelling in January 2015 and salt-intake reduction in March 2016, were conducted in the same population.

2. Methodology

This was an 18 months serial cross-sectional survey-based study. A total of three research visits were done throughout the project period from November 2014–March 2016.

2.1. Sampling and Study Subject

Representatives of village households (age 18 years or older) were invited for the needs assessment (2014) and the interventions (2015 and 2016). Only one participant was invited from each household. Due to the lack of community information such as household maps, convenience sampling was used for recruiting respondents for the needs assessment and interventions in the village. Recruitment was promoted through household visits, broadcasting promotion messages by the village head, delivering leaflets, and poster distribution. There were 140 registered households with 608 residents in the ManBangTang village during the study period. There were 52 respondents (37.41% of all households) in the needs assessment (2014); 40 (25.15% of all households) participated in the first intervention in 2015 and 45 (28.13% of all households) participated in the second intervention in 2016.

2.2. Evaluation Tool and Data Collection

The 2014 health needs assessment tool was a questionnaire combining eight health topics (including chronic disease management, food and cooking safety (including food labelling and salt intake), personal hygiene, water supply and quality, waste management, disaster risk reduction, first-aid training, and local climate change), sociodemographic details and environmental assessments were surveyed to collect the perception and practices of the villagers. The needs assessment were developed based on the guidance report from the WHO for building a healthy village [29].

For the food labelling (2015) and salt-intake reduction intervention (2016), pre- and post-intervention questionnaires assessing knowledge, attitude, and practices (intention to practice) (KAP) of the relevant topics and sociodemographic information were used for intervention evaluations. The needs assessment results were intended to also be used to design intervention. Thus the questionnaires also included the messages delivered in the interventions (knowledge, attitude and practice (KAP)). Interventions content were adopted from relevant sources: for the salt intake standard, it was adopted from the Chinese Nutritional Society [30]; the food label standard was referenced to the Standard for the Labeling of Prepackaged Food of the China Food and Drug Administration [31]. Table 1 shows the food-related health questions in this study.

Table 1. Questions used in assessing food labelling and salt consumption awareness, attitude and behaviour in the visits (2014, 2015 & 2016).

2014 Visit: Needs Assessment	2015 Visit: Food Labelling	2016 Visit: Salt Consumption
Food labelling related information	Pre- & post- intervention question	Pre- & post- intervention question
Have you ever brought package food before? (exclude rice, oil, and salt) (Answer: Yes/ No)	Do you agree: "I understand that consuming expired food will affect my health."? (Answer: Yes/ No)	Do you think you consume enough salt per day? (Answers: Not enough, enough, more than enough)
What kinds of packaged food you usually buy? (Answers: multiple choice with various food type)	Do you agree "I can distinguish whether the food is expired or not."? (Answer: Yes/ No)	Do you think high salt consumption will cause hypertension? (Answer: Yes/ No)
How often do you read the food label on packaged food before consuming it? (Answer: Always, sometimes and never)	Is the following packaged food expired? (3 Yes/No questions with their local food package images)	Do you think cure food is high in salt? (Answer: Yes/ No)
Why don't you check food labels on packaged foods? (Answer: Multiple choices)	Do you agree "I will check the food label before purchasing the packaged food."? (Answer: Yes/ No)	Do you think hypertension causes cardiovascular disease? (Answer: Yes/ No)
What information on the food label will you usually pay attention to? (Answer: Multiple choices)	Will you check the food label before consuming the packaged food? (Answer: Yes/ No)	Do you think hypertension causes stroke? (Answer: Yes/ No)
Have you ever encountered any food label that you didn't understand? (Answer: Yes/ No)	Do you agree "I will not purchase and consume any expired packaged food."? (Answer: Yes/ No)	Do you know the recommended daily salt consumption level for adults? (Answer: Yes/ No with an open answer on the salt amount)
If you encounter a food label that you don't understand, what will you do? (Answer: Multiple choices)	I will remind my family and friends to check the food labels and pay attention to expired food. (Answer: Yes/ No)	Do you know the function of a salt restriction spoon? (Answer: Yes/ No)
Salt-consumption related question	Post-intervention only question	Do you know the function of a salt restriction bottle? (Answer: Yes/ No)
Please estimate your daily salt consumption. (3 answers: less than, approximately and more than 1 teaspoon)	Do you agree "I am confident to build a habit of checking the food labels on packaged food."? (Answer: Yes/ No)	Can you control your daily salt consumption at less than 6 g in the next month? (Answer: Yes/ No)

Table 1. *Cont.*

2014 Visit: Needs Assessment	2015 Visit: Food Labelling	2016 Visit: Salt Consumption
Food safety related questions Have you experienced any food safety problem before? (Answer: Yes/ No)		Can you consume less cure food in the next month? (Answer: Yes/ No)
Have you got sick or suffered from food poisoning after experiencing the above food safety problem? (Answer: Checklist)		
Which factor will you consider to determine whether the food has gone bad or not? (Answer: Multiple choices)		

Translators were recruited to facilitate communication with the study respondents who could not speak Mandarin (6.25% out of the attendees in the second visit). Verbal consent was obtained from all study respondents prior to administering the questionnaire. All questionnaires were administered face-to-face by field researchers and local translators.

2.3. Statistical Analysis

The data were double entered by trained research staff. Descriptive analysis of sociodemographic information of study subjects was generated and compared to the 2010 Yunnan population census. Chi-squared test was used to compare results from pre- and post-intervention questionnaires for the effectiveness of health interventions. The significant level of this study was set at $p < 0.05$. All statistical analyses were conducted using SPSS version 21.0 (IBM Corp., Armonk, NY, United States). Ethics approval was obtained from the Joint Chinese University of Hong Kong- New Territories East Cluster Clinical Research Ethics Committee.

3. Results

Results are presented in three sections. The first section describes the sociodemographic characteristics of the respondents. The second part presents the results of 2014 needs assessment which included perception and practice of food labelling, general salt intake, and other food safety issues were described. The third section examines the effectiveness of the education intervention in 2015 and 2016 which targeted food labelling and salt reduction respectively.

3.1. Sociodemographic Characteristics of the Sample among the Three Visits

A total of 52 (37.41%), 26 (18.57%) and 34 (24.29%) households were recruited in the 2014 needs assessment, 2015 food labelling intervention and the 2016 salt-intake reduction intervention, respectively (Table 2). The sample in 2015 was younger than the population recruited in 2014 and 2016 ($p < 0.05$), while the proportion of respondents with lower education level was higher in the 2014 sample. The ethnic minority samples were not comparable to the general Yunnan population ($p < 0.05$). The study sample had a high proportion of female and people with lower education level.

Table 2. Sociodemographic characteristics of the households participating in the 2014 to 2016 field visits in ManBangTang Village, Yunnan, China.

	ManBangTang Village			Yunnan [a]
	2014	**2015**	**2016**	**2010**
N	52	26	34	NA
Age *	30.0 (24.25–40.0)	20.0 (18.0–37.25)	35.0 (24.0–48.0)	NA
Female	20 (38.5%)	13 (43.3%)	11 (34.4%)	48.11%
Male-to-female ratio	1:0.63	1:0.76	1:0.52	1:0.9273
Education level *				
Illiterate/Non-formal Education	7 (13.7%)	3 (11.5%)	9 (26.5%)	14.97%
Primary school	30 (58.8%)	6 (23.1%)	10 (29.4%)	43.39%
Junior secondary	13 (25.5%)	17 (57.7%)	14 (41.2%)	27.48%
Senior secondary	1 (2.0%)	2 (7.7%)	1 (2.9%)	8.38%
Tertiary	0 (0.0%)	0 (0.0%)	0 (0.0%)	5.78%

[a] Sources: the Sixth National Population Census report in 2010 [32]; * $p < 0.05$.

3.2. *General Food-Health-Related Practices and Experiences*

3.2.1. Food Labelling

Among the 52 respondents, 36 of them (69.23%) reported the practice of buying packaged food. Snacks (52.8%, 19/36) and meat (33.3%, 12/36) were the most commonly brought packaged foods. As for the practice of reading the food labels before consuming packaged food, 60.0% (21/35) reported that they would read the food label. Among this group, 37.1% (13/21) claimed they always read the labels. The expiry date was the type of information on food labels that most respondents paid attention to; 95.2% among those that would read food labels would pay attention to expiration dates. Among those who did not practice reading food labels (14/35), about half of them (6/14) stated that they did not understand the label. Among respondents who practiced reading food labels on packaged food (n = 21), half of them (11/21) reported seeing confusing food labels before. About half (10/21) would ignore the label if they could not understand it.

3.2.2. Salt Consumption

Out of 52 respondents, 39 had reported their daily salt consumption. Among these, 56.8% (21/39) claimed they consumed one teaspoon or more of salt per day, only 27.0% (10/.39) claimed they consumed less than one teaspoon of salt per day.

3.2.3. Food Safety Problems

Out of the 52 respondents, 42 answered the question "had you encountered any food safety problem before" (Table 3). Among them, 23.8% (10/42) had encountered food safety problems before. Among those had encountered food safety problems, 40% were related to expired food (4/10) while 50% were associated with food quality problems (5/10). Thirty percent (3/10) had reported feeling sick or suffering from food poisoning as a result of the food quality problem.

Table 3. Needs assessment results related to food labelling, salt consumption, and food safety problems.

Questions (*N*)	Items/Choices	*N* (%)
Food Labelling [a]		
Type of food packages they bought (n = 36)		
	Fish	2 (5.6%)
	Meat	12 (33.3%)
	Fruit	6 (16.7%)
	Cereal	5 (13.9%)
	Milk/Product	3 (8.3%)
	Egg	2 (5.6%)
	Snacks	19 (52.8%)
	Others	4 (11.1%)
Check the food label before consuming the packaged food (n = 35)		
	Always	13 (37.14%)
	Sometimes	8 (22.86%)
	Never	14 (40 %)
Reasons for not checking the food labels on the packaged food (n = 14) [b]		
	Do not know there is a food label on the packaged food	1 (7.1%)
	Do not understand	6 (42.9%)
	Never thought about this before	2 (14.3%)
	Don't know	1 (7.1%)
	Rejected Answer	4 (28.6%)
Types of food labels subject pay attention to (n = 21)		
	Nutrition **	4 (19.0%)
	Expiration date	20 (95.2%)
	Way of Storage	2 (9.5%)
	Manufacture location	3 (14.3%)
Had you met the confusing food labels (n = 21)		
	Always	4 (19.0%)
	Sometimes	7 (33.3%)
	Never	5 (23.8%)
	Don't Know	3 (14.3%)
	Refuse to answer	2 (9.5%)
What will you do if you meet any un-understandable food label (n = 21)		
	Ignorance	10 (47.6%)
	Ask others for information	2 (9.52%)
	Not to purchase/eat	6 (28.57%)
	Don't know	2 (9.52%)
	Refuse to answer	1 (4.76%)
Salt consumption		
Daily Salt intake(n = 39)		
	1 teaspoon or above	21 (53.85%)
	Less than 1 teaspoon	10 (25.64%)
	Cannot estimate the salt intake	8 (20.51%)
Food safety related problem		
Encountered any Food safety problem (n = 52)		
	Yes, usually	2 (4.76%)
	Yes, but not often	8 (19.05%)
	Never	32 (76.19%)

Table 3. *Cont.*

Questions (*N*)	Items/Choices	*N* (%)
Encountered what kinds of food safety problem (n = 10) [c]		
	Food expired	4 (40%)
	Counterfeit food	1 (10%)
	Food spoilage	5 (50%)
	Usage of illegal additive	1 (10%)
	Would you get any food poisoning due to food safety problem	3 (30.0%)
Factors to define whether the food is gone bad or not (n = 44)		
	Taste	8 (16.3%)
	Smell	6 (12.2%)
	Appearance	21 (42.9%)
	Feeling	6 (12.2%)
	Date/Food Label	3 (6.1%)

** One respondent specifically mentioned protein and fat; [a] Respondents were also asked if they had bought Cereal and Beans, but none replied they had; [b] No respondent replied "No label on the packaged food" and "not important" as the reason for not checking the food label; [c] No respondents report they had encountered "wrong/misleading instruction" as a food safety problem.

The most common methods used by the respondents to determine whether the food had gone bad or not were checking the appearance (42.9%, 21/44), followed by tasting (16.3%, 8/44), smelling (12.2%, 6/44), personal feeling (12.2%, 6/44) and reading the food label (6.1%, 3/44).

3.2.4. Associating Factors of the Food-Health-Related Practices (Food Labelling and Salt-Intake Reduction)

The association between sociodemographic characteristics and the practice of reading food labels and salt consumption were explored using the needs assessment data (2014). The chi-squared test showed that higher education level was associated with more frequent use of reading food label (p = 0.046), where 80% of those with secondary education; 59.1% of those with primary education and 0.0% of those receiving no formal education would always or sometimes read the label. Age and gender were not shown to be associated with the practices of reading food labelling or salt consumption related behavior.

3.3. *Evaluation of Health Education Intervention Effectiveness*

There were 26 (81.25%) valid pre-and post-intervention questionnaires in the 2015 health intervention on food labeling topic and 40% (N = 18) valid pre- and post-intervention questionnaires in the 2016 health intervention on the salt-intake reduction topic. The dropout rate was due to the open-to-public format of the interventions. Some respondents left before completing the post-questionnaire or arrived after the intervention had started. Only those who had completed a pre- and a post-questionnaire were considered attending the whole intervention. This group of respondents could reflect the interventions' effect better and therefore were considered in the evaluations. The pre- and post-questionnaires were compared using pairwise McNemar's test to evaluate the changes in knowledge, awareness, and behaviors on both topics after the intervention. Table 4 shows the evaluation results of both interventions.

Table 4. Key findings on the effectiveness of pre-and post-intervention in the 2015 Food Labelling.

2015 Health Intervention on Food Labelling ($N = 26$)			
	Pre- (%)	Post- (%)	p value
Food Labelling awareness and knowledge			
Understand that eating expired package food will affect health	73.1%	100.0%	0.004 *
Able to distinguish if the food is expired	46.2%	88.5%	<0.001 *
Question sample 1 (Able to distinguish if the food is expired)	36.0%	72.0%	0.012 *
Question sample 2 (Able to distinguish if the food is expired)	44.0 %	48.0%	0.780
Question sample 3 (Able to distinguish if the food is expired)	24.0%	54.0%	0.023 *
Food Labelling behavior			
Will not eat or buy any expired food	69.1%	76.9%	0.532
Check the expiry date every time before buying	34.6%	80.8%	0.001*
Check the expiry date every time before consuming	30.8%	76.9%	0.001 *
Remind my family and friends keep checking the expiry date	69.2%	92.35	<0.035 *
Confident enough to cultivate the habits of reading food labels	-	100%	-

* $p < 0.05$.

3.3.1. 2015 Health Intervention on Food Labelling

In the 2015 health intervention, 26 valid sets of pre- and post- questionnaires were analyzed. Ten questions, including the food labelling awareness, knowledge, and behaviors, were asked (Table 4). Significant improvements in knowledge and awareness towards food labelling were observed after the intervention (four out of five questions). After the intervention, more respondents understood expired food could affect health (from 73.1 % to 100%, $p < 0.001$, McNemar's test). Three food label samples were presented to test if the respondents were able to tell whether the food was expired based on the information on the food label. Significant improvements were found in two out of the three questions after the interventions (Table 4). Changes in attitude towards reading food labelling were also observed after health intervention (two out of four questions). The number of respondents who indicated that they would check the expiry date before buying and consuming packaged food increased from 34.6% to 80.8% ($p = 0.002$, McNemar's test) and 30.8% to 76.9% ($p = 0.002$, McNemar's test), respectively.

3.3.2. 2016 Health Intervention on Salt-Intake Reduction

In the 2016 visit, 18 sets of valid pre- and post-questionnaires were collected (Table 5). Significant improvement was found in three out of six awareness and knowledge questions after the intervention. The proportion of respondents who knew high salt intake would cause hypertension increased from 50% to 88.9% ($p = 0.039$, Chi-square test). More respondents (from 44.4% to 88.9%) were aware that hypertension might cause heart disease ($p = 0.012$, Chi-square test). Although only half of the respondents could tell the correct suggested amount of daily salt consumption after the intervention, the improvement was statistically significant (from 11.1% to 50%, $p = 0.039$, Chi-square test).

After the intervention, the proportion of respondents who understand the function of the salt-reduction spoons and bottles increased from 11.1 % to 83.3% ($p < 0.001$, Chi-square test) and 11.1% to 72.2% ($p = 0.001$, Chi-square test), respectively. No significant changes were found for the attitude towards cutting down the daily salt-intake to the suggested standard or decreasing cured food consumption were observed.

Table 5. Key findings on the effectiveness of pre-and post-intervention in 2016 Salt Reduction.

2016 Health Intervention on Salt Reduction (N = 18)			
	Pre- (%)	Post- (%)	p value
Salt reduction awareness and knowledge			
Consume enough salt on a daily basis	61.1%	55.5%	1.000
High salt diet cause hypertension	50%	88.9%	0.039 *
Cured food contains high salt amount	61.1%	72.2%	0.375
Chronic hypertension cause heart disease	44.4%	88.9%	0.012 *
Chronic hypertension cause stroke	38.9%	72.2%	0.065
Understand the suggested amount of daily salt consumption	11.1%	50%	0.039 *
Salt reduction behavior			
Understand the function of salt-restriction spoon	11.1%	83.3%	<0.001 *
Understand the function of salt-restriction bottle	11.1%	72.2%	0.001 *
Control the consumption of salt below 6g daily in future month	66.7%	94.4%	0.063
Control the consumption of cured food in future month	72.2%	94.4%	0.125

* $p < 0.05$.

4. Discussion

This study examined the behavioral patterns in the 2014 needs assessment (including reading food labels and salt consumption), the effectiveness of health education interventions on food labeling (in 2015) and salt-intake reduction (in 2016) among an ethnic minority-based community (the Kunge population) in rural China. Results indicated about 60% of respondents who consumed packaged food would read the food label and most of them read the food label for expiry date information. Those who had a higher education level were more likely to read the food label. However, about half of them had found food labels confusing to comprehend. About half of the respondents also reported a daily salt intake level higher than the WHO's recommended amount [3] and about 24% of respondents reported experiencing some form of food safety problems. For both food labelling and salt-intake interventions, significant improvements in knowledge, including the health effects of consuming expired food, how to read the expiry date in a food label, the suggested amount of daily salt intake for adults, the association among high salt intake, hypertension and heart diseases, and the function of the salt-restriction-spoon and bottle, were observed after the interventions. In terms of attitude towards behaviors, more respondents indicated that they would check the expiry date before buying and eating packaged food and would control their salt consumption after the interventions, though the changes in attitude for salt consumption control was not statistically significant.

Only 60% of the respondents who had bought packaged food would pay attention to the food label. This figure was lower compared to another similar research from India. The study from Puducherry in India [33] reported that 90% of the respondents would pay attention to the food labels on packaged food. The relatively lower rate found in the Kunge respondents might be associated with the lack of relevant health education and education level in the community. As mentioned in the introduction, there are many incidents of problematic food products in rural areas [7–9]. This suggested that the awareness of food safety was insufficient in these areas, which increases the vulnerability in this population. Our needs assessment's result found that respondents with a higher education level had greater awareness of reading food labels. This supports the need, and potential value, to raise the food-health-related awareness in the community. The evaluation results showed that education interventions were effective in increasing awareness as well as their attitude towards the corresponding behaviors. A larger scale of education programmes and evaluation of the long-term impact of such programmes should be considered for the community.

High salt intake appeared to be common in the Kunge population in Yunnan. Nearly 60% of the respondents consumed one teaspoon or more per day, which exceeded the suggested standard for adults by the WHO (under one teaspoon) [3]. The result was consistent with those found in studies of other minority groups from rural China communities [16,17]. High salt intake was also found in another ethnic minority, the Yi, in Yunnan [34]. About 80% of them preferred preserved food which was suggested to be one of the underlying causes of a high prevalence of hypertension (37%) among the Yi population. Hence, salt-intake reduction should be promoted in rural community in Yunnan, in particular for ethnic minority communities, to reduce the risk of relevant health problems.

Among those who have encountered food safety problems (23.8%), food spoilage (50%) and expired food (40%) were the top two food safety problems reported. This finding is different from that of a study conducted in urbanized regions, Beijing and Nanjing, in China [35]. The greatest concerns found in the urban study were about food hygiene and food poisoning while expiry date only ranked the 4th among the food safety issues. The differences in food safety concerns between rural and urban regions may be related to the food surveillance systems as spoilage food was more commonly found in the food markets in rural areas due to the less efficient surveillance of food quality [7].

Significant improvement in knowledge and intention to practice the behavior were identified in both the salt reduction and food labelling interventions. Despite the improvements in the understanding of the effects of consuming expired food and the ability and willingness to read the food label, the proportion of respondents that claimed they would not purchase or consume expired food (76.9%) was still lower than that reported in another Chinese study conducted in 31 provinces (89.4%) [36]. This may be related to the economic status among the rural village. Our needs assessment in 2014 found that the study community was under the poverty line. For financial reasons, respondents might still consume expired food even if they understood the potential adverse health effects. Improving the quality of local food supply and encouraging the community to purchase packaged food when needed (to avoid overstocking) might help to reduce the chances for the community to consume expired food. More studies are warranted for drafting effective policies to tackle the problem. Similarly, improvement in salt intake-related knowledge did not imply a change of behavior in salt-intake and consumption of cured food. More research will be needed to understand the economic, cultural, and behavioral challenges.

There were a few limitations in this study. First, only immediate effects of the interventions could be measured due to the project nature. Evaluation of long-term effects should be considered whenever possible to assess and achieve sustainability of the knowledge transferred. Second, this study did not cover the entire food-related behavior topic. Among food safety and consumption pattern, only salt consumption and food labelling of expiration date were investigated. There are other important dietary behaviors such as sugar and oil consumption and food-safety related behavior like storage or information seeking [5] to be explored in future studies. Third, the sample size for evaluating the effectiveness of the intervention was small which may not represent the whole community, especially for the salt-intake reduction. This limited the power of analysis and did not allow subgroup analysis and special consideration should be paid when interpreting the results for scaling up of related programs. Furthermore, there is also a lack of published or official documentation about this minority group for data triangulation. Lastly, language barrier was another limitation. For that, translators were invited to assist during data collection to minimize the barrier. Yet, despite of these limitations, this article will provide information about food and diet, two important aspects of H-EDRM for this special minority group in China.

5. Conclusions

This study identified the food-related Health-EDRM issues in a rural ethnic minority (Kunge) village in Yunnan, China. Not checking expiry dates of packaged food and a high salt diet were the most common problems in the Kunge community. Education interventions were found effective in improving food-related health knowledge despite the small sample sizes. These included the adverse health effects of consuming expired food, how to read the food label for expiry date information, the association among high salt intake, hypertension and heart health, the suggested maximum amount of salt intake for adults, and the function of salt-restriction-spoon and bottle. These interventions were also shown to be effective in changing attitudes toward some behaviors, such as willingness to read the food labels before buying and consuming packaged food. However, no significant improvements were found for the attitudes toward not consuming expired food, control salt-intake and decreased consumption of cured food. This suggests that although health education was effective in raising awareness and promoting health knowledge in a rural ethnic minority community, other elements, including economic status, culture and local food policy, should be considered when promoting changes of health behavior [37]. Special attention should be paid when interpreting the results for the representativeness of the small sample size.

Author Contributions: Conceptualization, E.Y.Y.C.; Methodology, H.C.Y.L.; T.K.C.L., C.K.P.W.; Validation, H.C.Y.L.; Formal analysis, E.S.K.L., S.N.S.T.; Investigation, E.Y.Y.C., H.C.Y.L., E.S.K.L., S.N.S.T., T.K.C.L., C.K.P.W.; Data curation, E.S.K.L., S.N.S.T.; Writing-Original Draft Preparation, E.Y.Y.C., E.S.K.L., S.N.S.T.; Writing—Review & Editing, E.Y.Y.C., H.C.Y.L., E.S.K.L., S.N.S.T.; Project Administration, E.Y.Y.C., T.K.C.L., C.K.P.W.; Funding Acquisition, E.Y.Y.C.

Funding: This research is funded by I.CARE Social Service Projects Scheme, Wu Zhi Qiao Charitable Foundation, Medical Humanitarian Response and Disaster Development Fund and Hong Kong Jockey Club Disaster Preparedness and Response Institute.

Conflicts of Interest: The authors declare no conflict of interest.

References

1. World Health Organization. Food Safety Overview. Available online: http://www.searo.who.int/entity/foodsafety/topics/overview/en/ (accessed on 11 March 2019).
2. Xue, J.; Zhang, W. Understanding China's food safety problem: An analysis of 2387 incidents of acute foodborne illness. *Food Control* **2013**, *30*, 311–317. [CrossRef]
3. World Health Organization. Salt Reduction. Available online: https://www.who.int/news-room/fact-sheets/detail/salt-reduction (accessed on 26 February 2019).
4. World Health Organization. Food Safety. Available online: https://www.who.int/news-room/fact-sheets/detail/food-safety (accessed on 11 March 2019).
5. World Health Organization. Food Safety: What You Should Know. Available online: http://www.searo.who.int/entity/world_health_day/2015/whd-what-you-should-know/en/ (accessed on 26 February 2019).
6. Adebowale, O.; Kassim, I.O. Food safety and health: A survey of rural and urban household consumer practices, knowledge to food safety and food related illnesses in Ogun state. *Epidemiol. Biostat. Public Health* **2017**, *14*, e12568-1–e12568-7.
7. Liu, J. Woguo shao shu minzz shipin anquan wenti ji qi zhìli (The food safety problem and mangement in China). *Guizhou Soc. Sci.* **2013**, *285*, 150–154. (In Chinese)
8. People's Daily Online. Renmin ribao shenghuo manbu: Nongcun bushi guoqi shipin qingxiao de (Rural village is not a expired food market). Available online: http://opinion.people.com.cn/n/2014/0418/c1003-24911122.html (accessed on 26 Febeuary 2019). (In Chinese).
9. Oriental Daily News. Shenzhou guancha wenti shipin gong nongcun chrngxisng you bie liang chong tian (Observation in China: Problematic food supply in rural village, distinctive difference of food problem between urban and rural area). Available online: https://hk.on.cc/hk/bkn/cnt/commentary/20140209/bkn-20140209011401057-0209_00832_001.html (accessed on 26 February 2019). (In Chinese).
10. Ministry of Commerce of the People's Republic of China. 2008 Nian liutong lingyu shipin anquan diaocha baogao.Doc (2008 safety investigation report of food product flow in China). Available online: http://doc.mbalib.com/view/f23fae622d72c5315bf7749cf74dc288.html (accessed on 26 February 2019). (In Chinese)
11. Lozano, R.; Naghavi, M.; Foreman, K.; Lim, S.; Shibuya, K.; Aboyans, V.; Abraham, J.; Adair, T.; Aggarwal, R.; Ahn, S.Y.; et al. Global and regional mortality from 235 causes of death for 20 age groups in 1990 and 2010: A systematic analysis for the Global Burden of Disease Study 2010. *Lancet* **2012**, *380*, 2095–2128. [CrossRef]
12. Wei, Q.; Sun, J.; Huang, J.; Zhou, H.Y.; Ding, Y.M.; Tao, Y.C.; He, S.M.; Liu, Y.L.; Niu, J.Q. Prevalence of hypertension and associated risk factors in Dehui City of Jilin Province in China. *J. Hum. Hypertens.* **2015**, *29*, 64–68. [CrossRef]

13. Shao, S.; Hua, Y.; Yang, Y.; Liu, X.; Fan, J.; Zhang, A.; Xiang, J.; Li, M.; Yan, L.L. Salt reduction in china: A state-of-the-art review. *Risk Manag. Healthc. Policy* **2017**, *10*, 17–28. [CrossRef] [PubMed]
14. Chinese National Knowledge Infrastructure. Zhongguo jingji yu shehui fazhan tongji shujuku: Diaocha diqu jumin manxingbing huan bing lu (%) (Survey of chronic disease prevalence (%) among residents in various regions). Available online: http://tongji.cnki.net/kns55/Navi/result.aspx?id=N2015110062&file=N2015110062000236&floor=1 (accessed on 11 March 2019). (In Chinese).
15. Wang, Z.; Chen, Z.; Zhang, L.; Wang, X.; Hao, G.; Zhang, Z.; Shao, L.; Tian, Y.; Dong, Y.; Zheng, C.; et al. Status of hypertension in China: Results from the China hypertension survey, 2012–2015. *Circulation* **2018**. [CrossRef]
16. Hipgrave, D.B.; Chang, S.; Li, X.; Wu, Y. Salt and sodium intake in China. *J. Am. Med. Assoc.* **2016**, *315*, 703–705. [CrossRef] [PubMed]
17. Mente, A.; O'Donnell, M.; Rangarajan, S.; McQueen, M.; Dagenais, G.; Wielgosz, A.; Lear, S.; Ah, S.T.L.; Wei, L.; Diaz, R.; et al. Urinary sodium excretion, blood pressure, cardiovascular disease, and mortality: A community-level prospective epidemiological cohort study. *Lancet* **2018**, *392*, 496–506. [CrossRef]
18. Wong, J.; Sun, W.; Wells, G.; Li, Z.; Li, T.; Wu, J.; Zhang, Y.; Liu, Y.; Li, L.; Yu, Y.; et al. Differences in prevalence of hypertension and associated risk factors in urban and rural residents of the Northeastern region of the people's republic of China: A cross-sectional study. *PLoS ONE* **2018**, *13*, e0195340. [CrossRef]
19. Wang, Q.; Xu, L.; Sun, L.; Li, J.; Qin, W.; Ding, G.; Zhang, J.; Zhu, J.; Xie, S.; Yu, Z.; et al. Rural-urban difference in blood pressure measurement frequency among elderly with hypertension: A cross-sectional study in Shandong, China. *J. Health Popul. Nutr.* **2018**, *37*, 25. [CrossRef]
20. Li, J.; Shi, L.; Li, S.; Xu, L.; Qin, W.; Wang, H. Urban-rural disparities in hypertension prevalence, detection, and medication use among Chinese Adults from 1993 to 2011. *Int. J. Equity Health* **2017**, *16*, 50. [CrossRef]
21. Yuan, F.; Qian, D.; Huang, C.; Tian, M.; Xiang, Y.; He, Z.; Feng, Z. Analysis of awareness of health knowledge among rural residents in Western China. *BMC Public Health* **2015**, *15*, 55. [CrossRef]
22. Chan, E.Y.Y.; Huang, Z.; Lam, H.C.Y.; Wong, C.K.P.; Zou, Q. Health Vulnerability Index for Disaster Risk Reduction: Application in Belt and Road Initiative (BRI) Region. *Int. J. Environ. Res. Public Health* **2019**, *16*, 380. [CrossRef]
23. Chan, E.Y.Y.; Man, A.Y.T.; Lam, H.C.Y. Scientific evidence on natural disasters and health emergency and disaster risk management in Asian rural-based area. *Br. Med. Bull.* **2019**, *129*, 91. [CrossRef]
24. Chan, E.Y.Y.; Ho, J.Y.; Huang, Z.; Kim, J.H.; Lam, H.C.Y.; Chung, P.P.W.; Wong, C.K.P.; Liu, S.; Chow, S.; Man, A.Y.T.; et al. Long-Term and Immediate Impacts of Health Emergency and Disaster Risk Management (Health-EDRM) Education Interventions in a Rural Chinese Earthquake-Prone Transitional Village. *Int. J. Disaster Risk Sci.* **2018**, *9*, 319–330. [CrossRef]
25. Pickering, C.J.; O'Sullivan, T.L.; Morris, A.; Mark, C.; McQuirk, D.; Chan, E.Y.; Guy, E.; Chan, G.K.; Reddin, K.; Throp, R.; et al. The Promotion of "Grab Bags" as a Disaster Risk Reduction Strategy. *PLoS Curr.* **2018**, *10*.
26. Jiang, G.; Shi, J. Kun Ge Hua Yin Xi (phonetic System of Kunge). *J. Chongqing Univ. Technol.* **2015**, *29*, 302.
27. Jiang, G.; Shi, J. Kun Ge Ren Yu Yan Shi Yung Xian Zhuang Diao Cha (A Field Investigation of Language Use of the Kunge Ethnic Group). *J. China West Norm. Univ. Pilos. Soc. Sci.* **2013**, *1*, 80–85. (In Chinese)
28. The World Bank. The International Poverty Line Has Just Been Raised to $1.90 a Day, but Global Poverty Is Basically Unchanged. How Is That Even Possible? Available online: http://blogs.worldbank.org/developmenttalk/international-poverty-line-has-just-been-raised-190-day-global-poverty-basically-unchanged-how-even (accessed on 26 February 2019).
29. Howard, G.; Bogh, C.; Prüss, A.; Goldstein, G.; Shaw, R.; Morgan, J.; Teuton, J. *Healthy Villages: A Guide for Communities and Community Health Workers*; World health organization: Geneva, Switzerland, 2002.
30. Ge, K. The transition of Chinese dietary guidelines and the food guide pagoda. *Asia Pac. J. Clin. Nutr.* **2011**, *20*, 439–446.
31. China Country Commercial Guide. China—Labeling/Marking Requirements. Available online: https://www.export.gov/article?id=China-Labeling-Marking-Requirements (accessed on 11 April 2019).
32. National Bureau of Statistics of China. Yunnan sheng 2010 nian di liu ci quanguo renkou pucha zhuyao shuju gongbao (Main statistics report of Yunnan province of the Sixth National Population Census). Available online: http://www.stats.gov.cn/tjsj/tjgb/rkpcgb/dfrkpcgb/201202/t20120228_30408.html (accessed on 26 February 2019). (In Chinese)

33. Jain, S.; Gomathi, R.; Kar, S. Consumer awareness and status of food labeling in selected supermarkets of Puducherry: An exploratory study. *Int. J. Adv. Med. Health Res.* **2018**, *5*, 36.
34. Chen, L.; Zong, Y.; Wei, T.; Sheng, X.; Shen, W.; Li, J.; Niu, Z.; Zhou, H.; Zhang, Y.; Yuan, Y.; et al. Prevalence, awareness, medication, control, and risk factors associated with hypertension in Yi ethnic group aged 50 years and over in rural China: The Yunnan minority eye study. *BMC Public Health* **2015**, *15*, 383. [CrossRef]
35. Liu, A.; Niyongira, R. Chinese consumers food purchasing behaviors and awareness of food safety. *Food Control* **2017**, *79*, 185–191. [CrossRef]
36. Yim, L.P.; Li, Y.; Tong, W.; Lu, W.; Hu, Z.F.; Huang, P. Zhongguo chengxiang jumin anquan ren zhi nengli he jijiu zijiu nengli fenxi (Safety cognitive ability and first aid capacity in emergency event among urban and rural residents in China). *China J. Public Health* **2015**, *31*, 842–845. (In Chinses)
37. Chan, E.Y.Y.; Shaw, R. *Public Health and Disasters: Health Emergency and Disaster Risk Management in Asia*; Springer: Singapore, 2019; in press.

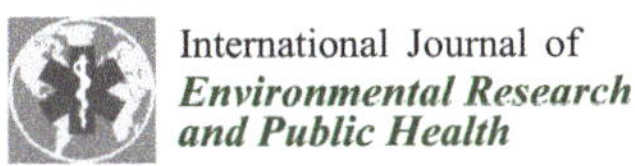
International Journal of
Environmental Research and Public Health

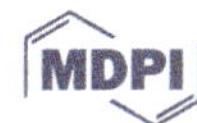

Article

Post-Traumatic Stress among Evacuees from the 2016 Fort McMurray Wildfires: Exploration of Psychological and Sleep Symptoms Three Months after the Evacuation

Genevieve Belleville *, Marie-Christine Ouellet and Charles M. Morin

School of Psychology, Laval University, Quebec, QC G1V 0A6, Canada;
marie-christine.ouellet@psy.ulaval.ca (M.-C.O.); cmorin@psy.ulaval.ca (C.M.M.)
* Correspondence: genevieve.belleville@psy.ulaval.ca; Tel.: +418-656-2131 (ext. 4226)

Received: 25 February 2019; Accepted: 3 May 2019; Published: 8 May 2019

Abstract: This study documents post-traumatic stress symptoms after the May 2016 wildfires in Fort McMurray (Alberta, Canada). A sample of 379 evacuees completed an online questionnaire from July to September 2016, and a subsample of 55 completed a psychiatric/psychological diagnostic interview. According to a self-report questionnaire, 62.5% of respondents had a provisional post-traumatic stress disorder (PTSD). The interview confirmed that 29.1% met criteria for PTSD, 25.5% for depression, and 43.6% for insomnia; in most cases, insomnia was definitely or probably related to the fires. Traumatic exposure may elicit or exacerbate sleep problems, which are closely associated with PTSD after a disaster.

Keywords: post-traumatic stress disorder; psychological distress; mental health; sleep

1. Introduction

Exposure to a natural disaster is a type of traumatic event that may lead to the development of post-traumatic stress disorder (PTSD). The wildfires that began on 1 May 2016 in Fort McMurray (Alberta, Canada) destroyed 1595 buildings, which contained 2600 housing units, and led to massive displacement of approximately 88,000 people. The fire, which was officially put out in August 2017, after 458 days, devastated a total of 5895 km^2. Although it caused no direct human fatality, during the evacuation, many individuals faced direct or potential threat to their life or health, or significant losses. Damage was estimated at $3.58 billion, making it the most expensive natural disaster in Canadian history. The inhabitants of the city were displaced at least one month. The city started rebuilding in June 2016, a process expected to take three to four years. Three months after the evacuation, families were still living through ongoing adversity and uncertainty as they adapted to new or temporary homes, schools and workplaces. Beyond the individual experience of the disaster, entire communities have experienced it collectively, facing a variety of challenges at the social, community and economic levels (e.g., housing issues, insurance claims, rebuilding). Both individual and collective stressors are known to contribute to psychological adjustment after a disaster [1].

Specific data on the consequences of major forest fires are not only rare, but their generalizability to other communities may be questioned. Data collected from victims of the 2003 California fires have revealed that two-thirds of the respondents had feared for their lives or the life of a loved one; three months later, a quarter met the criteria for PTSD, and a third met the criteria for major depression [2]. Another study with victims of the Australian bushfires of 1983 demonstrated that health conditions related to stress, including mental disorders, were much more common in this population than conditions unrelated to stress [3]. Three to four years after the Victorian Black Saturday bushfires in Australia (2009), 16–22% of highly affected communities had PTSD and 13% had major depression [4]. To date, two published studies have reported significant issues related to the mental health impacts of the Fort McMurray wildfires. One case-controlled study conducted 18 months after the wildfires showed elevated prevalence of probable self-reported mental health diagnoses (depression, anxiety, alcohol/substance use) in children [5]. The only study reporting mental health indicators in adults was conducted 6 months after the wildfires and focused on self-reported anxiety and alcohol/substance use: Almost 20% of the 486 surveyed participants had a probable diagnosis of generalized anxiety disorder, 14% had high risk of alcohol dependence, and 10% had high risk of drug dependence [6].

Most studies examining the mental health impacts of fires have focused on PTSD, depression, anxiety and substance use [7–9]. However, sleep problems—mostly in the form of insomnia and recurrent nightmares, but also sleep-related movement and breathing disorders—are closely associated with both PTSD [10] and depression [11]. Of the 160 studies on the impacts of disasters reviewed by Norris and collaborators (2002), only 10 measured sleep [12]. There is accumulating evidence that persistent sleep problems constitute an important predictor of psychopathology after a traumatic event [13]. Moreover, sleep disturbances appear to be among the most common reactions after a traumatic event: Severe problems with sleep were the most frequently reported complaints two to three weeks after the explosion of a fireworks storage facility in Enschede, The Netherlands, among a vast array of physical and mental health concerns including problems with daily functioning, pain, anxiety and depression [14].

Most people exposed to a disaster experience intense psychological reactions but will remit after some time [15,16]; in parallel, continued stressors contribute to enduring psychological distress, including PTSD [17,18]. Individual factors, such as appraisals of the event and coping strategies, may also influence mental health after a disaster. Ehlers and Clark's cognitive model suggests that post-traumatic symptoms persist when individuals process information in a way that produces a sense of imminent threat [19]. Two processes are thought to feed this perception of current threat: Recurrent negative appraisals of the trauma and its consequences and the disturbance of autobiographical memory. The latter process is potentiated by unhelpful coping strategies, such as avoidance. Avoidance may concern stimuli that are external (places, people) or internal (memories, thoughts); self-medication with alcohol or other substances may also be a form of avoidance. Sleep difficulties, such as insomnia and nightmares, may play a role as they contribute to physiological arousal and strong emotions, two aspects that may promote the perception of current threat.

In sum, both the wide range of symptoms (e.g., PTSD, anxiety, depression, sleep) and the timeline (e.g., when they occur, how long they persist) are important aspects to consider in the assessment of the mental health impact of a disaster on the affected community. Moreover, due to their unpredictable nature, it is exceptionally difficult to obtain empirical data about the impact of natural disasters. Methodological challenges must be faced: The main bias is often related to the retrospective nature of the data collected, i.e., when we ask people to remember their immediate post-traumatic reactions weeks or even years after the traumatic event [20] and the lack of baseline information on premorbid status. The objective of this research was thus to rapidly document post-traumatic stress symptoms, mental disorders and psychological difficulties in a sample of evacuees of the 2016 Fort McMurray wildfires. The goal was to collect data in the immediate aftermath, i.e., three months after the evacuation, to support self-reported symptoms with standardized clinical interviews, and to assess common mental health disorders (PTSD, depression, anxiety, substance use) as well as sleep problems. We also wanted to examine the associations between symptoms of post-traumatic stress and depression, sleep problems, post-traumatic cognitions and coping strategies. We wished to explore the differential contribution of sleep difficulties in post-traumatic stress severity once the severity of depression was accounted for, as well as the influence of cognitions and coping strategies once the severity of depression and sleep problems were accounted for.

2. Method

The Laval University institutional review board approved the research protocol, and participants provided informed consent.

2.1. Participants and Procedure

A sample of evacuees from the 2016 Fort McMurray wildfires were asked to complete an online questionnaire. To participate, they had to be aged 18 or older and be fluent in English. A subsample of these volunteers also underwent a standardized clinical interview. The clinical interviews were conducted in the business meeting room of a local hotel.

Two research assistants—doctoral students in clinical psychology—went to Fort McMurray from 25 July to 16 August 2016 to recruit participants and conduct the clinical interviews. They recruited volunteers in various public places (e.g., mall, grocery store). They distributed invitations to complete the online questionnaire, printed on business cards, and also participated in local radio broadcasts to discuss the project and its recruitment. The online questionnaire remained open from 25 July 25 to 5 September 2016. Appointments were taken with individuals interested to participate to the clinical interview, either later in the same day or in the following days. A snowball sampling methodology was also used where participants were invited to refer to the research team other potentially interested acquaintances. The research assistants were easily joinable by phone or email for the whole time of their stay in Fort McMurray.

The research assistants were supervised by the principal investigator (GB), a psychologist specialized in PTSD. They had access to phone supervision as needed for the entire duration of their stay.

2.2. Measures

The clinical interview merged two validated standardized diagnostic instruments: The Clinician-Administered PTSD Scale (CAPS) [21] to assess current PTSD, and the Mini International Neuropsychiatric Interview (MINI) [22] to assess current major depression, panic, agoraphobia, generalized anxiety, social phobia and obsessive-compulsive disorders, as well as drug and alcohol use disorders. These instruments provided a stringent examination of the fifth edition of the Diagnostic and Statistical Manual of Mental Disorders (DSM-5) [23] criteria for each disorder. Questions related to the CAPS item #E6 (sleep disturbance) were given a special attention, in order to be able to diagnose insomnia. An insomnia diagnosis was assigned to participants who met the following five criteria: (1) Difficulties falling or staying asleep or waking up too early, and these were (2) present at least three times a week, (3) associated with daytime disturbances, (4) present for at least three months, and (5) occurred despite adequate opportunity for sleep. Questions probing personal antecedents were asked at the end of the interview, i.e., "We just did an overview of the symptoms you have/might have had since the fires. Now I wonder if you have ever experienced problems similar in the past, before the fires. Have you ever had Depression/Insomnia/Recurrent Nightmares/Anxiety Disorder before?".

The online questionnaires were presented as aimed at studying post-traumatic stress among victims of the Fort McMurray fire. The first questions were open-ended and asked participants to describe their personal experience of the fire and the evacuation, as well as their consequences. Participants then proceeded to complete the PTSD Symptoms Checklist (PCL-5) [24], the Patient Health Questionnaire [25], the Insomnia Severity Index [26], the Pittsburgh Sleep Quality Index and its Addendum for PTSD (PSQI; PSQI-A) [27,28], the Post-Traumatic Cognitions Inventory (PTCI) [29] and the Ways of Coping Questionnaire (WCQ) [30].

The PCL-5 is a 20-item self-report measure that assesses PTSD symptoms in the past month. In this study, we used the PCL-5 to assess symptom severity and to make a provisional PTSD diagnosis. The symptom severity score ranges from 0–80, higher scores indicating more severe symptoms. A provisional PTSD diagnostic may be assigned to respondents who endorse 1 B item (questions 1–5),

1 C item (questions 6–7), 2 D items (questions 8–14), 2 E items (questions 15–20). A cutoff score of 33 is also proposed to discriminate between people with or without probable PTSD [31].

The PHQ is a 59-item questionnaire that was used as a screening tool for mental health disorders of depression, anxiety, alcohol, eating, and somatoform during the past four weeks. From the PHQ, we also used the PHQ-9, a subscale composed of 9 summed items to assess the severity of depressive symptoms [25].

The ISI is a 7-item questionnaire designed to assess the severity of both nighttime and daytime components of insomnia in the past month. Total score ranges from 0–21, higher scores indicating more severe insomnia. A cutoff score of 10 is optimal to detect insomnia in a community sample [32].

The PSQI is an 18-item questionnaire that assesses seven components of sleep quality in the past month: Subjective sleep quality, sleep latency, sleep duration, sleep efficiency, sleep disturbances, use of sleep medication, and impairment of daytime functioning. A global sleep quality score ranging from 0–21 is obtained by summing the seven component scores, higher scores indicating poorer sleep quality. A global sleep quality score higher than 5 is interpreted as poor sleep.

We also used the 7-item addendum to the PSQI, the PSQI-A, to assess the frequency of trauma-related sleep disturbances (hot flashes, general nervousness, memories or nightmares of traumatic experience, severe anxiety or panic not related to traumatic memories, bad dreams not related to traumatic memories, episodes of terror or screaming during sleep without fully awakening and episodes of acting out dreams) in the past month. Total score ranges from 0–21, higher scores indicating more frequent trauma-related sleep disturbances.

The PTCI is a 33-item questionnaire which assessed the degree to which respondents endorsed several post-traumatic cognitions (thoughts) in general on a 1–7 Likert-type scale. Three subscales constitute the PTCI. The Negative cognitions about the self subscale includes 21 items which depict a negative overall opinion of oneself, including a perception of the self as being incapable and weak (e.g., *I am a weak person*), permanently and negatively altered by the event (e.g., *I worsened forever*) and without hope for the future (e.g., *I have no future*). The Negative cognitions about the world/others subscale includes 7 items highlighting the world as a dangerous place and people as inherently unreliable (e.g., *You cannot trust anyone*). The self-blame subscale includes 5 items assessing blame for the occurrence of the traumatic event (e.g., *The event occurred because of the way I acted*). Each subscale score is the average 1-to-7 answer per statement.

Finally, a short version of the WCQ assessed the frequency of use of three coping strategies in the past week: Seeking social support (6 items), positive reappraisal/problem solving (9 items) and distancing/avoidance (6 items). Each item is rated on a 0–3 Likert-type scale. Subscale scores are computed by summing the score of each item, and higher scores indicate more frequent use of the strategy.

2.3. Data Analyses

To document post-traumatic stress symptoms, mental disorders and psychological difficulties, frequencies were computed for categorical variables, and means and standard deviations were computed for continuous variables. Lower and upper limits of 95% confidence interval for each mean and for each proportion were computed. Correlations between variables were examined by calculating Pearson's coefficients. To avoid overlap on the various questionnaires in the correlation and regression analyses, the PCL-5 total score was computed excluding the two sleep items (#2—repeated, disturbing dreams, and #20—trouble falling or staying asleep) and the PHQ-9 total score was computed excluding its sleep item (#3—trouble falling or staying asleep, or sleeping too much). To document the factors associated with the severity of PTSD symptoms, a hierarchical multiple regression analysis was performed, with PTSD symptom severity (PCL-5 total score) as the predicted variable. The observation of the Gaussian distribution of the studentized residuals along with a non-statistically significant Shapiro–Wilk test suggested that the residuals were normally distributed. The first block consisted of gender and age, and was entered with the standard method as a control for the potential effect of these sociodemographic characteristics on PTSD severity. The second block of variables was entered with the standard method and was composed of depressive symptoms (PHQ-9 total score excluding the sleep item). The third block was entered with the standard method and was composed of insomnia severity (ISI total score), global sleep quality (PSQI total score), and trauma-related sleep disturbances (PSQI-A total score). The fourth and final block was entered with the standard method and was composed of negative cognitions about the self (PTCI subscale), negative cognitions about the world (PTCI subscale), self-blame (PTCI subscale), seeking social support (WCQ subscale), problem-solving/positive reappraisal (WCQ subscale) and distancing/avoidance (WCQ subscale). Correlation and regression analyses were performed with SPSS 13.0 for Windows (SPSS Inc., Chicago, IL, USA).

3. Results

3.1. Sample Description

Three hundred and ninety-four (394) respondents registered to complete the online questionnaire, i.e., went on the website describing the study and clicked to begin the questionnaire. Fifteen questionnaires (3.8%) remained completely or mostly unanswered. Among the 379 completed questionnaires, between 0.02 and 8.4% of data were missing, depending on the question/variable. Missing data were not replaced. Participants were mostly female (77%). Mean age was 40.10 years old (SD = 12.20). Almost three quarters were married or in a common-law relationship (72%); 18% were single, and 7% were either separated, divorced or widowed. Most participants (61%) had children. Residence status in the regional municipality of Wood Buffalo (which includes the city of Fort McMurray) was permanent for 88% and temporary for 7%. Before the fires, most participants worked part or full time (77%); 4% were retired, 3% were on a sick or invalidity leave, and 2% were students. Nearly one participant in four (23%) reported a change in work status since the fires.

Fifty-six (56) respondents participated to the interview. One interview was excluded from the analyses because of incomplete responses: The interviewer suspected that the participant was intoxicated and/or suffering from psychotic symptoms, and redirected the interview to ensure the participant's safety and access to local mental health resources. The final subsample of 55 participants was practically equally distributed between males (49%) and females (51%). Mean age was 43.07 years old (SD = 14.67). About half were married or in a common-law relationship (49%); 31% were single, and 16% were either separated, divorced or widowed. Most participants (62%) had children. Residence status in the community of Wood Buffalo (which includes the city of Fort McMurray) was permanent for 95% and temporary for 4%. Before the fires, most participants worked part or full time (76%); 4% were retired, 18% were unemployed, and 2% were students. One participant in six (16%) reported a change in work status since the fires.

Although all participants of the clinical interview were invited to complete the online questionnaire, thirty-five (35) did so, representing 9.2% of the sample of completed questionnaires. Compared to respondents who only completed the online questionnaire (344), participants who completed the interview and the online questionnaire (35) were more likely to be male and older, and they showed an overall portrait of less severe mental health problems. They were less likely to have self-reported PTSD, somatoform disorder and major depressive disorder. They showed lower scores on measures of post-traumatic, insomnia and depressive symptoms. They reported less use of avoidance-based coping strategies, less endorsement of cognitions regarding the self, the world or self-blame, and better sleep quality.

3.2. Main Results

Data from the online survey showed that, three months after the fires, roughly 60% suffered from significant post-traumatic stress, i.e., they had a provisional PTSD diagnosis according to the PCL-5 or a PCL-5 score of 33 or higher (see Table 1). The most frequently reported symptoms were repeated disturbing memories, feeling upset when reminded of the stressful experience, and trouble falling or staying asleep. Table 2 presents scores obtained on the other self-report questionnaires. The PHQ showed high proportions of respondents endorsing the diagnostic criteria of major depressive disorder (33.1%), somatoform disorder (27.0%) and anxiety disorders other than panic (27.0%). High rates of panic disorder (17.4%), alcohol abuse disorder (17.1%) and binge eating disorder (15.1%) were also observed. Results showed overall high severity of depressive symptoms, insomnia and post-traumatic sleep disturbances, as well as poor sleep quality.

Data from the clinical interviews showed that in this subsample of 55 volunteer participants, 29.1% met the clinical diagnostic criteria for PTSD and 25.5% met the clinical diagnostic criteria for major depression disorder (see Table 3). Among the anxiety disorders, panic disorder and generalized anxiety disorder were the most frequent. Substance use disorders, especially drug use disorder, were diagnosed in 16.7% of the sample. The most frequently encountered diagnosis in this sample was insomnia disorder, with a proportion of 43.6%. Participants were asked whether their sleep difficulties started or got worse after the fires; in most cases, the insomnia disorder was definitely (68%) or probably (16%) related to the fires. Most people with current insomnia (78%) reported having experienced insomnia in the past. PTSD was associated with current insomnia ($X^2(1) = 17.65$, $p < 0.001$), but not with insomnia antecedents ($X^2(1) = 0.432$, $p = 0.511$).

Table 4 presents the associations between the different variables under study. More severe PTSD symptoms was associated with more severe depression and insomnia symptoms, poorer sleep quality and more severe trauma-related sleep disturbances, stronger endorsement of negative cognitions concerning the self, others and self-blame, and with more frequent use of avoidance strategies. PTSD symptom severity was also negatively correlated with age, that is, more severe in younger people.

Results from hierarchical multiple regression analyses indicated that the final model accounted for 77.0% of PTSD symptom severity variance, $F(8, 340) = 146.722$, $p < 0.001$ (Table 5). Sex and age did not contribute significantly to the model (although age was positively associated with symptom severity when no other variable than sex was included in the model). Significant predictors included depressive and insomnia symptoms, trauma-related sleep disturbances, post-traumatic cognitions concerning the others or the world as untrustworthy or dangerous, avoidance-based coping strategies and problem-solving/reappraisal coping strategies.

Table 1. Proportion of respondents reporting post-traumatic stress disorder (PTSD) symptoms according to the PTSD symptoms checklist (PCL-5) (n = 374–379 [a]).

Symptom	Number of Respondents Who Endorsed the Symptom (Rated as 2 = "Moderately" or Higher)	Proportion of Respondents Who Endorsed the Symptom (Rated as 2 = "Moderately" or Higher)	95% CI
1. Repeated, disturbing memories (n = 376)	291	77.39	[72.90–81.35]
2. Repeated, disturbing dreams (n = 374)	203	54.28	[49.21–59.26]
3. Suddenly feeling as if the stressful experience was happening again (n = 376)	206	54.79	[49.74–59.75]
4. Feeling very upset when reminded of the stressful experience (n = 377)	289	76.66	[72.13–80.65]
5. Strong physical reactions when reminded of the stressful experience (n = 377)	250	66.31	[61.40–70.90]
6. Avoidance of memories, thoughts or feelings related to the stressful experience (n = 375)	247	65.87	[60.93–70.49]
7. Avoidance of external reminders of the stressful experience (n = 376)	226	60.11	[55.08–64.93]
8. Trouble remembering important parts of the stressful experience (n = 374)	167	44.65	[39.69–49.72]
9. Strong negative feelings about oneself, other people or the world (n = 377)	145	38.46	[33.69–43.46]
10. Blaming oneself or someone else for the stressful experience (n = 376)	155	41.22	[36.36–46.26]
11. Strong negative feelings (n = 376)	225	59.84	[54.81–64.67]
12. Loss of interest (n = 378)	229	60.58	[55.57–65.38]
13. Feeling distant or cut off (n = 378)	253	66.93	[62.04–71.48]
14. Trouble experiencing positive feelings (n = 378)	197	52.12	[47.09–57.11]
15. Irritable behaviors (n = 376)	226	60.11	[55.08–64.93]
16. Taking too many risks (n = 377)	72	19.10	[15.45–23.37]
17. Being "superalert" (n = 377)	265	70.29	[65.49–74.68]
18. Easily startled (n = 378)	229	60.58	[55.57–65.38]
19. Difficulty concentrating (n = 378)	262	69.31	[64.49–73.75]
20. Trouble falling or staying asleep (n = 378)	274	72.49	[67.78–76.75]
Provisional PTSD diagnosis [b] (n = 379)	237	62.53	[57.55–67.25]
PCL-5 Total Score 33 or higher (n = 379)	226	59.63	[54.62–64.45]

Note: [a] On each of the 379 completed PCL-5, between 1 and 5 questions were left unanswered. Missing data were not replaced. [b] Proportion of respondents who have endorsed 1 B item (questions 1–5), 1 C item (questions 6–7), 2 D items (questions 8–14), 2 E items (questions 15–20).

Table 2. Results on self-report questionnaires (n = 347–378 [a]).

Questionnaire	n	%	95% CI
PHQ—Somatoform Disorder (n = 378)	102	26.98	[22.75–31.67]
PHQ—Major Depression Disorder (n = 378)	125	33.07	[28.52–37.96]
PHQ—Panic Disorder (n = 379)	66	17.41	[13.92–21.55]
PHQ—Other Anxiety Disorder (n = 378)	102	26.98	[22.75–31.67]
PHQ—Bulimia (n = 377)	14	3.71	[2.22–6.13]
PHQ—Binge Eating Disorder (n = 377)	57	15.12	[11.86–19.09]
PHQ—Alcohol Abuse (n = 375)	64	17.07	[13.06–21.21]
	M	SD	95% CI
Depressive Symptoms (PHQ-9) (n = 378)	10.72	6.65	[10.05–11.39]
Insomnia Symptoms (ISI) (n = 375)	15.50	7.75	[14.72–16.28]
Trauma-Related Sleep Disturbances (PSQI-A) (n = 375)	5.52	4.72	[5.04–6.00]
Global sleep Quality (PSQI) (n = 375)	11.76	4.98	[11.26–12.26]
Sleep Quality (PSQI) (n = 375)	1.90	0.85	[1.81–1.99]
Sleep Latency (PSQI) (n = 375)	2.01	1.10	[1.90–2.12]
Sleep Duration (PSQI) (n = 370)	1.76	1.03	[1.66–1.86]
Sleep Efficiency (PSQI) (n = 370)	1.61	1.28	[1.48–1.74]
Sleep Disturbances (PSQI) (n = 375)	1.92	0.76	[1.84–2.00]
Use of Sleep Medications (PSQI) (n = 374)	0.99	1.28	[0.86–1.12]
Daytime Dysfunction (PSQI) (n = 375)	1.62	0.95	[1.52–1.72]
Post-Traumatic Cognitions (PTCI) (n = 347)	48.05	43.06	[43.55–52.55]
Self (PTCI) (n = 359)	1.40	1.43	[1.25–1.55]
World (PTCI) (n = 359)	2.25	1.66	[2.08–2.42]
Self-Blame (PTCI) (n = 359)	0.55	0.99	[0.45–0.65]
Seeking Social Support (WCQ) (n = 358)	6.70	4.02	[6.28–7.12]
Problem-Solving / Positive Re-Appraisal (WCQ) (n = 358)	10.24	6.07	[9.61–10.87]
Distancing / Avoidance (WCQ) (n = 359)	6.82	4.15	[6.39–7.25]

Note: [a] Among the 379 completed questionnaires, between 1 and 32 data were missing per variable. Missing data were not replaced. M = mean; PHQ = Patient Health Questionnaire; SD = standard deviation.

Table 3. Proportions of respondents diagnosed with PTSD or other mental disorders according to clinical interviews [a] (n = 54 or 55 [b]).

Diagnosis	Number of Respondents	Proportion of Respondents	95% CI
PTSD (n = 55)	16	29.09	[18.77–42.14]
Major Depression Disorder (n = 55)	14	25.45	[15.81–38.30]
Panic Disorder (n = 55)	13	23.64	[14.37–36.35]
Agoraphobia (n = 55)	7	12.73	[6.31–24.02]
Generalized Anxiety Disorder (n = 55)	13	23.64	[14.37–36.35]
Social Phobia (n = 55)	5	9.09	[3.95–19.58]
Obsessive-Compulsive Disorder (n = 55)	0	0.00	–
Drug Use Disorder (n = 54)	7	12.96	[6.42–24.42]
Alcohol Use Disorder (n = 54)	2	3.70	[1.02–12.53]
Insomnia Disorder (n = 55)	24	43.64	[31.38–56.73]

Note: [a] PTSD diagnosed with the Clinician-Administered PTSD Scale for DSM-5 (CAPS), Insomnia Disorder diagnosed with questions from the Insomnia Interview Schedule adapted according to the DSM-5 criteria, all other disorders diagnosed with the Mini International Neuropsychiatric Interview (MINI). [b] One participant did not provide information to assess alcohol use and another one did not provide information to assess alcohol use.

Table 4. Correlation coefficients between variables (n = 354–374).

	PTSD	Sex	Age	Depression	Insomnia	Sleep Quality	Sleep Disturbances	Self	World	Self-Blame	Support	Problem-Solving
PTSD												
Sex	0.088											
Age	−0.122 *	−0.177 **										
Depression	0.808 **	0.023	−0.056									
Insomnia	0.673 **	0.082	−0.022	0.726 **								
Sleep Quality	0.564 **	0.107 *	0.044	0.624 **	0.803 **							
Sleep Disturbances	0.702 **	0.118 *	−0.033	0.671 **	0.634 **	0.592 **						
Self	0.730 **	0.028	−0.166 **	0.733 **	0.529 **	0.425 **	0.639 **					
World	0.638 **	−0.042	−0.116 *	0.568 **	0.408 **	0.347 **	0.543 **	0.768 **				
Self-Blame	0.501 **	−0.094	−0.056	0.508 **	0.353 **	0.289 **	0.462 **	0.680 **	0.596 **			
Support	0.053	0.150 **	−0.054	0.100	0.088	0.066	0.115 *	−0.025	0.064	0.043		
Problem-Solving	−0.096	0.012	0.078	−0.090	−0.053	−0.052	0.010	−0.180 **	0.022	−0.014	0.622 **	
Avoidance	0.532 **	0.153 **	−0.248 **	0.464 **	0.414 **	0.351 **	0.444 **	0.505 **	0.445 **	0.351 **	0.196 **	0.134 *

* $p < 0.05$; ** $p < 0.01$; Note: Avoidance: distancing/avoidance (WCQ subscale); Depression: depressive symptoms (PHQ-9 total score excluding the #3 sleep item); Insomnia: insomnia severity (ISI total score); Problem-Solving: problem-solving/positive reappraisal (WCQ subscale); PTSD: post-traumatic symptom severity (PCL-5 total score excluding the #2 and #20 sleep items); Sleep Disturbances: trauma-related sleep disturbances (PSQI-A total score); Sleep Quality: global sleep quality (PSQI total score); Self: negative cognitions about the self (PTCI subscale); Self-Blame: self-blame (PTCI subscale); Support: seeking social support (WCQ subscale), World: negative cognitions about the world (PTCI subscale).

Table 5. Multiple regression analyses predicting PTSD symptom severity (excluding sleep items) ($n = 344$).

	Variables	B	SE B	β	Adjusted R^2	R^2 Change
Step 1					0.023 **	0.23 **
	Sex	4.778	2.377	0.102		
	Age	−0.176	0.077	−0.123 *		
Step 2					0.680 **	0.654 **
	Sex	2.403	1.363	0.055		
	Age	−0.125	0.044	−0.087 **		
	Depressive symptom severity (PHQ-9 excluding sleep item)	2.439	0.092	0.811 **		
Step 3					0.721 **	0.043 **
	Sex	0.853	1.296	0.019		
	Age	−0.126	0.042	−0.088 **		
	Depressive symptom severity (PHQ-9 excluding sleep item)	1.732	0.138	0.576 **		
	Global sleep quality (PSQI)	−0.141	0.173	−0.040		
	Insomnia symptom severity (ISI)	0.291	0.126	0.128 *		
	Post-traumatic sleep disturbances (PSQI-A)	0.932	0.154	0.249 **		
Step 4					0.753 **	0.035 **
	Sex	1.555	1.263	0.035		
	Age	−0.064	0.041	−0.045		
	Depressive symptom severity (PHQ-9 excluding sleep item)	1.393	0.153	0.465 **		
	Global sleep quality (PSQI)	−0.121	0.164	−0.034		
	Insomnia symptom severity (ISI)	0.287	0.119	0.126 *		
	Post-traumatic sleep disturbances (PSQI-A)	0.646	0.155	0.173 **		
	Negative cognitions about the self (PTCI)	0.227	0.736	0.018		
	Negative cognitions about the world/others (PTCI)	1.827	0.463	0.172 **		
	Self-blame (PTCI)	0.046	0.681	0.002		
	Seeking social support (WCQ)	−0.166	0.157	−0.038		
	Positive reappraisal/Problem solving (WCQ)	−0.107	0.107	−0.037		
	Distancing/Avoidance (WCQ)	0.461	0.145	0.109 **		

* $p < 0.05$; ** $p < 0.01$. B = beta weight; SE B = standard error of the beta weight.

4. Discussion

The objective of this study was to rapidly document post-traumatic stress symptoms, mental disorders and psychological difficulties in a sample of evacuees in the immediate aftermath of the 2016 Fort McMurray wildfires. Result showed that roughly 60% of respondents to an online questionnaire reported significant post-traumatic stress symptoms, or could be given a provisional PTSD diagnosis according to their responses to a validated self-report questionnaire (PCL-5). This is similar to what was observed among the residents of Enschede, The Netherlands, two or three weeks after the explosion of a fireworks storage facility in a residential area, where more than 50% reported anxious and depressive symptoms of anxiety and sleeping problems, and nearly 75% reported disaster-related reactions of intrusion and avoidance [14]. Four months after a devastating tornado struck the town of Albion, PA in 1985, 76% of its residents also showed high levels of post-traumatic stress [33].

The most frequently reported post-traumatic stress symptoms were repeated disturbing memories (reported by 77.4% of the sample), feeling upset when reminded of the stressful experience (76.7%), and trouble falling or staying asleep (72.5%). The widespread presence of sleep disturbances is a finding consistent with that of studies with larger and more representative samples exposed to a disaster: Rates of severe problems with sleep were threefold that of the general population in the residents of Enschede, The Netherlands, after the fireworks storage facility explosion [14].

Self-report questionnaires suggested alarmingly elevated rates of clinically significant symptoms of major depressive disorder (one in three respondents), but also of somatoform, anxiety and panic disorders, alcohol abuse and binge eating. Respondents reported overall high severity of depressive symptoms, insomnia symptoms and trauma-related sleep disturbances, as well as poor sleep quality. This highlights the relevance to include various outcomes in the assessment of the impact of a disaster on mental health. Because this study did not benefit neither from a comparison with a non-exposed control group nor from an estimation of pre-traumatic mental health of the Fort McMurray population, we cannot directly attribute the observed symptoms to the experience of the fires and of the evacuation. However, all of the observed values were largely greater than prevalence rates of mental health disorders reported in the general population: For example, according to the 2002 Canadian Community Health Survey on Mental Health and Well-Being, the 12-month prevalence of any anxiety disorder is 4.8%, and any mood disorder is 5.3% [34].

We also analyzed data from a subsample of 55 evacuees who participated in a clinical interview where a stringent examination of DSM criteria was conducted. This more rigorous and conservative approach indicated that 29.1% fulfilled the DSM-5 criteria for PTSD. Prevalence of PTSD was somewhat more elevated than that assessed with a DSM-IV-based clinical interview in a sample of individuals three months after an earthquake in North China (18.8%) [35]. However, in the latter study, when researchers calculated the prevalence of PTSD without the requirement for presence of both avoidance and numbing symptoms (DSM-IV's Criterion C), as is it now the case in DSM-5, they obtained an estimated closer to the one we obtained (27.4%). Almost half of participants with PTSD in the present study (43.6%) could be considered as having an insomnia disorder (recurrently having significant trouble falling or staying asleep). This is about three times higher than in the general Canadian population where the prevalence of insomnia disorder is estimated to be 13.4% [36]. Moreover, although 78% of the subsample reported having had insomnia episodes before the fires, the current insomnia episode was presumably trauma-related, i.e., definitely/probably started or got worse after the fires, in 84% of the cases.

We also wanted to explore the association between of symptoms of post-traumatic stress, and depression, sleep problems, post-traumatic cognitions and coping strategies as assessed three months after the fires. After controlling for sex and age, significant factors associated with post-traumatic stress symptom severity included, depressive symptoms, trauma-related sleep disturbances, post-traumatic cognitions (perceiving other people or the world as untrustworthy or dangerous), insomnia symptoms, avoidance-based coping strategies and problem-solving/reappraisal coping strategies. The observed associations were consistent with the role of cognitions and coping strategies in producing a sense of imminent threat that contribute to maintain and exacerbate post-traumatic stress symptoms [19]. These preliminary findings also suggest that sleep problems, either sleep disturbances or insomnia, are closely associated with PTSD in the aftermath of a disaster, beyond the expected association due to the presence of depressive symptoms. Sleep difficulties may be present before the traumatic event or occur as a result of trauma, and their persistence several days or weeks after the traumatic event may act as a specific risk factor for PTSD [37]. They may constitute symptoms of PTSD, but they may also develop into difficulties concomitant with PTSD, but still different in their nature and their response to treatment [38,39]. Inversely, the treatment of trauma-related sleep problems may have a positive impact on other post-traumatic stress symptoms [40,41]. Interventions to protect or restore sleep after exposure to a disaster are likely to be useful, but the efficacy of sleep management strategies to prevent the development of other mental health problems after traumatic exposure has yet to be studied.

These findings are to be interpreted with caution, as they were assessed very early in the aftermath of the fires and the evacuation, i.e., approximately three months after the evacuation. Some of the respondents had not yet returned home. Furthermore, it is possible that individuals feeling distress could have been more motivated to participate compared to persons with no particular mental health symptoms. Previous findings have shown that resilience, namely the ability to maintain at a stable, healthy level of psychological and physical functioning [15], is to be expected in the majority of individuals. In a study of the aftermath of Hurricane Ike [42], it was found that 75% of the population never developed PTSD when they were evaluated in the 18-month period following the disaster. In addition, between 45–58% did not develop depression, functional impairment, or report days of poor health. Recovery, whereby persons may experience some levels of psychopathology (such as anxiety, depression or sleep problems) but gradually return to pre-event levels of functioning [16], is another common trajectory, where some level of psychological symptoms could be expected as a "normal" reaction to a severely abnormal event, but where symptoms eventually subside. Data collected three to four years after the Victorian Black Saturday bushfires in Australia (February 2009) indicated that more than 80% recovered from symptoms of psychological distress without developing significant mental health problems in the long run [4]. However, studies of resilience and recovery have focused on PTSD and depression, and have not included the assessment of sleep difficulties. Longitudinal follow-ups of the Fort McMurray community will be needed to assess the longer-term evolution of the all of the psychological impacts that were highlighted in these results.

5. Conclusions

This study represented a preliminary effort to guide future investigations on the mental health of the Fort McMurray community. A study of the natural history of PTSD, depression and sleep disorders is currently in progress to document the prevalence of psychopathology in the long-term (e.g., three years post-disaster), and to examine the impact of sociodemographic characteristics (e.g., sex/gender, age, ethnicity, income and membership in a First Nation) and degree of loss caused by the fires on prevalence rates. This ongoing study will examine the longitudinal predictors of the course of post-traumatic adaptation, by determining the sociodemographic, psychopathological, cognitive, behavioural and social factors longitudinally associated with not only distress, but also resilience and post-traumatic growth. Finally, we perceived an urgent need in our pool of respondents to be heard about their mental health service needs. Although evidence has shown that patients usually prefer psychological treatment to medication to treat anxiety and depression problems, gender, age and ethnicity greatly influence beliefs and perceived needs in terms of mental health [43]. Data on mental health needs after a disaster from the patients' perspective are needed to guide the development of large-scale interventions that are accessible and relevant to the affected community.

Author Contributions: Data curation, G.B.; Formal analysis, G.B.; Funding acquisition, G.B., M.-C.O. and C.M.M.; Investigation, G.B.; Methodology, G.B., M.-C.O. and C.M.M.; Project administration, G.B.; Supervision, M.-C.O.; Writing—original draft, G.B.; Writing—review & editing, G.B., M.-C.O. and C.M.M.

Funding: This research was funded by Institute for Catastrophic Loss Reduction.

Conflicts of Interest: The authors declare no conflict of interest.

References

1. Norris, F.H.; Friedman, M.J.; Watson, P.J.; Byrne, C.M.; Diaz, E.; Kaniasty, K. 60,000 disaster victims speak: Part I. An empirical review of the empirical literature, 1981–2001. *Psychiatry* **2002**, *65*, 207–239. [CrossRef] [PubMed]
2. Marshall, G.N.; Schell, T.L.; Elliott, M.N.; Rayburn, N.R.; Jaycox, L.H. Psychiatric disorders among adults seeking emergency disaster assistance after a wildland-urban interface fire. *Psychiatr. Serv.* **2007**, *58*, 509–514. [CrossRef] [PubMed]
3. Clayer, J.R.; Bookless-Pratz, C.; Harris, R.L. Some health consequences of a natural disaster. *Med. J. Aust.* **1985**, *143*, 182–184.
4. Bryant, R.A.; Waters, E.; Gibbs, L.; Gallagher, H.C.; Pattison, P.; Lusher, D.; MacDougall, C.; Harms, L.; Block, K.; Snowdon, E.; et al. Psychological outcomes following the Victorian Black Saturday bushfires. *Aust. N. Z. J. Psychiatry* **2014**, *48*, 634–643. [CrossRef] [PubMed]

5. Brown, M.R.G.; Agyapong, V.; Greenshaw, A.J.; Cribben, I.; Brett-MacLean, P.; Drolet, J.; McDonald-Harker, C.; Omeje, J.; Mankowsi, M.; Noble, S.; et al. After the Fort McMurray wildfire there are significant increases in mental health symptoms in grade 7–12 students compared to controls. *BMC Psychiatry* **2019**, *19*. [CrossRef]
6. Agyapong, V.I.O.; Hrabok, M.; Juhas, M.; Omeje, J.; Denga, E.; Nwaka, B.; Akinjise, I.; Corbett, S.E.; Moosavi, S.; Brown, M.; et al. Prevalence rates and predictors of generalized anxiety disorder symptoms in residents of Fort McMurray six months after a wildfire. *Front. Psychiatry* **2018**, *9*. [CrossRef] [PubMed]
7. Fergusson, D.M.; Horwood, L.J.; Boden, J.M.; Mulder, R.T. Impact of a major disaster on the mental health of a well-studied cohort. *JAMA Psychiatry* **2014**, *71*, 1025–1031. [CrossRef] [PubMed]
8. Goldmann, E.; Galea, S. Mental health consequences of disasters. *Annu. Rev. Public Health* **2014**, *35*, 169–183. [CrossRef] [PubMed]
9. Laugharne, J.; Van de Watt, G.; Janca, A. After the fire: The mental health consequences of fire disasters. *Curr. Opin. Psychiatry* **2011**, *24*, 72–77. [CrossRef] [PubMed]
10. Miller, K.E.; Brownlow, J.A.; Woodward, S.; Gehrman, P.R. Sleep and Dreaming in Posttraumatic Stress Disorder. *Curr. Psychiatry Rep.* **2017**, *19*, 71. [CrossRef]
11. Murphy, M.J.; Peterson, M.J. Sleep disturbances in depression. *Sleep Med. Clin.* **2015**, *10*, 17–23. [CrossRef]
12. Norris, F.H.; Sherrieb, K.; Galea, S. Prevalence and consequences of disaster-related illness and injury from Hurricane Ike. *Rehabil Psychol* **2010**, *55*, 221–230. [CrossRef]
13. Babson, K.A.; Feldner, M.T. Temporal relations between sleep problems and both traumatic event exposure and PTSD: A critical review of the empirical literature. *J. Anxiety Disord.* **2010**, *24*, 1–15. [CrossRef] [PubMed]
14. van Kamp, I.; van der Velden, P.G.; Stellato, R.K.; Roorda, J.; van Loon, J.; Kleber, R.J.; Gersons, B.B.; Lebret, E. Physical and mental health shortly after a disaster: First results from the Enschede firework disaster study. *Eur. J. Public Health* **2006**, *16*, 253–259. [CrossRef] [PubMed]
15. Bonanno, G.A. Loss, trauma, and human resilience: Have we underestimated the human capacity to thrive after extremely aversive events? *Am. Psychol.* **2004**, *59*, 20–28. [CrossRef] [PubMed]
16. Bonanno, G.A.; Mancini, A.D. Beyond resilience and PTSD: Mapping the heterogeneity of responses to potential trauma. *Psychol. Trauma* **2012**, *4*, 74–83. [CrossRef]
17. Math, S.B.; Nirmala, M.C.; Moirangthem, S.; Kumar, N.C. Disaster Management: Mental Health Perspective. *Indian J. Psychol. Med.* **2015**, *37*, 261–271. [CrossRef] [PubMed]
18. Tempest, E.L.; Carter, B.; Beck, C.R.; Rubin, G.J. Secondary stressors are associated with probable psychological morbidity after flooding: A cross-sectional analysis. *Eur. J. Public Health* **2017**, *27*, 1042–1047. [CrossRef]
19. Ehlers, A.; Clark, D.M. A cognitive model of posttraumatic stress disorder. *Behav. Res. Ther.* **2000**, *38*, 319–345. [CrossRef]
20. Frissa, S.; Hatch, S.L.; Fear, N.T.; Dorrington, S.; Goodwin, L.; Hotopf, M. Challenges in the retrospective assessment of trauma: Comparing a checklist approach to a single item trauma experience screening question. *BMC Psychiatry* **2016**, *16*. [CrossRef]
21. Blake, D.D.; Weathers, F.W.; Nagy, L.M.; Kaloupek, D.G.; Gusman, F.D.; Charney, D.S.; Keane, T.M. The development of a Clinician-Administered PTSD Scale. *J. Trauma Stress* **1995**, *8*, 75–90. [CrossRef]
22. Sheehan, D.V.; Lecrubier, Y.; Sheehan, K.H.; Amorim, P.; Janavs, J.; Weiller, E.; Hergueta, T.; Baker, R.; Dunbar, G.C. The Mini-International Neuropsychiatric Interview (M.I.N.I.): The development and validation of a structured diagnostic psychiatric interview for DSM-IV and ICD-10. *J. Clin. Psychiatry* **1998**, *59* (Suppl. 20), S22–S33.
23. American Psychiatric Association. *Diagnostic and Statistical Manual of Mental Disorders: DSM-5™*, 5th ed.; American Psychiatric Publishing, Inc.: Arlington, VA, USA, 2013.
24. Forbes, D.; Creamer, M.; Biddle, D. The validity of the PTSD checklist as a measure of symptomatic change in combat-related PTSD. *Behav. Res. Ther.* **2001**, *39*, 977–986. [CrossRef]
25. Kroenke, K.; Spitzer, R.L.; Williams, J.B. The PHQ-9: Validity of a brief depression severity measure. *J. Gen. Intern. Med.* **2001**, *16*, 606–613. [CrossRef]
26. Bastien, C.H.; Vallieres, A.; Morin, C.M. Validation of the Insomnia Severity Index as an outcome measure for insomnia research. *Sleep Med.* **2001**, *2*, 297–307. [CrossRef]
27. Buysse, D.J.; Reynolds, C.F.; Monk, T.H.; Berman, S.R.; Kupfer, D.J. The Pittsburgh Sleep Quality Index: A new instrument for psychiatric practice and research. *Psychiatry Res.* **1989**, *28*, 193–213. [CrossRef]

28. Germain, A.; Hall, M.; Krakow, B.; Shear, M.K.; Buysse, D.J. A brief sleep scale for Posttraumatic Stress Disorder: Pittsburgh Sleep Quality Index Addendum for PTSD. *J. Anxiety Disord.* **2005**, *19*, 233–244. [CrossRef]
29. Foa, E.B.; Ehlers, A.; Clark, D.M.; Tolin, D.F.; Orsillo, S.M. The Posttraumatic Cognitions Inventory (PTCI): Development and validation. *Psychol. Assess.* **1999**, *11*, 303–314. [CrossRef]
30. Folkman, S.; Lazarus, R.S. *Manual for the Ways of Coping Questionnaire*; Consulting Psychologists Press: Palo Alto, CA, USA, 1988.
31. Weathers, F.W.; Litz, B.T.; Keane, T.M.; Palmieri, P.A.; Marx, B.P.; Schnurr, P.P. The PTSD Checklist for DSM-5 (PCL-5). National Center for PTSD; 2013. Available online: https://www.ptsd.va.gov/professional/assessment/adult-sr/ptsd-checklist.asp (accessed on 27 February 2019).
32. Morin, C.M.; Belleville, G.; Belanger, L.; Ivers, H. The insomnia severity index: Psychometric indicators to detect insomnia cases and evaluate treatment response. *Sleep* **2011**, *34*, 601–608. [CrossRef]
33. Steinglass, P.; Gerrity, E. Natural disasters and post-traumatic stress disorder: Short-term versus long-term recovery in two disaster-affected communities. *J. Appl. Soc. Psychol.* **1990**, *20*, 1746–1765. [CrossRef]
34. Statistics Canada. Canadian Community Health Survey: Mental Health and Well-Being 2003. Available online: https://www150.statcan.gc.ca/n1/daily-quotidien/030903/dq030903a-eng.htm (accessed on 27 February 2019).
35. Wang, J.; Smailes, E.; Sareen, J.; Fick, G.H.; Schmitz, N.; Patten, S.B. The prevalence of mental disorders in the working population over the period of global economic crisis. *Can. J. Psychiatry* **2010**, *55*, 598–605. [CrossRef]
36. Morin, C.M.; LeBlanc, M.; Bélanger, L.; Ivers, H.; Mérette, C.; Savard, J. Prevalence of insomnia and its treatment in Canada. *Can. J. Psychiatry* **2011**, *56*, 540–548. [CrossRef]
37. Koren, D.; Arnon, I.; Lavie, P.; Klein, E. Sleep complaints as early predictors of posttraumatic stress disorder: A 1-year prospective study of injured survivors of motor vehicle accidents. *Am. J. Psychiatry* **2001**, *159*, 855–857. [CrossRef]
38. Belleville, G.; Guay, S.; Marchand, A. Persistence of sleep disturbances following cognitive-behavior therapy for posttraumatic stress disorder. *J. Psychosom. Res.* **2011**, *70*, 318–327. [CrossRef]
39. Galovski, T.E.; Monson, C.; Bruce, S.E.; Resick, P.A. Does cognitive-behavioral therapy for PTSD improve perceived health and sleep impairment? *J. Trauma Stress* **2009**, *22*, 197–204. [CrossRef]
40. Casement, M.D.; Swanson, L.M. A meta-analysis of imagery rehearsal for post-trauma nightmares: Effects on nightmare frequency, sleep quality, and posttraumatic stress. *Clin. Psychol. Rev.* **2012**, *32*, 566–574. [CrossRef]
41. Talbot, L.S.; Maguen, S.; Metzler, T.J.; Schmitz, M.; McCaslin, S.E.; Richards, A.; Perlis, M.L.; Posner, D.A.; Weiss, B.; Ruoff, L.; et al. Cognitive behavioral therapy for insomnia in posttraumatic stress disorder: A randomized controlled trial. *Sleep* **2014**, *37*, 327–341. [CrossRef]
42. Lowe, S.R.; Joshi, S.; Pietrzak, R.H.; Galea, S.; Cerdá, M. Mental health and general wellness in the aftermath of Hurricane Ike. *Soc. Sci. Med.* **2015**, *124*, 162–170. [CrossRef]
43. Prins, M.A.; Verhaak, P.F.; Bensing, J.M.; van der Meer, K. Health beliefs and perceived need for mental health care of anxiety and depression—The patients' perspective explored. *Clin. Psychol. Rev.* **2008**, *28*, 1038–1058. [CrossRef]

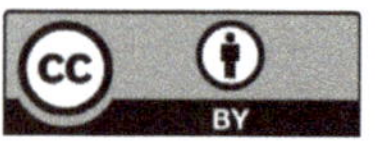

MDPI
St. Alban-Anlage 66
4052 Basel
Switzerland
Tel. +41 61 683 77 34
Fax +41 61 302 89 18
www.mdpi.com

International Journal of Environmental Research and Public Health Editorial Office
E-mail: ijerph@mdpi.com
www.mdpi.com/journal/ijerph

www.ingramcontent.com/pod-product-compliance
Lightning Source LLC
LaVergne TN
LVHW070204170726
843515LV00007B/1999

9783039363148